Praise for *Heart & Hands*

"An impressive and deeply caring book . . . reveals a shrewd and compassionate sensitivity to women's needs in pregnancy and childbirth."
—Sheila Kitzinger
Author of *The Complete Book of Pregnancy and Birth*

"Here is a book of great beauty that uniquely combines traditional midwifery teachings with the most up-to-date obstetrical theories and techniques."
—Don Creevy, MD, FACOG
Clinical Assistant Professor of Gynecology and Obstetrics
Stanford University School of Medicine

"A beautifully written and comprehensive guide . . . speaks to the need to protect the baby's rights and health."
—Mike Witte, MD
Board Certified Pediatrician
Medical Director for the Point Reyes Clinic

"Detailed and compassionate, *Heart & Hands* offers childbearing women, midwives, and doctors a wealth of practical information. It provides a view of pregnancy and birth not as a purely medical, mechanical event, but as a complex physical, emotional, social, and spiritual experience. Elizabeth Davis loves and respects women, and her work places childbearing where it belongs— in the strong and capable hands of mothers and midwives."
—The Boston Women's Health Collective
Authors of *The New Our Bodies, Ourselves*

"*Heart & Hands* conveys the essence of midwifery! To supplement today's abundant scientific and technological information, it literally describes the missing dimension— a commitment to the art of midwifery."
—Dorothea M. Lang, CNM, MPH

"Provides a rich assortment of anecdotes and remedies for common problems. . . . The author is to be commended for her emphasis on the fourth trimester, the important three-month period when mothers and babies are recovering from birth and becoming acquainted. It is fortunate for midwives and prospective parents that this book has been expanded and updated."
—John Kennell, MD
Professor of Pediatrics
Rainbow Babies' and Children's Hospital
University Hospitals of Cleveland

"Portrays well the beauty and power of birth. It honors the central role of the midwife in prenatal care, birth, and postnatal care, precisely the role recommended repeatedly by the World Health Organization for all the countries of the world. This book should be read by all birth attendants. . . ."
—Marsden Wagner, MD
Neonatologist, Perinatal Epidemiologist
Author of *Born in the U.S.A*

"Emphasizes pregnancy as wellness . . . this book parallels the family-centered approach that I advocate in established medical and nursing practices."
—Celeste R. Phillips, RN, EdD

"The elements of caring for and caring about women are so maturely thought out and articulated that I readily recommend the book to all midwifery students of any type of educational program, for any practice setting."
—Mary V. Widhalm, CNM, MS
Director of Midwifery
Lincoln Medical and Mental Health Center
Bronx, New York

"Elizabeth Davis has done her profession a very valuable service by providing a textbook that is eminently readable and that gives the aspiring midwife the benefit of having a friend and mentor in the form of a book—and that is no small accomplishment! She delves into the area of judgment, which is the acid test for any midwife. She is the Wise Woman speaking, the Sage Femme who can cut through the morass of information, the current standards, and the new theories, and take us to the heart and kernel of what this work is all about."
—Tish Demmin, LM
Former President
Midwives Alliance of North America

Heart & Hands

ALSO BY ELIZABETH DAVIS

Orgasmic Birth: Your Guide to a Safe, Satisfying, and Pleasurable Birth Experience

The Women's Wheel of Life

Women's Sexual Passages: Finding Pleasure and Intimacy at Every Stage of Life

Women's Intuition

Energetic Pregnancy: A Guide to Achieving Balance, Vitality & Well-Being from Conception to Birth & Beyond

Heart & Hands

A Midwife's Guide to Pregnancy and Birth
5th Edition

ELIZABETH DAVIS

Illustrations by Linda Harrison

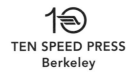

TEN SPEED PRESS
Berkeley

Reader, please note:
The medical and health procedures in this book are based on the training, personal experiences, and research of the author as well as on recommendations of responsible medical sources. But because each person and situation is unique, the author and publisher urge the reader to check with a qualified health professional before using any procedure when there may be any question as to its appropriateness. The publisher does not advocate the use of any particular birth-related technique but believes this information should be available to the public. Because there are risks involved, the author and publisher are not responsible for any adverse effects or consequences resulting from the use of any of the suggestions, preparations, or procedures in this book. Please do not use these unless you are willing to assume these risks. Feel free to consult a physician or other qualified health professional. It is a sign of wisdom, not cowardice, to seek a second or third opinion.

Copyright © 1981, 1987, 1992, 1997, 2004, 2012 by Elizabeth Davis

Published in the United States by Ten Speed Press, an imprint of the Crown Publishing Group,
a division of Random House, Inc., New York.
www.crownpublishing.com
www.tenspeed.com

Originally published as *A Guide to Midwifery: Heart & Hands* by John Muir Publications, Santa Fe, in 1981, and in a subsequent mass-market edition by Bantam Books in 1983. New editions of this work were published as *Heart and Hands: A Midwife's Guide to Pregnancy and Birth* by Celestial Arts, Berkeley, in 1987, 1997, and 2004 with an updated edition in 1992.

Ten Speed Press and the Ten Speed Press colophon are registered trademarks of Random House, Inc.

Photos on pages xii and 63 by Stacie Nunes, copyright © 2004, 2012
Photos on pages 2, 6, 14, 19, 71, 77, 89, 121, 201, 212, 215, 233, 250, 252 by Kati Molin, copyright © 2012
Photos on pages 113, 122, 128 by Pedro Gonzales, copyright © 2004, 2012
Photos on pages 8, 55, 57 by Amy Swagman, copyright © 2012
Photos on pages 11, 35, 62, 85, 91, 101, 109, 124, 125, 180, 198, 206, 225, 229, 244, 253 by Suzanne Arms,
    copyright © 1981, 1987, 1992, 1997, 2004, 2012
Photos on pages 37, 94, 108, 110, 143, 151, 166, 217, 224 by Judith Halek, copyright © 2012
Photos on pages 55, 57 by Amy Swagman, copyright © 2012
Photos on pages 100, 129 by Katy Raddatz, copyright © 1981, 1987, 1992, 1997, 2004, 2012
Photo on page 136 by Paivi Laukkanen, copyright © 2012
Photo on page 140 by Ed Buryn, copyright © 1981, 1987, 1992, 1997, 2004, 2012
Photos on pages 155, 218 by Gary Yost, copyright © 1981, 1987, 1992, 1997, 2004, 2012
Photo on page 174 by Doris Silva, copyright © 2012

Library of Congress Cataloging-in-Publication Data
Davis, Elizabeth, 1950–
  Heart & hands : a midwife's guide to pregnancy and birth / Elizabeth Davis ; illustrations by Linda Harrison. — 5th ed.
    p. ; cm.
  Heart and hands
  Includes bibliographical references and index.
  I. Title. II. Title: Heart and hands.
  [DNLM: 1. Midwifery. 2. Pregnancy. WQ 160]

  618.2—dc23
                              2012014041

ISBN 978-1-60774-243-2
eISBN 978-1-60774-244-9

Printed in the United States of America

Front cover photograph copyright © Molka/iStockphoto
Design by Colleen Cain
Illustrations by Linda Harrison

10 9 8 7 6 5 4 3 2 1

Fifth Edition

Contents

Acknowledgments

I begin by thanking my teacher Tina Garzero for her patience and love in teaching me this wonderful art and way of being. To John Walsh, I will always remember your humor and guidance.

To all my midwifery students, thank you for your inspiration, insights, critiques, and the push to help me stay current.

To Shannon Anton, thank you for your excellent sections on homeopathy and herbs in pregnancy, birth, and postpartum, as well as the unforgettable account of Liam Andrew.

To Linda Harrison, thanks again for the stunning illustrations. For the use of their lovely photos, I thank Suzanne Arms, Pedro Gonzales, Stacie Nunes, Ed Buryn, Katy Raddatz, Gary Yost, Judith Halek, Paivi Laukkanen, Kati Molin, Amy Swagman, and Doris Silva.

And to all the parents and children pictured throughout the book and the midwives who appear here or who assisted the families pictured, my humble gratitude.

To the staff at Ten Speed Press, especially Julie Bennett, Sara Golski, Colleen Cain, Ellen Cavalli, and Ken DellaPenta, my deep thanks and appreciation. And in memory of my former publisher, David Hinds—I will always be grateful for your friendship and unfailing commitment to making *Heart & Hands* as technically complete and aesthetically pleasing as possible.

At last, my thanks to my children Orion Davis, Celeste Nava, and John Shebalin, for teaching me about the Mystery of Birth and loving me no matter what.

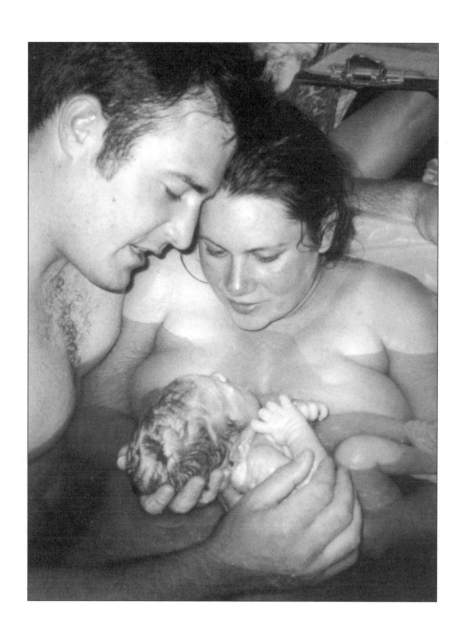

Preface to the Fifth Edition

I am so grateful to have had yet another opportunity to revise *Heart & Hands*. This process has recast not only the content and style of the text but also my understanding of and approach to my work. This is invaluable to me as a midwifery educator, and I hope the results benefit all my readers.

If you are an expectant or new mother, I thank you for your interest in this detailed information. Although I have attempted to provide a mixture of facts, stories, and opinions, you must infuse this with your personal experience. Your intuition and innate sense of what is right for you must always come first.

I take the revision process seriously and can honestly state that every line in the book has been reconsidered as per its timeliness and accuracy. This edition is much more detailed than the last. Controversies on the routine use of ultrasound, treatment for group B streptococcus, diagnosis of gestational diabetes, vaginal birth after cesarean (VBAC), and induction for postdates are fully addressed. New ways to structure apprenticeship have been added to chapter 7, Becoming a Midwife. Sections in chapter 8, The Midwife's Practice, feature updated guidelines for charting, maintaining client confidentiality, and structuring practice to help prevent burnout. Sections on psychosocial issues have been greatly expanded, particularly with regard to the impact of sexual abuse and other traumas on the

birthing process. Along these lines, questions on this subject originally found in the Medical/Health History form (see appendix C) are now found in the Mother's Confidential Worksheet (appendix D), to be kept separate from the mother's records to protect her privacy.

Thanks to expanded opportunities for international teaching and learning, I have incorporated midwifery techniques from Australia, Bulgaria, Canada, China, Costa Rica, France, Germany, Guatemala, Hungary, Italy, Mexico, New Zealand, Russia, and the United Kingdom on many topics, including comfort measures in birth, prolonged labor, breech birth, and shoulder dystocia. That birth is an event in which mothers and babies may experience human rights violations is increasingly acknowledged internationally, a subject explored at length in chapter 1.

The most sweeping philosophical changes occur in chapter 4, Assisting at Births. As I reviewed this material, I saw that it bore remnants of the medicalized view that birth needs to be managed, with someone on hand to suggest positions to the mother, massage her perineum, prevent tears, promote bonding, and so on. I realized that, in the evolution of our work, we are transitioning from one developmental phase to the next. In the early years of our renaissance, we rediscovered the power of birth but were often in denial of our own birth traumas. As a consequence, we tended to overdo our involvement in labor so that mothers would never feel abandoned, or suffer the indignities of episiotomy, or know the pain of separation from their babies as we had. But with new information on the physiology of birth, it is clear that the less we do, the better. Calm, undisturbed mothers know what to do, and when. The more we learn, the more it seems our early vision has been realized: birth works, and we can trust it!

It is interesting that while we were busy figuring this out, a grassroots movement for unassisted birth sprang up internationally. Although monetary factors are part of this choice for some mothers, other factors, like a desire for privacy, self-determination, and the freedom to be fully intimate with partner and other supporters rate much higher. This movement is indicative of many things, not the least of which is that professionalism in health care tends to breed elitism or complacent self-interest. In much the same way that midwives unwilling to be told what to do by medicine formed their own movement and articulated their own goals and visions, mothers unwilling to be told what to do by midwives are taking a stand, and we would be wise to take heed.

On the other hand, as midwifery develops its own body of research, we find that many of our practices and beliefs are well founded, with solid support for the physiology of water birth, delayed cord clamping, baby-led breastfeeding, and so on. Some of this evidence is new, and some so old as to be nearly forgotten. I am thrilled to incorporate the latter in this edition of *Heart & Hands*, with gratitude to all the midwives who have shared their wisdom with me. I particularly want to thank midwife, author, and friend Anne Frye for her outstanding contributions, and Maria Iorillo for her help on the Medical/Health History form.

Perhaps all these factors together are responsible for a new surge of interest in autonomous practice, a rekindled desire to offer full-scope care "from womb to tomb" as we have done throughout the ages. Everywhere in the world, I see midwives struggling with the medicalization of birth and institutionalized disregard of women, being reduced to mere baby catchers while being hopelessly overworked and underpaid. But some are finding the strength to speak up and get organized. At the 2011 Midwifery Today conference in Germany, in response to a passionate desire of the participants (and many years of discussion across the globe), I announced the formation of the International Alliance of Autonomous Midwives. Although still in the early stages, this organization is long overdue and could make a huge difference not only for midwives but also for the women and families they serve. At the same time, I am excited to see midwifery students organizing internationally to advocate their rights to humane, connected, and respectful education, as I believe that a new wave of autonomous practitioners will result.

This is particularly critical in light of the cesarean epidemic and resulting rise in maternal mortality. A multilayered, multilevel approach is needed to address this, but at the core, deep reverence for what is truly natural in birth must be restored to all cultures, and in this, midwives have their work cut out for them. I once wrote an article for *Midwifery Today* on this subject, titled "Wild, Beautiful Birth," in which I used the contrast between a beautiful, clear running river in the Alaskan wilderness and a lifeless, polluted creek in California as a metaphor for the loss of purity and wildness in ourselves, in birth, in the care we provide the women we serve. It may take courage and more than a little effort to rekindle our original passion for this work, but the time has come. The personal is political: we must practice what we preach about birth and let the beauty of birth shine through and inform all we do.

Preface to the First Edition

The purpose of this book is to offer a practical guide to midwifery—to instruct those women interested in becoming midwives and to convey the realities of practice. Midwifery is a lost and found art, finding its place in our time via its links to feminism and expanding consciousness. It also appeals to a growing do-it-yourself resourcefulness. Women who want to be midwives have usually experienced birth firsthand and want to share and facilitate a new awareness of the power of being female. Most are seeking to extend their relationships with other mothers and babies. Many women who think that midwifery is their calling will read this book and realize that there are many other related areas that need development, such as birth education, postpartum support, and family counseling.

This book is intended to demystify the medical elitism surrounding a very basic, natural body process. There are other books that give more detailed information on obstetrics, but none explains how to adapt this information to individual women and how to bend the rules to fit each situation. This is a book on practical midwifery, with a special focus on creative management of complications. Thus it provides some answers for parents who want more than just good quality care and are seeking to understand the various alternative solutions to problems that may arise in pregnancy and birthing. This information is also intended for midwives practicing in remote areas with little or no medical consultation.

However, this manual is only a partial guide to midwifery practice, as nothing can substitute for experience—the educated intuition that comes from attending many births. But at least the suggested practices and procedures may stimulate the aspiring midwife to question and study, and may also inspire dedicated practitioners to break ground with new, responsible methods. If this book moves parents and health professionals alike to innovative thought and humanistic understanding, the heart of its purpose will be realized.

Thanks be to the midwives—a positive, loving, bright, and pioneering bunch of women—for freely sharing skills and information without which this book would not have been written.

CHAPTER 1

The Midwife: A Profile

From the very beginning, women have helped one another give birth. One particularly attuned to this task emerged as the village midwife, wielding the skills of her time and culture. It is the midwife, not the physician, who has attended birth for most of human existence. In modern-day cultures of Norway, the Netherlands, Denmark, Germany, and Sweden, midwife-assisted birth is still the norm. In fact, the six countries with the lowest perinatal mortality rates in the world all make generous use of midwives, who attend 70 percent of all births. In the United States, where midwives assist only 5 to 8 percent of births due to political constraints, perinatal mortality is alarmingly high: we rank thirtieth internationally (meaning that twenty-nine countries lose fewer babies than we do).[1] Our maternal mortality rating is even worse; we are forty-second.[2]

Despite the efficacy of the midwifery model, midwives have been persecuted throughout history, particularly in the West. During the Inquisition and the subsequent period known as the "burning times," the main targets were the midwives. Healing by way of nature and aligned with the wisdom of the body, it's no wonder the *Malleus Maleficarum*, handbook of the Inquisition, declared: "No one

does more harm to the Catholic Church than do the midwives."

In the United States, attacks against midwifery accelerated in the early 1900s, when medicine became a profession for profit and the newly emerged male physician became eager for the revenues of childbirth. Women were barred from university, thus those wanting to attend childbirth could not acquire the requisite credentials. At this point, midwifery was nearly eradicated, so vehement was the campaign of male physicians to discredit midwife practitioners who were portrayed as slovenly, immoral, drunken, promiscuous, and perverse, "whores with dirty fingers." In medieval times, midwives were branded consorts of the devil; now they became "loose women" intent on their own healing methods, in contrast to "good girls" who pursued nursing and accepted roles subservient to the physician.

Unsurprisingly, physician-attended birth proved to be both expensive and unsafe. The high incidence of childbed fever linked to hospital birth in the early 1900s not only cost women their lives but also tapped their families for a tidy sum. Still, women who could not afford to be in the hospital continued to rely on midwives and their skills in preventive medicine, with an emphasis on cleanliness, good nutrition, and the use of natural healing modalities. Thus midwives of the past fostered their clients' strength by providing education and counseling on a variety of health-related issues, much as they do today. The midwife's scope of practice has traditionally been care "from womb to tomb" with a holistic, community health approach to treating a spectrum of women's diseases and afflictions.

For midwives to continue to assert their time-honored scope of practice meant war with the increasingly powerful medical profession: a war that continues to this day. Left to their own devices, midwives would not have survived this struggle; they were poor, politically powerless, and disorganized. Midwifery exists today for one reason only: women's insistence on midwifery care.

Although traditional midwives trained by apprenticeship have practiced almost continuously in the United States, the development of nurse-midwifery is fairly recent. The Frontier Nursing Service began training midwives in 1939, using a model developed in England. There are now more than forty programs preparing nurse-midwives, although barriers to practice are considerable. Physician reactions to the nurse-midwife are mixed: on the one hand, she can be a valuable adjunct to a busy practice; on the other, if she wants to practice independently with her own caseload, she is a threat, an economic competitor. That the physician expects the nurse to be subordinate is rooted in cultural suppression of women healers and the tenets of technocratic medicine. But the midwife's responsibilities require the autonomy to make her own decisions and use interventions, maneuvers, and procedures in case of emergency that inadvertently cross into the physician's self-proclaimed scope of practice—and herein lies the conflict.

The question of how to forge legitimacy within the medical system has caused sharp divisions between nurse-midwives who align more strongly with nursing than midwifery and those who identify more with midwifery than nursing. Internationally, the debate continues as to whether training in nursing is truly relevant. It is noteworthy that in the Netherlands, applicants to midwifery schools lose points for a nursing background, as it is understood that a nurse's conditioning to follow doctors' orders is contrary to the independent thought and action essential for competent midwifery practice. With the one exception of South Africa, the United States is the only country in the world that utilizes the title "nurse-midwife."

Nurse-midwifery does enjoy fully secure legal status in the United States, whereas direct-entry midwifery (midwifery without a nursing background) is still illegal in many states. Although direct-entry midwives have struggled to legalize their practice, they continue to meet with bitter opposition from the wealthiest and most powerful lobby in the country, the American Medical Association (AMA). In California alone, seven legislative attempts were

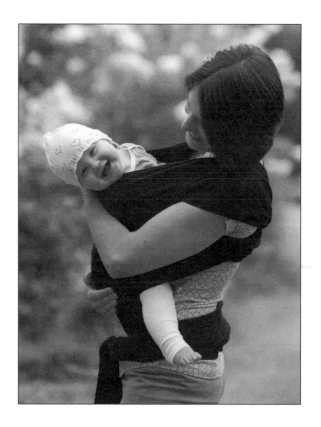

made over ten years, during which more than fifty midwives were investigated, with a number arrested and prosecuted. Direct-entry midwives once numbered 350 in the Golden State, but a decade later, their ranks had dwindled to 60 or so.

How did this happen? In 1974, a pregnant agent from the District Attorney's office visited Santa Cruz midwife Kate Boland. Wired for sound, she garnered evidence to the effect that Boland was found guilty of practicing medicine without a license. Thus in California (as in other states), the practice of midwifery was defined as a misdemeanor. Misdemeanor practices resulting in death or injury—regardless of whether the death or injury was unpreventable—are subject to felony charges of manslaughter or murder. It has cost midwives a tremendous sum (tens of thousands of dollars) to defend themselves and their colleagues against unfounded counts of murder. This money has been hard to come by and would have been better spent to fund legalization efforts or the founding of midwifery schools and public education campaigns. We do not exaggerate in calling this modern-day war against midwives a "witch hunt."

And yet, the continued threat of criminal prosecution has motivated the effort to legalize midwifery in the States. It is a testament to the fortitude and vision of direct-entry midwives that they have been able to survive the costs—not only financial, but personal as well—of these seemingly endless and agonizing legal battles. We owe the evolution of our profession to the persistence of our founding mothers and to the next generation that fought so hard to secure these gains. As a result, licensing (LM) or certification (CM) is now available in twenty-six states, with eight more actively pursuing legalization (in the rest, the practice is unregulated).

How was this accomplished? By 1980, midwives had begun writing their own standards of practice, particularly in states where midwives were not prosecuted. Then in 1982, the Midwives Alliance of North America (MANA) was founded to help

midwives "of every stripe" articulate their visions and find support in their struggle for legitimization.

Shortly after the first edition of *Heart & Hands* was published in 1981, I was asked to serve on the first MANA Executive Board. By then, several other board members had already passed progressive legislation in their respective states. After an intense day of meetings, several of them approached me and asked me point-blank, "So, Liz, what are you going to do to organize California?" Honestly, the thought had not crossed my mind, especially in light of how underground we were at the time. When I asked their advice, they suggested we devise a process of self-certification. When I questioned the necessity of this obviously huge undertaking, they pointed out that if we did not regulate ourselves, the state would step in and do it for us. With the help of my students and colleagues, this dream became a reality in 1986.

Several historic events bear mentioning at this juncture. In 1985, MANA members first considered the possibility of national certification. But the notion was shelved for fear that setting national standards might negatively impact individual states' self-determination in regulations. Then, in 1991, the Carnegie Foundation funded a task force of both direct-entry and nurse-midwives to address the future of midwifery education. This group produced a document entitled *Midwifery Certification in the United States*, which outlined identical competencies and scope of practice for all midwives regardless of training route. Before long, there was renewed discussion of national certification for direct-entry midwives.

Some years earlier, in response to members' desire to have a means of demonstrating their competence, the North American Registry of Midwives (NARM) was founded by MANA to develop and administer a national registry exam. In light of the Carnegie findings, NARM decided to move ahead with national certification in 1993. To facilitate this, I called the first national planning and development meeting, inviting midwives from every state who had expertise in formulating legislation or regulations. Together, we formed the Certification Task Force (CTF), charged with developing the certification process and providing technical assistance to NARM on its implementation. This process was approved by the MANA membership, and in 1995, the first certified professional midwife (CPM) was recognized by NARM.

NARM certification is unique in that it is *competency based*. The candidate may complete an accredited program or a portfolio process based on independent study, but in either case, she must demonstrate entry-level midwifery knowledge and skill via

1. verification of requisite clinical experience;
2. verification of requisite skills and caregiving abilities;
3. verification of good character (letters of recommendation); and
4. verification of knowledge (comprehensive written examination).

Once certified, she must agree to fulfill continuing educational requirements, keep CPR and neonatal resuscitation skills updated, work within the scope defined by the MANA core competencies, and uphold MANA standards and ethics of practice. (In contrast, the American College of Nurse-Midwives [ACNM] offers certification only to those who have completed an accredited program.)

How does the CPM credential interface with state licensure or certification? In time, it seems likely that the CPM process will be adopted state by state as the universal process for assessing direct-entry competence. Midwives in states with unduly restrictive practice guidelines might use national certification as a rationale for regulatory changes. Many states already utilize the NARM test as their licensing or certification board exam. As more and more states adopt the national process in its entirety, reciprocity will be increasingly available for midwives wishing to relocate, and the entire profession will benefit from increased self-regulation.

Across the globe, self-regulation is the point where battle lines have been drawn between midwives and the medical profession. With cesarean rates in the United States at 33 percent; in China, 46 percent; in Vietnam, 36 percent; in Paraguay, 42 percent; and in Italy and Mexico, 40 percent, the need for health-promoting, noninterventive midwifery care has never been clearer.[3] The question is how to generate more midwives and how they should be trained to address this crisis. Some nurse-midwives believe that higher education, or master's-level midwifery, is the key to greater professional autonomy. Conversely, most direct-entry midwives believe that no credential will be enough as long as physicians are the ruling class and that midwives must define midwifery on its own terms, rather than jumping through an endless series of legitimacy hoops. Despite these differences, I believe that midwives must unite behind the issue of autonomous practice. The fight for autonomous midwifery now rages internationally; there is not a country in the world where midwives are not restricted in caregiving. In some, they can give prenatal care but cannot assist births; in others, the situation is the opposite.

To address this worldwide struggle of midwives to take their rightful place in the health care system, the International Confederation of Midwives (ICM) drafted the *International Definition of a Midwife*. The World Health Organization (WHO) and the International Federation of Gynecology and Obstetrics (FIGO) adopted this in 1972. Here is the 2005 revision:

> A midwife is a person who, having been regularly admitted to a midwifery educational program, duly recognized in the country in which it is located, has successfully completed the prescribed course of studies in midwifery and has acquired the requisite qualifications to be registered and/or legally licensed to practice midwifery.
>
> The midwife is recognized as a responsible and accountable professional who works in partnership with women to give the necessary support, care, and advice during pregnancy, labor and the postpartum

period, to conduct births on the midwife's own responsibility and to provide care for the newborn and the infant. This care includes preventative measures, the promotion of normal birth, the detection of complications in mother and child, the accessing of medical care or other appropriate assistance, and the carrying out of emergency measures.

The midwife has an important task in health counseling and education, not only for the woman, but also within the family and the community. This work should involve antenatal education and preparation for parenthood and may extend to women's health, sexual or reproductive health, and childcare.

A midwife may practice in any setting including the home, community, hospitals, clinics, or health units.[4]

This definition is remarkable not only for what it says, but for what it leaves unspoken. Nowhere do we find any stricture regarding the risk status of clients or any attempt to limit the practice to **well-women** or **interconceptional care**, terms commonly used in statutes to restrict scope of practice. Particularly powerful are the assertions that a midwife conducts births on her own responsibility and may execute emergency measures. Unfortunately, the description of educational preparation often leaves traditional midwives out of the loop (reflecting an ongoing controversy within the ICM). More inclusive documents have been generated by the MANA membership, including *MANA Statement of Values and Ethics*, *MANA Core Competencies for Midwifery Practice*, and *MANA Standards and Qualifications for the Art and Practice of Midwifery* (see appendix A).

Yet another organization that has contributed to the professionalization of midwifery is the Midwifery Education Accreditation Council (MEAC), which is recognized by the U.S. Department of Education. MEAC was created by a group of midwifery educators who wanted to promote better learning experiences for students by linking their programs to the accountability mechanisms and funding opportunities of accreditation. MEAC's founding principle is to preserve a variety of educational routes to practice, particularly apprenticeship. Contact info for MEAC,

MANA, ACNM, and NARM may be found in appendix B. At the grassroots level, Citizens for Midwifery (CFM) is the consumer arm of these organizations. In terms of public education, check out the consumer-oriented public education web page, Mothers Naturally, and also see the Big Push for Midwives, NARM's consumer activist site (see appendix B).

The organization of Midwifery Today bears special mention. With a magazine, e-zine, national and international conferences, and an international membership section, it plays a central role in fostering the next generation of midwives while drawing on the wisdom of those seasoned in practice. As a regular speaker on the Midwifery Today conference circuit, I can attest to the outstanding work of this organization and the deep inspiration to be found in learning about midwifery by sharing knowledge and skills in a supportive, international environment. (Again, see appendix B for more information.)

Considering the troubled past and the challenging present of midwifery, it is a miracle that it has survived. What makes midwifery so desirable to birthing women? Simply put, midwifery promotes well-being. It is an art of service, in that the midwife recognizes, responds to, and cooperates with natural forces. In this sense, midwifery is ecologically attuned, involving the wise utilization of resources and respect for the balance of nature.

Midwifery care is *personalized care*. Despite parameters of safety the midwife must uphold, she knows that wellness is an amorphous state with periodic deviations from normal. Her task is to decipher the unique and fluid patterns of each mother's health status. The more thorough and continuous her care, the more likely she is to detect a complication at its inception. And the better she and the mother communicate, the more readily they will be able to develop and implement a solution. She and the mother are a team, but the locus of responsibility is always with the latter. As the *MANA Statement of Values and Ethics* states, the mother is the "direct care provider for her unborn child" (see appendix A).

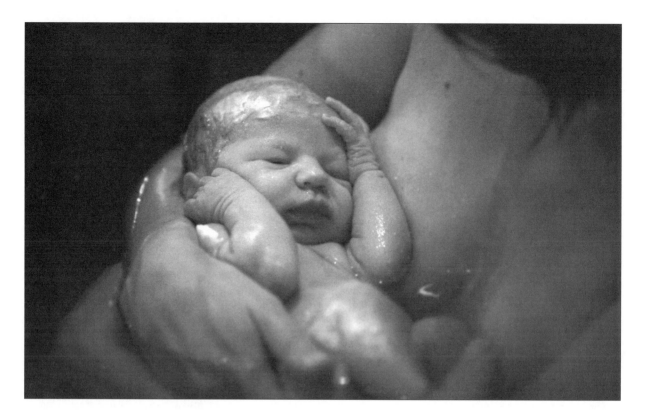

Birth is indeed a pinnacle event, but it is merely the finishing touch to a preestablished intimacy between the midwife, the mother and her supporters, and the baby. Every birth has some potential for complications, and the midwife is trained to respond to these, but her ability to do so is greatly enhanced by foreknowledge of those involved and their trust in her competence.

Thus the essence of midwifery care is to be humbly and fully available: an approach antithetical to that of medicine. Early in their training, medical students learn to control themselves through the rigors of residency and then to control their patients and outcomes through standardized procedures. They learn little of the art of caregiving, being taught instead to bypass personal involvement, mistrust their intuition, expect pathology, and fear death. It's no wonder they seek control, and as they do, there is no room for nature to take its course.

To better understand why practices and interventions vary so dramatically between home and hospital births, we must consider the paradigms of health care that largely determine these. Anthropologist Robbie Davis-Floyd has identified three such paradigms: technocratic, humanistic, and holistic.

- The **technocratic model** is based on beliefs that the body is a machine, that disease comes from without, that standardized care is best because it minimizes the risk of the unexpected, and that the practitioner knows best. In short, *it is a model based on control.*

- The **humanistic model** would modify the tenets of the technocratic model by making practices more humane, by allowing a bit more time for care, by emphasizing bedside manner and concern for the patient's needs and feelings. *It is a model based on kindness and good intentions.*

- The **holistic model** redefines the patient as a client and decision maker in the health care experience, the authority on her own health status, responsible for educating herself on her care options and for carrying out daily self-care, with her health a manifestation of emotional, psychological, and physical factors. *It is a model based on education and empowerment.*

In general, midwifery care incorporates humanistic or holistic tenets, whereas medical care is primarily technocratic.[5]

Technocratic, fear-based care has little appeal to women aware of other options. What women want is competent, sensitive attention to their entire being—care from the inside out. Defining our health as more than physical, we seek care that will enable us to be fully ourselves, at our greatest potential. This is precisely what midwives offer. Midwifery has been dubbed an art of invisibility because it is noninterventive except in rendering that which is needed to promote balance or restore harmony.

Who is today's midwife? No matter what her route to practice—or whether she is working openly, underground, or in or out of a hospital—she is ready and willing to go against the grain, that is, if she intends to practice independently. Illegal practice is especially difficult, for she must risk her own welfare to maintain that of her clients. This takes a strong, alert, and self-determined woman. And herein lies the secret to the midwife's notoriety: she is a rebel and a female one at that!

It is ironic that feminism has not more strongly aligned itself with midwifery, especially since reproductive self-determination is central to the feminist vision. Truly, what could be more feminist than the practice of midwifery? The most potent lesson of childbirth is the revelation of essential feminine force. Giving birth calls on a woman to shed her social skin and discover her ability to cooperate with and surrender to elemental forces. Birth can profoundly transform a woman, strengthening her faith and deepening her identity. Hence the midwife, guardian and facilitator of this process, is intrinsically feminist by the very nature of her work. She knows that women who labor on their own terms and triumph in spontaneous birthing will mother in a fiercely

independent fashion, with strength and inner certainty spilling into every other aspect of their lives.

Giving birth is more than just having a baby; it is a pivotal event in a woman's personal development. As mentioned earlier, midwives have traditionally cared for women throughout the life cycle, facilitating the physiologic milestones of menarche, birth, menopause, and death. These times of transition are more than biological; they are our Blood Mysteries. In them, we gain wisdom through our bodies that utterly transcends any rational process. Many indigenous cultures have deliberately created rites of passage for men involving sacrifice and suffering (such as the Native American Sundance) to replicate the growth and transformation rendered naturally to women through their Blood Mysteries.

Thus the cultural/evolutionary aspect of midwifery care motivates mothers to extend the power and joy of giving birth, to reach beyond the isolation of the nuclear family, to network and share their resources, and to raise their children cooperatively. In so doing, midwifery is also linked to innovations in child care, a renewed emphasis on extended family, and holism in other health care modalities as factors of nutrition, rest, exercise, and support are recognized as crucial to well-being. For the most part, women who choose midwifery seek connection; they long to rise above divisiveness and competition to establish support systems and create community.

Above all else, midwives advocate informed choice. They vigorously defend a mother's right to choose place and manner of giving birth, just as they fight for their own right to practice artfully and in any setting. Hospital privileges are often denied midwives and the physicians who support them. Here we see the deterioration of the art and science of obstetrics, with practice guidelines strictly inside the box, as runaway costs and frivolous malpractice claims mandate procedures for their own sake. We have lost some of our finest obstetricians to this crisis, those who could not, in good conscience, practice in a manner at odds with their patients' well-being. For midwives, this has meant a dearth of good backup and more urgency than ever to advance a mother/baby-centered model of perinatal care.

For these reasons, many women choosing midwifery care choose to give birth at home, seeking the comfort, privacy, and opportunity for family participation inherent in their own environment, with a minimum of interventions. The physiology of birth makes clear that the more relaxed and at ease a laboring woman feels, the more efficiently her body will function. If she is upset, she will release **stress hormones** (catecholamines) that inhibit cervical dilation. All birthing mammals behave thus: if denied privacy, moved, or threatened, an arrest of progress inevitably occurs. This is why Pitocin—a synthetic form of oxytocin, the hormone that causes labor contractions—is so frequently used in hospital births. However, Pitocin prompts contractions that are abnormally strong and painful so that women hoping for a natural childbirth often end up requesting pain relief. A vicious cycle ensues in that pain medications typically disrupt the forces of labor so that more Pitocin is needed. But there is a limit: if

the uterus is pushed too hard, it will not relax enough between contractions to permit healthy circulation, fetal distress will ensue, and a cesarean will become necessary. Known as the **cascade of interventions**, this chain of events drives the cesarean epidemic.

What are cesarean rates with midwifery care? For midwife-assisted births in hospital, rates are much less than with obstetric care. But what are the rates with homebirth? In 2005, the *British Medical Journal (BMJ)*, a prestigious and highly selective periodical, published the largest and most reputable study of homebirth in North America. In this study of 5,418 planned homebirths assisted by CPMs, only 12 percent of women transferred to the hospital, and of these, 4.7 percent had epidural anesthesia, 2.1 percent had an episiotomy, and 3.7 percent gave birth by cesarean section. No mothers died, and the intrapartum/neonatal mortality rate was 1.7 in 1,000, similar to rates in other studies of low-risk home or hospital birth. At six weeks postpartum, 95.8 percent of mothers in the study were still breastfeeding, 89.7 percent exclusively. Maternal satisfaction rates were high, at 97 percent.[6]

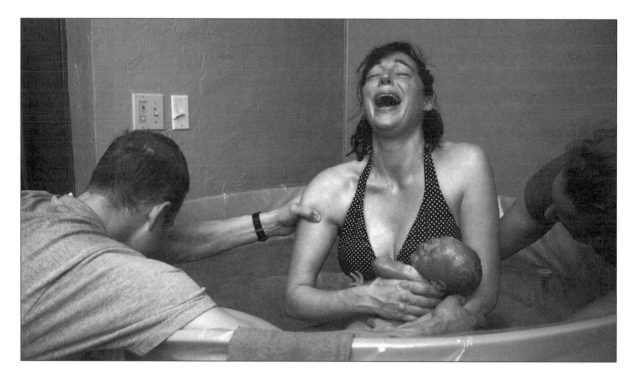

For Parents: Choosing a Midwife

1. How was she trained? Was it in a home, birth center, or hospital setting? Is she licensed and/or certified? If not, why not? Are former clients and community members available who can vouch for her? Is she active in, and well regarded by, her local midwifery community?

2. What is her experience? How many births has she attended since completing her training? Has she worked in a variety of settings and practices? Has she completed neonatal resuscitation recently? Does she regularly attend midwifery conferences, seminars, and workshops to further her education? Does she participate in peer review?

3. What do her services include? Do they include complete prenatal care? How long are the appointments? Does she do home visits (how many), sibling preparation, postpartum follow-up (how much), lab work, prepared childbirth classes?

4. What are her fees? Does she accept insurance, and what portion of her fee will be paid by your plan? What does her fee include? What if you move or change your mind during the pregnancy? Is her fee competitive? How does she want it to be paid?

5. Does she work alone, with a partner, or with assistants? If there are several assistants involved in the practice, can you choose one to be at your birth? What, exactly, is the assistant's role?

6. Does she have a ceiling on the number of births she attends per month? Is this in keeping with the amount of assistance she has? What would happen if two or more births were running simultaneously? Has she ever missed a birth? If so, what were the circumstances?

7. Who would back her up in case of personal emergency? Is it a midwife outside the practice? Will you have a chance to meet her before the birth?

8. What is her communications system like? Is she available twenty-four hours a day at all times? Is she planning to go on vacation during your pregnancy? If so, who will be on call, and how reachable is she? Can you get the same information on this backup midwife as you are now requesting in this interview? (This is especially critical if her vacation will take place during your third trimester.)

9. What experience has she had with complications, and which ones? Has she ever had to resuscitate a baby? How would she handle a hemorrhage or a stillbirth? Under what circumstances would she transfer care during pregnancy? Would she transport during labor?

10. What equipment does she bring to births: oxygen, IV fluids, resuscitation equipment for baby, medications for hemorrhage, homeopathy and herbs, vitamin K for baby? What does she offer for pain relief?

11. What is her medical backup like? Does she have a particular backup physician and hospital? Is this covered by your insurance? If not, what would be approximate costs to you? Do you have the option of transferring to a hospital that does take your insurance? If so, how is this arranged? If she has a particular backup physician and hospital, what are her privileges in that setting? If you do not have insurance, is there any type of retroactive coverage (state aid) available or pediatric backup?

12. What is her philosophy of care? Why is she a midwife? What are her basic beliefs about birth? Does she encourage family participation, father or partner participation, and how? What are her expectations of you regarding self-care in pregnancy?

13. Do you like her, feel comfortable in her presence? Can you be honest with her? Will she be honest with you? Can you trust her, and yet feel free to make your own decisions? Do you want her at your birth?

Two more studies from Canada show similar results. The first, from British Columbia, involved 2,899 planned homebirths with registered midwives, 4,604 planned hospital births with registered midwives, and 5,331 planned hospital births with physicians. The infant mortality rate for homebirth was 0.035 percent, compared to 0.057 percent for midwife-assisted births in hospital, and 0.095 percent in for physician-assisted births in hospital.[7] The second study, from Ontario, showed no significant difference in perinatal and neonatal mortality in 6,692 women who had planned homebirths and the same number who had planned hospital births, although rates of serious maternal complications were lower at home.[8] *When women are in charge of their environment, when they have the privacy to labor undisturbed, when they feel completely at ease and supported, outcomes are always superior.*

Thus the midwife's most basic task is to promote the mother's relaxation and peace of mind. Beyond her repertoire of medical techniques, her skills encompass less concrete abilities to intuit, evoke, and channel energy. Her hands are her most precious tools as she senses, heals, and blesses with her touch. She is infinitely patient—she waits and waits and waits some more. Yet she is ever attentive to the mother's condition and the baby's needs. Quietly aware, she serves as a mirror, reserving judgment but speaking the truth as the need arises. Above all, she keeps this dictum in mind: "It's not my birth." Upholding this core tenet of holistic care means surrendering her expectations to whatever the mother or baby and their supporters need or desire.

In this regard, midwives often speak of a laboring woman's ability to know what is best for herself and her baby. Research now shows this to be inherent in the physiology of birth (more on this in chapter 4). Thus we must never forget to ask the mother's opinion of how best to further her labor. Put simply, miracles happen in childbirth. The midwife must keep her senses alert but stand back, let birth happen, and gratefully bear witness.

If we hope to create a maternity-care system that implements midwifery and is truly mother/baby-centered, women and their supporters need access to information that will assist them in making informed choices regarding place of birth and practitioner with the personal qualities and competence to suit them. Midwives have an urgent obligation to educate the public and to stand firm in their support of holistic care. Why? Because whenever a woman reclaims her right to birth exactly as she desires, she opens the door to unprecedented joy and fulfillment for herself and her intimates while firmly reestablishing the primacy of motherhood in our culture.

Let us wait no longer to heed society's call for midwifery care!

Notes

1. United Nations Statistics Division, http://unstats.un.org.
2. World Health Organization, 2007, www.who.int.
3. World Health Organization. "Rising caesarean deliveries in Latin America: how best to monitor rates and risks," 2009. "Method of delivery and pregnancy outcomes in Asia: the WHO global survey on maternal and perinatal health," 2007–08. Organisation for Economic Co-operation and Development (OECD) Health Data 2010, June 2010.
4. www.internationalmidwives.org.
5. Robbie Davis-Floyd and Gloria St. John, *From Doctor to Healer: The Transformative Journey* (Piscataway Township, NJ: Rutgers University Press, 1998), 142–143.
6. Kenneth Johnson and Betty-Anne Daviss, "Outcomes of Planned Hospital Births with Certified Midwives: A Large Prospective Study in North America," *British Medical Journal* 330 (2005): 1416.
7. Patricia A. Janssen, Lee Saxell, Lesley A. Page, Michael C. Klein, Robert M. Liston, and Shoo K. Lee, "Outcomes of Planned Home Birth with Registered Midwife versus Planned Hospital Birth with Midwife or Physician," *Canadian Medical Association Journal* 181 (September 15, 2009): 377–83.
8. Eileen K. Hutton, Angela H. Reitsma, and Karyn Kaufman, "Outcomes Associated with Planned Home and Planned Hospital Births in Low-Risk Women Attended by Midwives in Ontario, Canada, 2003–2006: A Retrospective Cohort Study," *Birth* 36, no. 3 (September 2009): 180–89.

CHAPTER 2

Prenatal Care

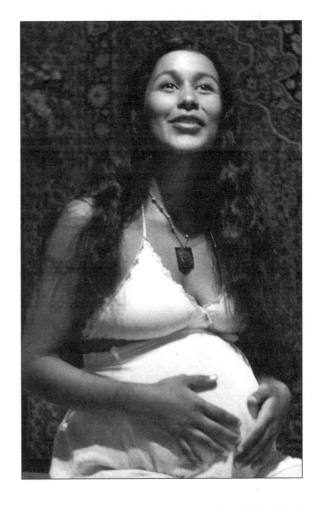

Midwives in independent practice offer comprehensive prenatal care. By so doing, they get to know clients well enough to have some sense of what to anticipate at the birth. In my experience, careful prenatal assessment is the cornerstone of safe and sustainable midwifery practice; the better we do our work prenatally, the less we are surprised by long, drawn-out labors. Every mother's condition is unique and is best appreciated with regular contact. In building rapport and a solid working relationship with our clients, we experience the benefits of **continuity of care**.

Assessment is important throughout pregnancy but is crucial during the last six weeks. At this point, the midwife can identify certain factors regarding the baby's position, size, and growth rate, and relate these to the mother's condition. On this basis, she can more realistically prepare the mother (and herself) for the labor, offering suggestions to prevent complications and make the birth easier. On a technical level, knowing the baby's and mother's norms enables the midwife to determine an acceptable range of normal during labor. For everyone concerned, prenatal care definitely proves its worth in terms of time, energy, and anxiety spared at births.

Prenatal care really means wellness care and as such involves knowledge of nutrition, exercise, non-allopathic healing options of herbology or homeopathy, and mind-body integration techniques like yoga and meditation. It also involves tests and procedures to screen for complications. Routine urinalysis, blood pressure evaluation, uterine/fetal palpation, fetal heart auscultation, and assessment of fundal height/fetal growth are detailed later in this chapter, as are lab work and interpretation of results. If any significant abnormality arises, medical consultation should be sought for guidance and prognosis.

The First Contact

Your first contact with a woman seeking your services will probably be by phone. Ask her how she became interested in having her baby at home and what she is looking for in a midwife. This will help you see how well founded her interest is and whether it is worth pursuing further. If you know each other already, put aside preconceived notions and be open to new impressions.

If this information checks out well, go ahead with questions about her current state of health, her relationship with her partner (if applicable), previous pregnancies, or any history of medical problems. This is the time to rule out any contraindications to homebirth (see the "High-Risk Factors in Pregnancy" sidebar, on page 20). Hopefully, she will have questions regarding your care: philosophy of practice, experience, backup, and so on. If you agree to meet, the initial visit should be scheduled within the following week or so, preferably at a time when her partner (if applicable) can also attend. Plan to spend at least two hours on this visit, as there will be plenty to discuss and, possibly, physical examinations to perform if you decide to work together.

Whatever you do, never try to talk a woman into working with you or giving birth at home. She must make these decisions on her own. To uphold principles of mother/baby-centered caregiving, the mother's responsibility must be established from the very beginning.

The Initial Interview

This very personal, in-depth meeting is your opportunity to understand the mother's ideals surrounding birth and parenting. If she has had other children, she will probably share her previous birth experience(s). If this is her first baby, she will be full of questions.

Your most important task in the initial interview is to determine whether you and the mother are suited to work together. The best way to do this is to be as relaxed and as open as possible. Follow the mother's energetic leads and physical pacing; match her timing and conversational style so she feels sufficiently at ease to disclose her deepest beliefs and concerns. If you gain her trust, any advice you feel compelled to offer will be taken seriously. Stay in a receptive mode, taking her in body and soul, and later, notice how this contact has affected you. If you feel uneasy or apprehensive, you may not be a match. Pay close attention to your first impressions: after thirty years of doing this work, I've had ample opportunity to hear midwives recount their unhappy outcomes, and in each and every case, they ruefully recalled feeling uncomfortable with the mother at the initial visit.

Elicit reasons for choosing homebirth from both the mother and her partner (if present). Notice priorities. Ask about the response of friends and family. Explore the choice as proactive versus reactive: For example, does the mother truly desire homebirth or simply fear birthing in hospital? Is cost an issue or determining factor?

To support mothers in doing what is best for them, it helps to understand the role of social and biological instincts. The need to belong—to be a member of a group and to be recognized by that group—is a social instinct. **Social instincts** lead us to make socially recognized choices. On the other hand, **biological instincts**, such as those for survival and self-realization, are more deeply rooted. These instincts connect us to our innermost feelings and biological competencies.[1] If biological instincts and social instincts are in conflict, problems can develop, as in the case of the woman wanting a homebirth when none of her friends or family approve. Women with strong biological instincts may break away from their group for a short time, but not without a certain amount of stress—something the midwife must take into account.[2]

In contrast, women with weak biological instincts need more social structure and approval. If planning homebirth, they may end up in the hospital and later feel very distressed because they didn't satisfy their biological instincts. Social and biological models are rarely aligned in hospital birth, thus women birthing within these systems often experience this conflict.[3]

To satisfy both instincts, a woman needs a group with values similar to her personal, instinctive model. This is why support of other homebirthing parents is so critical. It also explains why birth centers offer an effective middle ground for some women; they lessen the conflict because these centers are more accepted by society.[4] Draw on this perspective to understand the mother's response to questions about how her friends and relatives feel about her plans and, if they are not supportive, how she will deal with this.

Along the same lines, who will be at the birth? Ask to meet with her birth team as soon as possible to assess any social/biological conflicts in those hoping to attend, and on a practical level, to identify any gaps in her support system. Some mothers initially plan on having quite a party at the birth and then whittle down participants as the pregnancy progresses; you can help her fine-tune the choreography as the time draws near. Still, suggest that she ask everyone interested in being at the birth to commit to postpartum assistance. It is never too early to start lining up dinners, help with laundry or housework, and so on for the first few weeks after the baby comes.

Try to get a clear sense of how the mother defines your role in pregnancy, labor, and postpartum. Does she want guidance or self-determination? Are you comfortable with her ideals in this regard? Is she counting on support from her partner during the birth, or does she envision birthing mostly on her own? To what extent is she willing to accept routine assessments during labor? Are her assessments of the need for postpartum support realistic? As the mother expresses her hopes and desires, it becomes easier for you to anticipate her needs and make assessments and decisions regarding your participation.

Throughout this initial discussion, there may be moments when you feel like making suggestions. In keeping with the holistic model of care, take your prompts from the mother: let her define her needs and concerns. Ask questions based on what she tells you; for example, if she says she feels like she could use more support, ask her what kind of support might be most helpful (rather than suggesting what you consider best). It can't hurt to have lists of books, videos, websites, prenatal exercise or postpartum support groups, and so on, on hand, should she indicate interest.

And you are obligated to disclose your training, philosophy of care, style of practice, and your responsibilities toward and expectations of your clients. The easiest way to do this is with a take-home document: a "Professional Disclosure and Consent to Care" to be returned and signed in your presence.

This document should also include the standards of practice in your state (if applicable), conditions requiring consultation or referral, your relationship to the medical community, client rights (your state probably publishes a patient's bill of rights, which you might include in full or modify), risks of homebirth, and complications that might result in damage or death to mother or baby. Of course, you should stress that prenatal care and timely assessments in labor go a long way toward preventing complications, but make clear that some are unforeseeable. You also need to clarify what happens in the event that either of you decide to terminate care.

This document should further explain how the mother's health information will be protected (see the "Client Confidentiality and HIPAA Guidelines" section on page 243) and when information must at times be disclosed. In some states, midwives are required to break confidentiality and inform the appropriate agency or person (1) if they believe that their life or someone else's life, safety, or property is threatened or endangered; (2) if there is evidence or even suspicion of physical or sexual abuse or neglect of a minor child, other dependent, or a developmentally disabled adult or elderly person; and (3) if a judge orders certain information disclosed in a legal proceeding. In the event of a divorce custody battle, the attorney for the opposing side may have certain information subpoenaed. Make clear that you will inform your client of any subpoena: if they object to you complying, you may still be required to turn over the information, but only if ordered by a judge or otherwise required by law.

In many states, licensed/certified midwives are required by law to disclose whether they have malpractice insurance; in any case, you must disclose your legal status. Also make sure to list any students, assistants, and associates within the practice, including their names and respective roles, while informing clients that they may choose who will be involved in their prenatal care and birth and in what capacity. And explain what the mother can do if she wishes to register a complaint regarding your care.

The final paragraph (actual consent to care) should state that the client, in full knowledge of your philosophy of care, training, legal status, and standards of practice, voluntarily agrees to work with you, and with her signature, releases you and your associates from all liability. It is also wise to include a statement that in the event of a dispute, she will seek arbitration before filing suit.

As you review and discuss this form at the next visit, watch for anxious or negative reactions. Note any resistance to hospital transport or apprehension regarding life-threatening complications. If the mother or her partner seems unusually fearful, ask for her or his worst nightmare regarding the birth. This gives you an opportunity to assess their depth of commitment to homebirth and a chance to provide some background on how complications occur and how they might be forestalled. Emphasize the preventative role of prenatal care, both in terms of what you provide and what she will provide to herself and her baby.

Early in your caregiving, the two most serious emergencies—postpartum hemorrhage and fetal distress/need for resuscitation—require detailed discussion. Explain causes of postpartum hemorrhage and your procedures for handling it. Discuss methods for dealing with a distressed/depressed baby, including tools and techniques for resuscitation. Let the mother know that you will do your best to inform her of any unusual developments in the course of labor, but if emergencies develop, there may not be time for this. Make sure she understands this when she signs the consent to care.

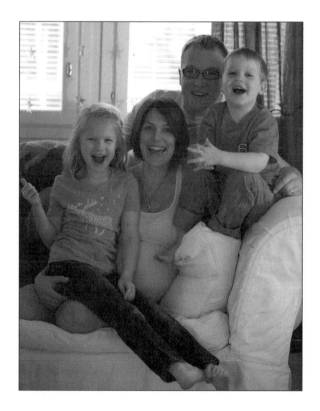

Medical/Health History

Medical/health history can be taken in person or provided by the mother via a take-home form (see appendix C). It should survey for all situations, conditions, and diseases that might impact this pregnancy. Preexisting diabetes or hypertension, thyroid disease (hyperthyroidism), chronic lung disease, severe asthma, clotting disorders, epilepsy, congenital heart disease (grades 2 to 4), kidney disease, and extreme obesity contraindicate homebirth. Conditions arising in pregnancy that rule out homebirth include Rh– with antibodies; severe anemia unresponsive to treatment; cancer (depending on treatment); acute viral infections such as rubella, cytomegalovirus, toxoplasmosis, chicken pox, or herpes (depending on when they occur); and any of the preexisting conditions listed above. Unresolved sexually transmitted disease, chronic malnutrition, drug addiction, moderate to frequent alcohol use, and smoking are also contraindications. Have a comprehensive obstetrical text available to evaluate any irregularities in the medical history, and seek the consultation of peers or medical backup whenever in doubt.

Obstetrical history is of foremost importance. Note any *history of emergencies* such as placental abruption, fetal distress, postpartum hemorrhage, shoulder dystocia, or neonatal asphyxiation, or, if the birth was out-of-hospital, history of transport for any reason. Investigate thoroughly and consider implications for the current pregnancy. *History of previous childbirth losses* requires attention to both physical factors and the mother's emotional recovery. Loss due to disappointing birth outcomes should also be discussed: Is there anything that the mother experienced with previous birthing that she wants to avoid this time, or something she wished for that didn't happen? To what extent has she processed these losses; how have they impacted her physical/mental health or that of other family members? Would it be appropriate to refer her to a counselor with expertise in this area?

Don't forget the issue of child spacing. If she has had a child within the past two years, explore the impact of close-set childbearing on her physical and psychological health.

Any *history of abortion* should be discussed whenever the mother is ready. What type of procedure was used? Was there any excess bleeding or infection? Suction is less traumatic to the uterine lining than **dilation and curettage** (**D&C**), which involves scraping the endometrium and may cause scarring that can interfere with placental implantation (as may **postabortion sepsis** [or infection]). How was the decision to have an abortion reached? What, if any, were the emotional side effects? Many women feel great loss after an abortion ("Like tearing your heart out," one woman said) and need to talk it over, either with you or with a specialist. The same is true of women with a *history of miscarriage*. If the mother had a saline, Cytotec (misoprostol), or prostaglandin-induced abortion, she experienced a version of labor and may link negative emotions with contraction sensations. Do your best to forestall difficulties in labor by discussing this thoroughly in advance.

What about *previous cesarean birth*? Now here is an area of controversy! For many years, the data on **vaginal birth after cesarean** (VBAC) with low transverse incision showed no significant dangers to mother or baby, with a uterine rupture rate of less than 1 percent. But in the past few decades, the use of Cytotec (misoprostol) as a labor stimulant—when in fact it is an ulcer medicine unapproved for this purpose—has increased the rate of uterine rupture to as much as 6 percent.[5] Consequently, the medical standard has changed from support for VBAC to a mandate for repeat cesarean. This is maddening, as midwives in the home setting don't use Cytotec (misoprostol) to stimulate labor anyway.

There are many potential consequences of cesarean birth of which most women are unaware. Cesarean section is, after all, major abdominal surgery. Risks include life-threatening sepsis, perforation of adjacent organs, scarring of the uterine lining that can lead to abnormal placental implantation and hemorrhage with subsequent childbearing, and the development of adhesions between the uterus and other organs that can cause problems years later, such as obstructed or twisted bowels that may require repeat surgery.[6] There is also an increased rate of maternal death with the procedure: 3.6 times higher than for vaginal birth.[7] In 1982, maternal death in the United States was at 7.5 per 100,000 live births; by 2005, the rate had doubled.[8]

Nevertheless, midwives in some states are now forbidden to assist VBAC at home; in others, they may do so. In New Hampshire, the following VBAC guidelines were instated in legal practice code 503.02:

A midwife shall accept as a client a woman who has had a previous birth by cesarean section only if:

a. The potential client has had only one previous cesarean section

b. The midwife can confirm through a review of the records of the previous delivery by cesarean section that the section was performed through a low transverse uterine segment incision

c. The potential client has had no other uterine surgeries

d. At least 18 months' time separates the date of the potential client's previous cesarean section and the due date of the current pregnancy

e. An obstetric ultrasound documents that the placenta is not in a low-lying anterior position

f. The potential client plans to give birth in a location no more than 20 minutes' drive from a hospital with obstetrical and anesthesia services on call 24 hours a day

There is also evidence to suggest that single-layer suturing of the cesarean incision (in contrast to the more thorough double-layer repair) quadruples the risk of rupture.[9] I've spoken about this to several of my obstetrician colleagues, who concur that it's less a matter of layers than thoroughness in uniting the endometrium so that no myometrium (inner muscle layer) remains exposed. But as single-layer repair has been practiced for years, and medical records seldom specify the method of incision

closure, the point is somewhat moot. Bottom line: the healthier the mother, and the greater the interval between cesarean and subsequent pregnancy, the less she is at risk.

Psychological issues for a mother desiring VBAC can be formidable. If she was told she needed surgery because her bones were too small, her hormone levels too low, or her baby too big, devastating emotional scars may remain and before vaginal birth is attempted, healing should take place. I have found hypnotherapy and eye movement desensitization and reprocessing (EMDR) to be highly effective for helping mothers regain confidence in themselves and their bodies. Psychotherapy has its place, but the trauma of cesarean is housed in the body and may thus be more responsive to therapies that go deeper. Group and individual support are also available through organizations like the International Cesarean Awareness Network (ICAN) (see appendix B).

Plans for out-of-hospital VBAC definitely require that the mother and her partner sign a detailed consent form. But because of all she must do to prepare herself, assisting a woman with a VBAC is truly a privilege.

Gynecological history is also of great significance in pregnancy. Check for *history of fibroids*, the prime symptom of which is painless bleeding with intercourse. These benign uterine masses vary in size but tend to grow considerably in pregnancy. If they are internal (growing inside the uterus rather than on the outside surface), they may reduce intrauterine space so that the baby's growth is restricted, or placental implantation may be abnormal and result in postpartum hemorrhage. An ultrasound is advisable to determine the exact size and location of fibroids. As for treatment, one study showed drinking green tea to be effective in eradicating fibroid lesions in animal subjects.[10]

Gynecological surgeries may also complicate pregnancy, depending on the procedure. If the mother has had a *cone biopsy* (to remove abnormal cervical cells), considerable scarring may retard dilation. Cervical cauterization and cryosurgery are less traumatic, but the cervix should still be checked for scarring. As the mother nears term, scar tissue may be softened by evening primrose oil massaged gently onto the cervix.

LEEP, a laser procedure similar in effect to cone biopsy, has been correlated to incompetent cervix and premature labor. Some midwives feel that any woman with a history of this procedure should be checked for cervical changes throughout pregnancy and must be carefully instructed regarding signs of premature labor.

Contraceptive history is also important. If the mother had an IUD prior to conception, she may be anemic due to excess menstruation and should be screened for this as soon as possible. The IUD can also cause scarring of the uterine lining, which predisposes to ectopic pregnancy, irregular implantation of the placenta, and third-stage hemorrhage. Pelvic inflammatory disease (PID) has the same effect. If scar tissue is discovered at the **cervical os** (cervical opening), massage with evening primrose oil (as described above) is recommended. Or if the mother used oral contraception or other hormonal methods immediately prior to pregnancy, she may be deficient in folic acid and should be advised to begin supplementation at once.

Family history is important for determining a propensity for hypertension, diabetes, heart disease, cancer, or other diseases that could impact pregnancy and may require additional screening from a specialist.

Spend plenty of time at this visit reviewing **symptoms experienced with this pregnancy.** Any *incidence of bleeding or spotting* is significant and should be closely tracked by both mother and midwife. If combined with nonrhythmic pain unaffected by position changes, consider the possibility of ectopic pregnancy (the window for rupture is ten to thirteen weeks) or, if in the last trimester, the possibility of placental abruption. In either case, the mother needs immediate transport for emergency care.

If bleeding is brown and chronic, rule out molar pregnancy and missed abortion (when the fetus has died but is retained). In late pregnancy, repeated episodes of painless bleeding suggest placenta previa (see chapter 3 for more on these conditions).

Generalized edema (affecting face and hands, not just ankles) prior to twenty-four weeks should be medically evaluated; if the mother is twenty-six weeks or more, rule out preeclampsia (see chapter 3). In either case, immediately have her eliminate processed foods, eat plenty of high-quality protein and fresh vegetables with salt to taste, and take ample fluids.

Particularly in early pregnancy, fluctuating hormone levels and circulatory changes may cause occasional *headaches*, but persistent headache, particularly in combination with signs of preeclampsia, indicates a medical crisis and the need for immediate referral. Visual disturbances or epigastric (upper abdominal) pain—especially on the right side—are urgent warning signs of preeclampsia (see page 79).

Any history of *flu-like symptoms*, such as swollen glands, extreme fatigue, or generalized body aches, should be noted, although the most devastating viral infections of pregnancy are frequently asymptomatic. **Cytomegalovirus** is a fairly common infection (60 percent of the general population has antibodies) but if contracted during pregnancy, is most damaging to the fetus in the first trimester. **Toxoplasmosis** too can cause severe neurological damage to the fetus. Although the baby's risk of becoming infected rises as pregnancy progresses (15 percent in the first trimester, 30 percent in the second trimester, and 60 percent in the third trimester), the severity is greatest if the baby is infected in the first trimester. A mother can minimize her chances of contracting toxoplasmosis by avoiding uncooked meat/fish, and if she has a cat, she must avoid any contact with cat feces (someone else should change the litter box). If she has a garden and the cat has access to it, she should garden with gloves and wash everything she harvests before eating. Even viral infections like **varicella** (chicken pox) can be extremely dangerous in pregnancy, so encourage all mothers to avoid possible exposure.

Any report of *painful vaginal sores* combined with flu-like malaise may indicate an initial outbreak of **herpes**. Immediately do a visual inspection and take cultures (the cervix should always be cultured, as herpes at this site can be asymptomatic). An initial outbreak in the first trimester can have serious consequences for the baby and requires immediate consultation. If there is a recurrence in pregnancy, repeat the cultures, and if cervical shedding is noted, plan to do a slide test (or at least a visual inspection) at the onset of labor to rule out current infection. With active lesions at the onset of labor, the standard of care is to perform a cesarean as neonatal infection can cause central nervous system damage and death. However, studies show the rate of neonatal infection to be much less with a recurrence at the onset of labor (3 percent) than with an initial outbreak (41 percent).[11] It appears that mothers who have a nonprimary outbreak while pregnant pass antibodies to their unborn fetuses. Therefore, if lesions are present externally (not in the immediate path of the baby), some midwives permit vaginal birth. Lesions must be covered with surgical adhesive film or spray-on bandage.

Any *history of vomiting* with the pregnancy should be carefully explored to rule out **hyperemesis gravidarium**. A mother with this condition has more than occasional nausea-related vomiting: it is chronic and self-perpetuating. This so disrupts her electrolyte balance that she cannot keep anything down and must be restabilized by intravenous replacement before she can eat or drink again. Hyperemesis gravidarium is one of the only conditions for which conventional medicine acknowledges emotional underpinnings, and some midwives have noticed a correlation between hyperemesis and psychological difficulties or conflicts regarding the pregnancy. Another theory is that liver irritation from elevated estrogen levels

may cause the condition, particularly in women with some degree of liver compromise. If counseling seems necessary, refer the mother, but at the same time, have her immediately take ginger root three times daily, either fresh grated in tea or ground in capsules. Continue to monitor her condition, and if vomiting persists beyond the first trimester, consult with a colleague or physician backup.

Fatigue is certainly common in early pregnancy (due primarily to elevated hormone levels), but fatigue combined with dizziness or nausea beyond the first trimester may indicate anemia (more on this condition in chapter 3).

Any report of *urinary tract problems* must be addressed immediately. During pregnancy, characteristic signs of urinary tract infection (UTI) such as stinging, urgency, and pain after urination may be nearly absent due to progesterone's softening effect on the urethra. This can lead to kidney infection, or pyelonephritis, which in turn can lead to premature labor. Any woman with a history of bladder infection must be alerted to these facts and should be told to call for screening with even the subtlest symptoms. In the meantime, have her immediately start drinking unsweetened cranberry juice or taking concentrate capsules. We used to think that the prime benefit of this was acidification of urine, but studies show that proanthocyanadin, a cranberry-based compound, prevents bacteria from adhering to uroepithelial cells.[12]

Also pay close attention to any report of *vaginal discharge or irritation*. Depending on her symptoms, screen for sexually transmitted diseases (STDs) at once, as some can negatively impact pregnancy (see the "Lab Work" section later in this chapter).

It is also crucial to note the use of any prescription or over-the-counter medications (OTCs) with this pregnancy. Thirty percent of mental retardation is of unknown etiology. The blood-brain barrier, which ordinarily protects the brain from harmful substances, is undeveloped in the fetus; thus pregnant women should confirm that prescription medicines are truly safe for pregnancy, and avoid OTCs with the same vigilance they do alcohol or recreational drugs.

Research has shown a correlation between Topamax (topiramate; taken for migraines and seizures) and anomalies of cleft lips or cleft palate. In addition, the FDA advises that babies whose mothers take antipsychotic drugs such as Haldol (haloperidol), Zyprexa (olanzapine), Seroquel (quetiapine), or Abilify (aripiprazole), may suffer withdrawal symptoms of agitation and difficulty with breathing and feeding for hours or days after birth. The Centers for Disease Control and Prevention further warns that taking opioid pain relievers (such as Vicodin [acetaminophin-hydrocodone], Oxycontin [oxycodone], and Tylenol [acetaminophin] with codeine) just before or in early pregnancy increases the risk of congenital heart defects, glaucoma, and other problems.[13] For more information, consult the *Physician's Desk Reference* (PDR), either a current volume of the text or the website www.pdr.net. Certain herbs are

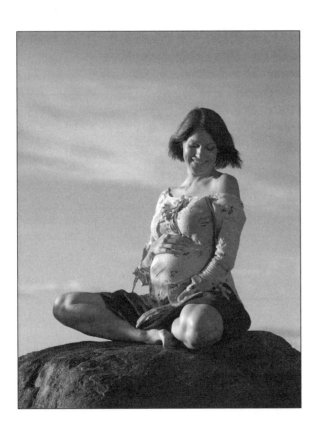

also dangerous in pregnancy as are high doses of some vitamins. Investigate herbal formulas by consulting an experienced herbalist, and make sure to document your findings (and the conversation) in the chart.

Certain household and workplace chemicals, and substances found in drinking water and food, may also be toxic and must thus be avoided. To investigate risks of specific environmental or work-related chemicals, consult Anne Frye's *Holistic Midwifery* (vol. 1). Any substance that can harm the fetus or cause fetal anomalies is called a **teratogen**. For more information, consult the Organization of Teratology Information Services (OTIS) at (866) 626-6847 or www.otispregnancy.org. Information is also available from the March of Dimes, at www.marchofdimes.com.

When reviewing the Medical/Health History form, pay close attention to the mother's response regarding ethnic, cultural, or religious preferences. If you have not had diversity training, consider taking a class or workshop on the subject. It is challenging to recognize your own cultural bias if you are white and part of the dominant culture. As Professor Peggy McIntosh states in her article "White Privilege: Unpacking the Invisible Knapsack":

> As a white person, I realized I had been taught about racism as something which puts others at a disadvantage, but had not been taught to see one of its corollary aspects, white privilege, which puts me at an advantage. . . . Many, perhaps most of our white students in the U.S. think racism doesn't affect them because they are not people of color: they do not see "whiteness" as a racial identity.[14]

For specific information on cultural and religious beliefs and preferences regarding pregnancy and birth, see the outstanding section on this subject in Frye's *Holistic Midwifery* (vol. 1).

A bonus in having the mother and her partner (if applicable) fill out the Medical/Health History at home is that the final set of questions prompt definitive statements regarding hopes, fears, and expectations. Responses to the possibility of damage or death to mother or baby speaks to perception of responsibility in the event of an unexpected outcome, level of emotional preparedness, and ultimately, commitment to homebirth. Responses regarding hospital transport are also important, as anything less than full willingness to consider the midwife's directives precludes a healthy working relationship. Likewise, responses regarding the midwife's role may reveal some incompatibility with your style of practice.

Occasionally you will encounter a woman unwilling to fill out take-home forms. She may profess enthusiasm for homebirth, yet in nearly every case I can recall, this stance has borne out an unwillingness to take responsibility. If any part of the history is incomplete, send it home to be finished up before accepting her into your practice.

Physical Examination

Every woman should have a complete physical exam early in pregnancy to rule out any conditions that might negatively impact her or the baby's health. Because the ability to perform physical assessment requires considerable hands-on training, I will not attempt to present this here. If you do not have this skill, another practitioner can perform the physical, but breast exams, pelvic exams, and the routine assessments described in this section are essentials of midwifery care. Learn more about physical examination from a comprehensive midwifery text, such as Frye's *Holistic Midwifery* (vol. 1) or Helen Varney's *Varney's Midwifery*.

Begin by establishing her **estimated date of delivery (EDD)**. Take the first day of her **last**

High-Risk Factors in Pregnancy

Medical and Health Factors

1. *Diabetes.* Preexisting diabetes is a definite contraindication to homebirth.

   Dangers: Fetal demise after thirty-six weeks, five times the normal incidence of fetal abnormalities, increased polyhydramnios, 30 to 50 percent higher incidence of preeclampsia, increased incidence of prematurity, and newborn respiratory difficulties.

2. *Thyroid disease, particularly hyperthyroidism.* Slight enlargement of the thyroid gland is normal in pregnancy, but persistent tachycardia or elevated levels of circulating thyroid hormone are symptoms of disease.

   Dangers: Thyroid medication has potential for causing severe fetal complications. Hyperthyroidism can cause miscarriage, premature labor, and fetal anomalies. Untreated hypothyroidism can lead to cretinism in the newborn.

3. *Active tuberculosis.* Refer to physician backup. If under treatment, prognosis for mother and baby is good, although the baby must be immediately separated from the mother if she is infectious.

   Dangers: There is a slightly higher risk of miscarriage or premature labor.

4. *Chronic lung disease.*

   Dangers: Mother is at risk for pulmonary complications, the baby for fetal acidosis and hypoxia.

5. *Severe asthma.*

   Dangers: Respiratory infections and stress may intensify attacks. Cardiopulmonary function could be reduced, affecting fetal growth and well-being. Certain medications used to treat asthma are contraindicated for pregnancy.

---

6. *Epilepsy.* There is controversy over whether or not this condition is exacerbated by pregnancy.

   Dangers: Anticonvulsant drugs may cause folic acid deficiency, which, when treated with folic acid, may cause seizures. The infant may develop deficiency of coagulation factors.

7. *Clotting abnormalities.* These include afibrinogenemia, hypo-fibrinogenemia, excessive fibrinalytic activity, or a combination.

   Dangers: Can lead to maternal blood loss, shock, or death.

8. *Rh– with antibodies.* Refer to physician backup.

   Dangers: Can result in hemolytic anemia, fetal or neonatal death (although intrauterine transfusion can avert this).

9. *Severe anemia.* Includes hereditary anemias such as thalassemia B or sickle cell, as well as nutritional anemias (iron, B-12, and folic acid deficiencies) unresolved at term.

   Dangers: Maternal infection, prolonged labor, hemorrhage, intrauterine growth restriction, or fetal hypoxia during labor may result.

10. *Acute viral infection.* These include rubella, mumps, cytomegalovirus, herpes, Coxsackie virus, pneumonia, hepatitis B or C, smallpox, severe influenza, and polio.

    Dangers: May cause birth defects; some of these cause fetal or maternal death.

11. *Congenital heart disease* (grades 2 to 4). Refer to physician backup. Condition requires clinical, electrocardiographic, and radiological surveillance.

    Dangers: Increased blood volume and weight put strain on impaired heart.

12. *Renal disease.* Impaired kidney function necessitates close medical surveillance in pregnancy. Signs of renal disease include protein in the urine, hypertension, edema, and elevated blood urea all before the twentieth week.

    Dangers: Acute renal failure may occur.

13. *Extreme obesity.* Preexisting condition, with history of medical problems, is a contraindication.

Dangers: Nearly two-thirds of extremely obese women have obstetrical complications, including diabetes, hypertension, pyelonephritis, uterine dysfunction, and hemorrhage.

Lifestyle and Personal Factors

1. *Tobacco use.* This is defined as more than ten cigarettes daily, although no amount can be considered without risk.

   Dangers: These include intrauterine growth restriction, miscarriage, congenital heart disease, fetal hypoxia in labor, and sudden infant death syndrome (SIDS).

2. *Malnutrition.* This is defined as extreme dietary deficiencies, which may be correlated to substance abuse, debilitating illness, or eating disorders.

   Dangers: Intrauterine growth restriction, preeclampsia, maternal or fetal infection, prematurity, stillbirth, dysfunctional labor, or hemorrhage may result.

3. *Drug addiction or chronic substance abuse.*

   Dangers: Intrauterine growth restriction, fetal hypoxia, respiratory distress syndrome (RDS), maternal malnutrition, infection, preeclampsia, dysfunctional labor, or hemorrhage may result. Newborns whose mothers are addicted to cocaine, crack or crank, heroin, or barbiturates will go through withdrawal within the first three days of delivery.

4. *Moderate to heavy alcohol use.* Periodic bingeing, or more than two drinks per day of alcohol, may cause damage or defects.

   Dangers: Fetal alcohol syndrome may result, with a 50 percent chance of mental retardation, 30 percent chance of anomaly, impaired eyesight, behavioral problems, or stillbirth.

5. *Heavy caffeine use.* This is defined as an excess of ten cups per day of moderately strong coffee, black tea, cola, or other caffeine-containing beverages.

   Dangers: Fetal malformations, heart defects, and reproductive problems may result.

menstrual period (LMP), count back three months, and add one week. This formula calculates ten lunar months (forty weeks), and is known as **Naegele's Rule**. Also record her **previous menstrual period (PMP)**, noting the interval between that and the LMP and comparing that with her average cycle length. A short interval (three weeks or less) suggests that the LMP was implantation bleeding, not a true period: recalculate the EDD accordingly.

A word of caution—don't take the EDD too seriously. The Mittendorf study showed the average length of human gestation to be forty-one weeks plus one day.[15] No wonder only 5 percent of women give birth on their due date! Frustrated by the confines of Naegele's Rule, midwifery professor Carol Wood Nichols developed a new method of calculating the EDD that takes variations in cycle length as well as previous childbearing into account. Here is her formula, known as **Nichols' Rule**:

- First-time moms with 28-day cycles: LMP + 12 months – 2 months, 14 days = EDD

- Second-time moms or more with 28-day cycles: LMP + 12 months – 2 months, 18 days = EDD

- Cycles longer than 28 days: EDD + (days in cycle – 28 days) = EDD

- Cycles shorter than 28 days: EDD – (28 days – days in cycle) = EDD[16]

Whatever the scope of your physical assessment, it provides an opportunity to earn the mother's trust. To do this, you must establish physical intimacy at a pace that is comfortable for her. Ask the mother's permission and obtain her consent. This may seem a formality to you after a while, but it is crucial in upholding her role as director of her care, and yours as her assistant.

Using the Prenatal Care Record (appendix E) to record your findings, begin by **checking her weight**, noting her pre-pregnant norm and total gain thus far. Assuming that her starting weight was normal for her height and frame, an average gain is about a pound per week. Many women are sensitive about their changing figure and should be reassured that an ample weight gain is both desirable and essential for the baby's health and their own endurance during labor and the immediate postpartum. It is noteworthy that most European midwives do not routinely check their prenatal client's weight, relying instead on hemoglobin levels, general vitality, and the baby's rate of growth as better determinants of well-being. Considering the degree to which women in the United States tend to be obsessed about their weight, easing up on this routine evaluation might benefit both mother and baby.

Then **check her urine** with a testing strip, looking for protein and glucose. Many midwives have cups and testing strips available in the restroom so mothers can do this on their own. After twenty-six weeks, anything over a trace of protein may indicate preeclampsia, although protein is also correlated to certain vaginal infections. Glucose in the urine is usually diet-related, but women with persistent positive readings in the first or second trimester may have an underlying diabetic condition and should be screened accordingly.[17]

If using a broad-spectrum strip, check also for blood, ketones, and nitrates. Blood or nitrates are suggestive of urinary tract infection; ketones signal inadequate food intake or dehydration (see page 70). Findings of either blood or protein require a clean-catch sample to rule out contamination from vaginal discharge. Always explain any unusual findings to the mother immediately.

Next **check her blood pressure**. Place the cuff firmly around the upper arm, position the gauge so you can see it, place the diaphragm side of your stethoscope over the **antecubital space** (bend at juncture of upper and lower arm) and hold it firmly with your thumb on top and fingers grasping elbow in back. Tighten the screw on the rubber bulb and pump the cuff to 160, then release the screw *very slightly* so that air flows out slowly enough that you can take a reading. The first sound you will hear is the **systolic reading**, which indicates the pressure in the arteries when the heart is actively pumping (note the corresponding number on the gauge), and the last sound you will hear is the **diastolic reading**, which indicates the pressure when the heart is at rest (again, note the number). Normal blood pressure during pregnancy ranges from 90/50 to 140/90, although readings higher than 130/80 or a steady rise from baseline are cause for concern.

In essence, diastolic pressure assesses baseline intravascular tension, whereas systolic pressure indicates cardiovascular tolerance for exertion. Medical texts claim that the systolic reading alone is influenced by emotional state, but I have found elevation in both to be fairly common at the initial visit, particularly if the mother is nervous. If so, I reassure her for the moment and take her blood pressure again before she leaves. If still high, I schedule a recheck in a few days. Women with consistent readings of 130/80 or more in early pregnancy may have undiagnosed essential hypertension. If readings are normal and later climb to this level, begin stress-reduction or other therapies in earnest (see page 77). Additional symptoms of generalized edema or proteinuria may indicate preeclampsia, for which the mother should be immediately referred to a physician.

Along with blood pressure, **check her pulse and temperature** to establish baselines. Since heightened reflexes can signal preeclampsia, it's also wise to **establish baseline reflexes** as soon as possible. Use a reflex hammer and note the degree of reflex irritability.

You should also **perform a breast exam**. Your goal is to determine the overall structure of her breast tissue and identify all masses within it, with bilateral symmetry the norm. Still, there is dramatic variation in structure from woman to woman. On occasion, I have been alarmed to find something quite unusual in one breast, only to be reassured by discovering the exact same tissue formation in the other. If the mother has had a breast reduction, see www.bfar.org/reduction.shtml; for breast augmentation, consult www.bfar.org/augmentation.php.

Of the several standard techniques for performing breast exam, I prefer the following:

1. Begin by observing the woman's breasts while she is sitting upright. Look for symmetry, note nipples pointing in an unnatural way, any puckering or pull around the areola, or irregularities in skin texture.

2. Have her lie down and continue your exam by checking the entire surface of the upper chest, collarbone down to the breasts, for accessory breast tissue. Do this with a pressing motion, sliding (rather than lifting) your fingers to be sure you don't skip an area. Normally, all you feel is a layer of muscle tissue with ribs beneath.

3. Continue the same pressing motion as you explore the breast tissue, quadrant by quadrant. It is okay to lift the breast and move it gently to one side or the other to accomplish this. Try using a combination of light, medium, and firm pressure in each area for a more precise assessment. If at any time you find a lump or mass, immediately check the same spot in the other breast (if structures match, everything is fine).

4. Focus on the upper, outer quadrant of the breast, as this contains the most tissue and is therefore the most likely site for abnormal growth. Feel more deeply into this area by using thumb and forefingers to reach in and grasp underlying tissue, rolling it to assess structure. In small- to moderate-sized breasts, the tissue forms a bar extending from armpit to nipple; larger breasts will have an extension of this bar down from the nipple to the bottom edge of the breast. Use this lifting and rolling motion on any area of the breast that has thick (or unusual) tissue. Again, if you find anything unusual, compare it with the other breast.

5. Feel directly beneath the nipple (there is a little crater there and the sensation is a bit strange, so warn the mother), and then squeeze the nipple gently to check for any secretion. Colostrum,

recognizable as a thick yellow discharge, may be evident after the first months of pregnancy. Occasionally women have greenish or bloody discharge that proves perfectly normal but should still be evaluated by an expert.

6. Finally, feel along the outer edge of the breast and into the armpit, feeling deeply for any lumps (likely to be enlarged lymph nodes).

7. Repeat the entire procedure on the other breast to establish symmetry.

Explain what you are doing step by step, and then have the mother repeat the exam in your presence. Many women give up on self-exam because they are alarmed to find their breasts lumpy instead of smooth. Reassure the mother that every woman's breasts are lumpy, so her best bet is to identify the lumps in one, and then compare with the other to be sure the lumps match. If her breasts are particularly dense or large, have her try leaning forward to palpate. This technique is thought to allow better access to deep breast tissue much the way mammogram screening does.

Also screen for **Paget's disease**, a rare form of breast cancer occurring on the outside of the breast, nipple, or areola. It first appears as a rash, with persistent redness, itching, or burning of the nipple/areola, progressing to oozing and crusting. If you suspect Paget's disease, immediately refer the mother to a specialist.

Pelvic assessment should not be performed until you and the mother have established trust. Of course you must ask permission before doing this exam, but for many women, weakened personal boundaries interfere with their ability to know what permission really means, particularly if they have experienced some kind of abuse (be it sexual, emotional, physical, obstetrical, or gynecological). Questions on the Mother's Confidential Worksheet (appendix D) address this issue, but you will not yet have this information. Every midwife should be aware of signs of abuse and how to respond appropriately (see page 102).

When the mother is ready for the exam, always ask her permission right before you begin. If you are doing it immediately after the breast exam and she has not put her shirt back on, see if she would like to do so and offer her a blanket or sheet to cover up. If her partner is present at the visit, don't assume she wants him or her there for this. Take your lead from her; she will invite her partner or ask if he or she can be present if this is what she desires.

I tell my students that when you touch a woman's vagina, you touch everything that has ever happened to her there. Therefore you must do the exam with sensitivity and reverence, following the mother's lead and ready to stop at any moment she verbally or physically indicates discomfort. Explain what you are doing as you go along, and warn her of sensations she will likely experience before they occur.

Ask her to position herself with knees bent, legs apart, and feet flat on the bed or exam couch so the small of her back is flat and her pelvis tips slightly upward. Put on a glove (you should have already washed your hands at this point), grasping the cuff with your nondominant hand and carefully inserting your dominant hand without touching the glove's outside surface. Once the glove is on, *do not touch anything but the vaginal area*. Using your other hand, apply lubricating jelly to your index and middle fingers, and ask permission to begin. As you do so, be guided by the mother's muscular reaction: never, ever force your way. Relax, don't be afraid to make eye contact if she is open to it, and continually reassure her by sharing your findings.

Begin by *checking her cervix*. Note its condition (consistency, length, patency), position (central, posterior, anterior), and any growths at or from the os, which may be, respectively, cysts or polyps. If growths are present or the cervix feels irregular in shape or texture, you will have an opportunity to visually assess when you do a Pap smear—although you should postpone this temporarily as lubricating jelly can contaminate results (see "Lab Work" on page 38).

If she is less than sixteen weeks pregnant, you may *confirm the EDD with a bimanual exam to size the uterus.* Place your fingers under the cervix and press up firmly while using your other hand to palpate the top of the uterus, or **fundus**. If this is difficult, place a finger on either side of the cervix and try pressing up that way. As you bring your hands together, you will get an idea of how large the uterus has grown. At ten weeks, the uterus is the size of a large orange or softball; at twelve weeks, the size of a grapefruit; at fourteen weeks, the size of a cantaloupe. (At sixteen weeks, bimanual exam is no longer necessary as the uterus can be palpated midway between the pubic bone and the umbilicus.)

If the uterus is not enlarged, do a pregnancy test before proceeding further. Or if uterine size does not seem to conform to the EDD, reevaluate the menstrual history. Women with irregular cycles may have incorrect dates, as may breastfeeding mothers who conceived before ever having a period. Others are uncertain of their dates because they continued to bleed after conception at the time menstruation would have ordinarily occurred. According to the current EDD, schedule a prenatal visit at twenty weeks to better determine dates by uterine size discrepancy (for details, see page 31).

Now you are ready to **perform pelvimetry**, or bony assessment. Explain to the mother what you are doing step by step (your partner or assistant can show points on a model pelvis).

To perform pelvimetry, measurements of your hand should be made be in advance. Measure first from the inside of your thumb joint to the tip of your middle finger. Then make a fist (tucking your thumb inside) and measure across your fingers. Note both these measurements in centimeters (cm).

Pelvimetry has five basic steps:

1. *Assess the depth of the sacral curve.* Begin by finding the coccyx. To do this, place your fingers (pad side down) a few inches inside the vagina, lift your wrist so fingers are perpendicular to the pelvic floor, and slowly but steadily press straight down as far as you can. When you feel the hardness of bone, keep pressure on this point and then rotate your thumb upward (so it faces the mother's chin). Keeping your fingertips firmly on the bone, trace the sacral curve up toward the sacral promontory. The sacral curve should drop deeply like a half-circle, so deeply that you may only be able to follow it for an inch or so. If it feels flat, note the possibility of an android pelvis. If you can feel the entire curve (and your fingers are not exceptionally long), note the possibility of a platypelloid or smaller gynecoid pelvis. Occasionally, a strong bulbocavernosus muscle (located about an inch or so inside the vagina) presents an obstacle to this maneuver. In this case, go in a bit further initially and then press fingers down perpendicularly, drawing your fingertips back toward you to find the coccyx.

2. *Assess the size of the pelvic inlet.* If the sacral curve is deep (no bone can be felt after a few inches), the inlet is clearly adequate. Otherwise, follow through until you reach the sacral promontory (your fingers should be at a horizontal plane). You are now in position to measure the **diagonal conjugate** (see illustration, page 28). For example, if the span from your thumb joint to fingertip is 13.5 cm, and 1 cm of your span remains outside the mother as you examine her, estimate the diagonal conjugate to be 12.5 cm. From this, subtract the 1.5 cm thickness of the pubic bone to obtain the actual inlet dimension the baby must negotiate, termed the **obstetrical conjugate**. A measurement of 10.5 cm or greater is considered adequate.

3. *Assess the contour of, and distance between, the ischial spines.* Withdraw your fingers until they are only a few inches inside the mother, bend them 90 degrees, and then press toward the pelvic sidewall until you feel bone. Move your fingertips slightly downward (if right handed, from nine to eight o'clock) and then hook them back toward you (see illustration, page 29). The

ischial spine is an attachment point for ligaments; it feels like a bump with a rubber band wound around it several times over. A definite indication that you have found it is the mother's response: she will flinch as you touch nerves in close proximity. Disregard the inclination to pull your fingers away, and press a bit more deeply (without poking) to see whether the prominence is blunt and barely noticeable or sharply pointed and protruding. Note the contour of one spine, then turn finger pads down and repeat the procedure for the other (at the four o'clock position). Sometimes one spine is prominent and the other is not. Complete your assessment by opening your fingers to measure the distance between the spines, or **bispinous diameter**, which should be at least 10.5 cm.

4. *Assess the angle, or width of the pubic arch.* Slowly turn your fingers pad side up and withdraw to leave an inch inside. Lift your palm about 45 degrees, press your fingers under the pubic bone, and assess the width of the pubic arch. You should be able to fit two fingers beneath the arch and spread them slightly apart.

5. *Assess the outlet dimension, or bituberous diameter.* Finally, take your fingers out to make this assessment: Find the low point on the ischial tuberosities (before they curve inward), make a fist, and press in between these points. If your fist is of average measurement—around 8.5 cm—it should fit comfortably, with some play side to side. (See illustration on page 30.)

This completes the pelvic exam. Chart your findings. Women occasionally ask if the shape or size of their hips has any bearing on labor. Explain that there is a difference between the **true pelvis**, which includes all dimensions from the inlet downward, and the **false pelvis**, which includes the iliac crests or hipbones, above. Though disconcerting, this terminology serves to illustrate that hip size is unreliable in predicting pelvic capacity.

In terms of **pelvic type**, refer to the diagrams on the opposite page. Basically, each type has certain ratios of depth (sacral curve and inlet) versus width (bispinous and bituberous dimensions, width of pubic arch). The **gynecoid** provides a round space, equally deep and wide, and is by far the most common. The **anthropoid** is notably deeper than it is wide, a tall oval with great depth in the sacral curve but more narrow in width than the average gynecoid (roomier at the bottom than at the top, it encourages the baby to enter the pelvis posteriorly). The **platypelloid** is wider than it is deep, a wide oval, with less depth in the sacral curve but more width than the average gynecoid. The **android** has all the quirks: prominent, close-set spines, tapering sidewalls, narrow pubic arch (less than 80 degrees), and close-set tuberosities. The android is sometimes called the funnel pelvis because it gets more and more narrow toward the outlet. Fortunately, pure android types are quite rare, although a woman may have a single android characteristic, like one prominent ischial spine.

Some midwives prefer to wait on pelvimetry until the last trimester, when hormone-induced softening of the four pelvic joints—the symphysis pubis joint, the sacrococcygeal joint, and the two sacroiliac joints—may dramatically increase any borderline aspect of the pelvis, particularly the transverse or outlet dimensions. I have personally found that doing pelvimetry early helps assuage the culturally induced fear of being "too small" to give birth vaginally. Ultimately, since an adequate pelvis is determined by the size of the baby, you can truthfully reassure any woman at this point that there is plenty of room. Don't worry if the tissues feel tight in early pregnancy, as changes during the third trimester are really quite remarkable.

Beginning midwives often find the **Three Ps** context of Passage, Passenger, and Powers helpful for appreciating the relative significance of pelvimetry. The **Passage** is defined as the bony pelvis and musculature, the **Passenger** is the baby and how it is

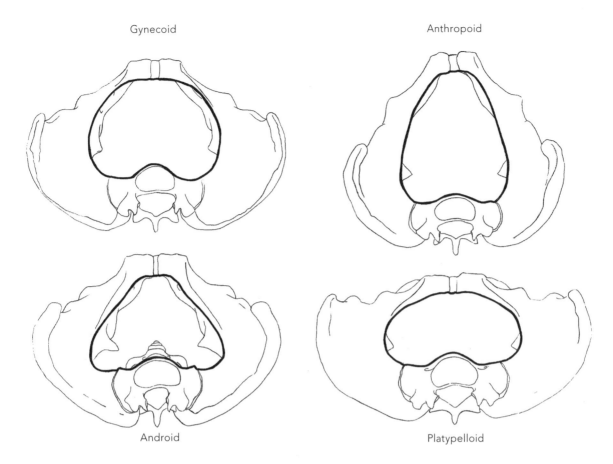

Gynecoid

Anthropoid

Android

Platypelloid

Basic Pelvic Types

presenting, and the **Powers** refer to uterine activity during labor (which reflect the mother's emotional and physical well-being).

Note that the term Passage refers not only to bone structure but also to vaginal muscle tone. According to research compiled by Frye in *Holistic Midwifery* (vol. 2), progress in labor is determined as much by flexibility in vaginal tissues as by pelvic type and size. Thus the importance of healing from sexual trauma cannot be overestimated. Particularly if you find that the mother tightens as you do the exam, or that the sacral curve is impossible to access because of tension in the pelvic floor, ask her about history of abuse and refer for counseling if indicated. Offer to teach her pelvic floor exercises and vaginal

awareness practices (see page 60) as soon as reasonably possible.

In terms of practical application of the Three Ps, a woman with a small Passage and medium-sized baby may nonetheless birth with ease if her tissues are relaxed and her Powers are strong. Then again, a woman with an ample Passage and average-sized baby might have difficulty if her Powers are weak due to poor health, history of abuse, or lack of support. Obstetrics rarely considers this equation; instead, it relies on forceps, vacuum extraction, and cesarean section: "If the baby doesn't deliver in time, we'll just pull or cut it out." Pelvimetry has thus become a lost art in obstetrics and, due to the fact that babies can be born vaginally 99 percent of the time when birth

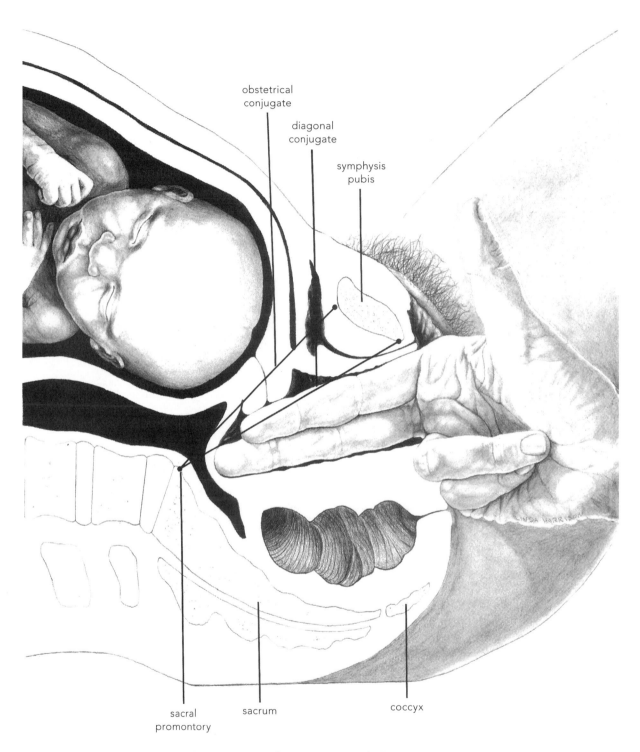

obstetrical
conjugate

diagonal
conjugate

symphysis
pubis

sacral
promontory

sacrum

coccyx

Measuring the Diagonal Conjugate

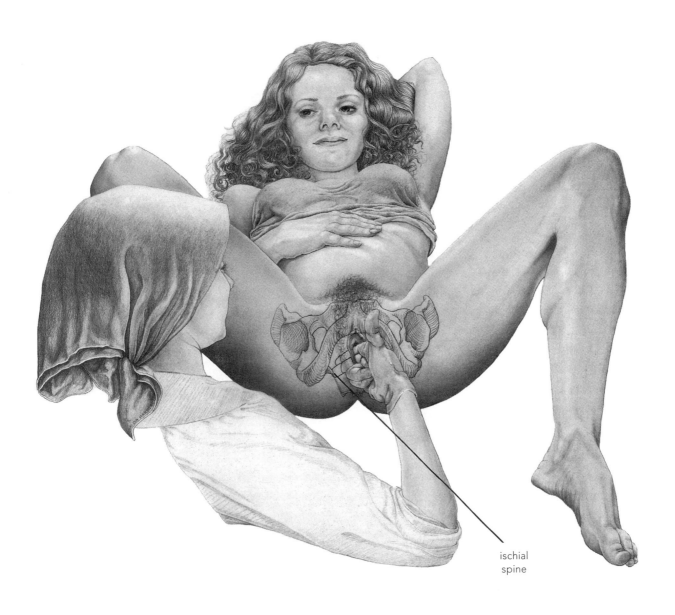

ischial
spine

Finding the Ischial Spines

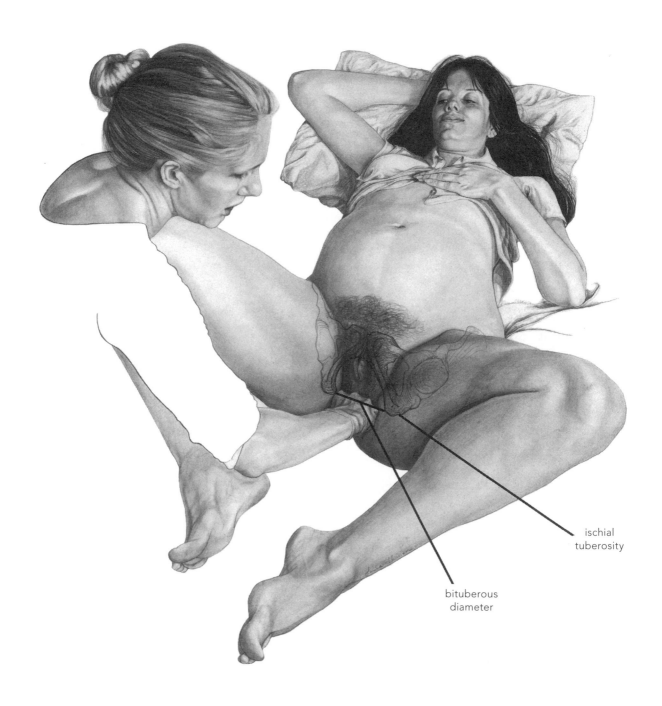

ischial
tuberosity

bituberous
diameter

Checking the Outlet Dimension

physiology is honored, some midwives have also abandoned the practice. Yet certain key midwifery skills, such as manually repositioning a malpresenting baby, or safely assisting a breech at home, depend largely on the mastery of pelvimetry.

If the mother is at least eighteen weeks pregnant, **measure the fundal height**. Using a soft tape measure, place one end at the upper edge of the pubic bone, then stretch the tape to the top of the uterus (the fundus). Record your measurement in centimeters. Make sure to dip in deeply at the very highest point, which may be slightly off-center, depending on the baby's lie. Give or take a couple of centimeters, the fundal height matches the baby's gestational age (GA), or the number of weeks pregnancy has progressed since the LMP.

As mentioned earlier, one of midwifery's "tricks of the trade" is to **schedule a prenatal visit at twenty weeks to confirm the EDD**, particularly if the LMP is in question. If the dates are correct, the uterus will be round and exactly at the level of the umbilicus, no matter if the mother is carrying twins, a baby destined to weigh 6 pounds (lb.), or one that will be 12 lb. at birth. If dates are off a month either way, it will be easy to tell. At sixteen weeks, the uterus is halfway between the umbilicus and pubic bone, a tall oval. At twenty-four weeks, it is several centimeters above the umbilicus, a wide oval reaching all the way out to the iliac crests. Palpate the uterus, and then adjust the EDD if necessary.

Performing uterine/fetal palpation is probably the most pleasurable and relaxing aspect of the exam for you and the mother, and it gives you both a chance to tune into the baby. From twenty-four weeks on, your evaluations include fetal lie, presentation, position, and attitude, plus assessments of fetal growth and responsiveness and amniotic fluid volume (AFV). The maneuvers used to palpate the baby are commonly known as **Leopold's maneuvers**.

Fetal lie—the relationship of the baby to the long axis of the mother's body—will be longitudinal, oblique, or transverse. Observe uterine contour: is it taller than it is wide or vice versa? Place one hand firmly at the side of the uterus (fingers pointing toward the mother's face), and with the whole surface of your other hand, feel the fundus to see if any obvious part can be identified. The head feels very hard and round; the butt is softer and irregular in contour. If nothing is immediately apparent in the fundus, feel along the sides of the uterus (with both hands, fingers pointing toward the mother's face). If the poles of the baby's body (head or butt) are at the sides, the baby is in a transverse or oblique lie. Although common at twenty-four weeks, the baby finds this lie increasingly confining as it grows and will generally seek the roomier, longitudinal aspect of the uterus by twenty-eight weeks.

If you've found the head or butt in the fundus, place your hands at the sides of the uterus as directed above and, exerting pressure from one hand to the other (moving the baby back and forth), feel for the back and small parts. Note on which side you feel the most mass; hold that hand firmly in place and with the opposite hand, press the baby to the steady hand, using it to determine if you have found the back. If at any point you feel a kick to one hand, expect the baby's back to be on the opposite side. If you cannot feel the back, the baby may be in a posterior position (see next page).

Next, determine the **presentation**. Open your hand in a wide C-shape, place it vertically just above the mother's pubic bone, press in several inches, and bring thumb and fingers together. If you feel the butt, the presentation is **breech**; if the head is there, the presentation is **cephalic**. If the lie is transverse, you have a **shoulder presentation**. Whatever the presentation, the part of it used to determine the position of the baby is called the **denominator**. For example, with a longitudinal lie, cephalic presentation, the denominator is the occipital bone at the back of the baby's head (see illustration "Fetal Skull," page 118). In breech presentation, the denominator is the sacrum, and with shoulder presentation, the acromion process (a bony prominence on the shoulder blade).

We base **fetal position** on the location of the denominator within the mother's pelvis. For example, if the baby is head down with its occiput and back on the mother's right side, this position is **right occiput transverse (ROT)**. Babies in transverse position are quite easy to feel; the back is distinct on one side with small parts on the other, and often a foot can easily be seen or felt. If the baby is head down with occiput and back on the mother's left but near her sacrum, we call this **left occiput posterior (LOP)**. Posterior babies are more challenging to palpate; there are lots of small parts and little more than an edge of back, but you may find a shoulder just above the pubic bone that will tell you more conclusively which side the baby is on. If the baby is breech with sacrum and back on the mother's left near her pubic bone, we call this position **left sacrum anterior (LSA)**. Anterior babies are "all back" with small parts tucked against the mother's back and out of range of feeling (see illustration "Fetal Presentation and Position" on opposite page for more examples).

Less commonly used is the term **presenting part**, which refers to the part of the presentation lying directly above the cervix. This is determined not by palpation but by internal exam.

Attitude is an assessment of the degree of head flexion. A well-flexed cephalic presentation will manifest a continuous C-curve of back and head from fundus to pubic bone. This is obviously more difficult to determine if the baby is posterior. Deflexion of the head can be corrected most effectively around thirty-five weeks gestation (see diagram on page 59).

Palpation is an art learned by experience. In some parts of Mexican Yucatán, the word for *prenatal visit* is the same as that for *massage*. Take your time while palpating; notice the mother's body language (her energy and tension levels), as well as the baby's responsiveness. Feel into the moment and take advantage of any opportunity to deepen communication. Teach the mother how to palpate herself, and if her partner is present, encourage him or her to feel the baby, too.

Few physicians palpate these days; it is yet another endangered art for which technology (ultrasound) has become a substitute. But if performed at each prenatal visit with continuity of care/care provider, palpation not only renders the assessments cited above but also provides clear evaluations of amniotic fluid volume and fetal growth and reactivity. These are especially critical if fetal growth restriction is suspected, if the uterus is large for dates, or if pregnancy is prolonged (see chapter 3).

As pregnancy advances, also try to **estimate fetal weight**. Learn this skill by palpating and guessing babies' weights in the last few weeks up to the time they are born, checking your estimate at the newborn exam. With the help of norms for fetal weight at each week of pregnancy (typically found on the EDD calculator wheel), you will soon be able to estimate quite accurately from about twenty-eight weeks onward.

Next, **take fetal heart tones (FHT)**, listening in the vicinity of the baby's back. With a fetascope, the heart should be audible by twenty weeks. Normal range is 120 to 160 beats per minute (BPM), although up to 170 BPM is normal for younger babies (the heart rate often slows 10 to 15 points as the baby grows). Invite the mother and her supporters to listen to the baby, too.

Once the baby is twenty-eight weeks, check for **variability** by listening for several fifteen-second increments, taking the BPM rate for each, and charting the overall range (e.g., 132 to 148 BPM). Variability typically occurs in response to stimulation (whether from palpation, uterine contractions, or the baby's own movements) and is a sign of neurological health. If you have any concerns, consult with backup.

It is noteworthy that since the first edition of *Heart & Hands* was published in 1981, the skills of fetal heart auscultation, pelvic assessment, fundal height assessment, and fetal/uterine palpation have been almost entirely replaced by ultrasound. Yet research has demonstrated repeatedly that neither maternal nor fetal outcomes are improved by

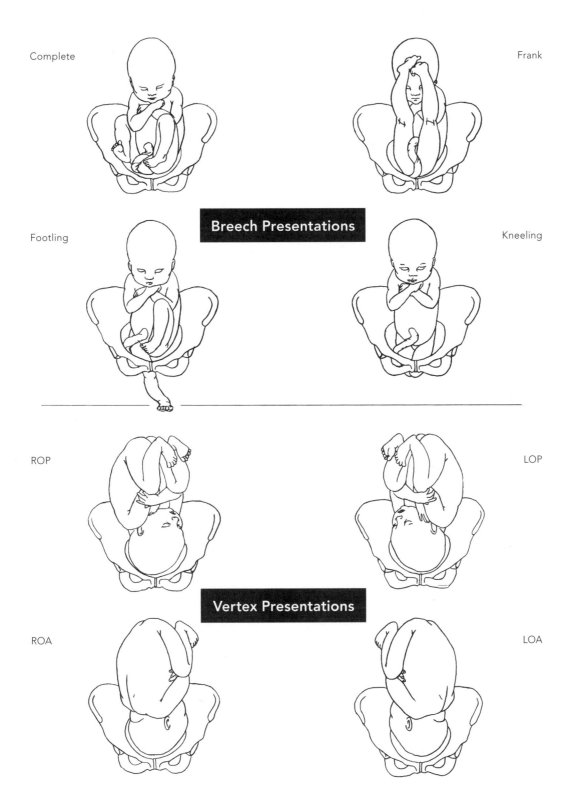

Complete

Frank

Breech Presentations

Footling

Kneeling

ROP

LOP

Vertex Presentations

ROA

LOA

Fetal Presentation and Position

the routine use of this technology.[18] In fact, serial ultrasound has been shown to induce fetal growth restriction.[19]

Perhaps the most alarming research showed abnormal neuron migration in mice at early stages of brain development with ultrasound exposure of thirty minutes or more, in which the authors saw a possible correlation to low birth weight, delayed speech, childhood epilepsy, developmental dyslexia, autism spectrum disorders, and schizophrenia.[20]

In cases with clear risk, ultrasound can be lifesaving. But in general, it is grossly overused for reasons that have nothing to do with good care; for example, to have hard copy records in case of lawsuit, to generate office revenues, or simply because the skill to do otherwise has been lost. Now studies are demonstrating what midwives have always known: the prenatal assessment skills described above are just as (or more) efficacious in determining fetal and maternal well-being.[21] Midwives must understand that they play a critical role in preserving these traditional skills and competencies.

Nutrition

Here is an area where paradigm of care really comes into play! In the technocratic paradigm, nutrition has little bearing on health and is seldom discussed. In the humanistic paradigm, a good care provider makes recommendations regarding optimal nutrition and what to avoid in pregnancy. But in the holistic paradigm, the care provider avoids making recommendations unless the mother requests them. Instead, she reviews the mother's diet and asks her questions: How does she feel physically and emotionally eating as she does? Are there any foods she would like to be eating that she is not? And if not, why not? Is money an issue? Does she have time to prepare food? Are there any foods she has been craving? What is her long-term relationship to food and nourishment? Having the mother articulate her own health status prompts her to become her own problem solver. Even if she asks your advice, resist the temptation to tell her what to do, asking instead what she thinks would work for her.

Make sure that she brings a three-day record of her food and fluid intake to the initial visit; this should include all supplements, herbs, and homeopathic formulas. Ask her to estimate portion size so you will be better able to determine exactly how much protein, calcium, iron, and so on, she is getting. You'll need a comprehensive reference to help you with this, such as the U.S. Department of Agriculture's *Composition of Foods*, available online at www.nal.usda.gov.

If the mother has symptoms that indicate deficiencies, help her improve the quality of the food she eats. Assimilation of supplements is unpredictable, and as normal doses for the mother are extremely high for the fetus, many must be taken with caution. Supplemental iron is routinely labeled with toxicity warnings, so doses should remain below 100 mg daily. The only safe quantities of vitamins A and D are the nonpregnant minimum daily requirements. Although nontoxic, high quantities of vitamin C taken near the time of delivery can cause newborn withdrawal symptoms, including scurvy. And if the mother ingests large amounts of calcium near term to raise her pain threshold in labor, neonatal **hypocalcemia** can result (see page 204).

Above all else, food comes first: supplements should be supplemental! Encourage the mother to buy organic whenever possible, as the nutritional value of most organic fruits and vegetables is higher than those commercially grown. Have her avoid dairy products with growth hormones; those clear of contaminants say "No bovine growth hormones" or "No BGH" on the label. Also suggest that she look for meat and eggs that are free of antibiotics. The reason for avoiding pesticides, hormones, and antibiotics should be obvious: these get to the baby at an alarming concentration relative to its size.

Make sure the mother is drinking at least 2 quarts of water daily, and double-check the source. A 2008 study showed disturbing effects from chlorine in tap water: at levels at 5 ig/L or less, no adverse effects were noted, but levels of 20 ig/L or greater showed a 50 to 100 percent correlation to cleft palate, ventricular septal defects (holes in the heart), and anencephalus (an absence of a major portion of the brain, skull, and scalp).[22] Have the mother contact her local water board for levels, or better yet, encourage her to buy bottled water or a filtering unit that removes chlorination.

Beyond a good quality, well-balanced diet, the following daily supplements may help compensate for devitalized soil, stress, air pollution, and so on:

- Vitamin E—400 units
- Vitamin C—500 mg

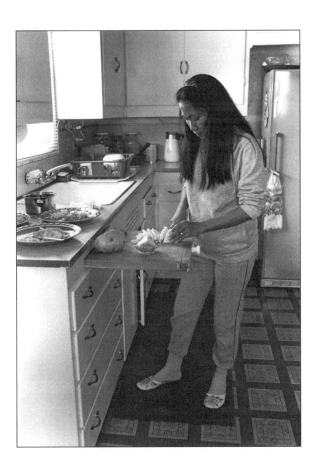

- Folic acid—800 mcg
- Iron—75 mg of a chelated, organic brand
- Calcium—1200 mcg
- Magnesium—600 mg
- Zinc—20 mg
- Fish oil—900 mg

Note that vitamin E is fat soluble so is best taken with foods containing fat. Vitamin C and iron can be taken together to enhance absorption of the latter. But calcium and iron counteract each other, so have the mother take them separately and avoid calcium-rich food or drink when taking iron pills.

Fish oil (with a vegan alternative in flaxseed oil) is a relatively new addition to the list of essentials. It contains omega-3 DHA and EPA fatty acids shown to have the following important benefits:

For baby
- Better brain development, higher intelligence
- Good nervous-system development
- Better eyesight, optimal retina formation
- Better sleep patterns
- Fewer behavioral problems

For mother
- Less chance of developing preeclampsia
- Less chance of preterm labor and cesarean
- Much lower risk of postpartum depression
- Greatly reduced incidence of breast cancer

Approximately 70 percent of Americans are deficient in omega-3 fatty acids, and 20 percent have blood levels so low they cannot be detected.[23] Fish oil supplements are clearly important, but pregnant women must keep an eye on quality, as cheaper brands may come from fish that is contaminated or from polluted waters. Advise the mother to be careful about the type of fish she eats as well, not only in pregnancy but also while nursing. To reduce potential exposure to mercury, she should avoid shark, swordfish, king mackerel, and tilefish. She should also avoid raw fish and shellfish (which may contain harmful bacteria or viruses) as well as smoked seafood, such as lox, which is high in sodium.

In terms of dietary requirements, the mother needs a minimum of 80 grams (g) protein daily. Dietary calcium is also critical, but dairy products are not always the best source; sesame butter (tahini) is excellent as are dark greens like kale and collards, and orange juice "plus calcium" (the acidity facilitates absorption). Iron is readily obtained from organ meats, but pumpkin seeds, dried fruits, almonds, and the aforementioned greens are also good sources. Adequate intake of calories is crucial for accelerated metabolic functions; pregnant women need at least 3,000 calories daily, and nursing mothers, 4,000 per day.

The vegan mother must be careful to ingest adequate B-12, without which a serious form of anemia may develop and cause neurological damage to both her and the baby. The best way for vegans to get B-12 is by supplement, with the vitamin in active form, that is, cyanocobalamin or hydroxocobalamin. Sublingual tablets are often best, as they absorb directly into the bloodstream. Although fermented soy products, shiitake mushrooms, seaweed, and spirulina have been touted to contain lots of B-12, they actually contain analogs of the vitamin that can block absorption of the real thing. Fortified fresh juices can be good sources; look for cyanocobalamin or hydroxocobalamin on the label.

Beyond these basics, how food is selected and when it is eaten also makes a difference. Every mother has an inner voice of hunger telling her what to eat, how much, and when. This may lead her to devour six oranges at one sitting or to crave a particular protein source to the exclusion of all others. Mothers with several children often recall that certain foods felt central to their well-being with each of their pregnancies (and not the same ones each time). Keep in mind, though that this inner voice of

hunger only operates in women free of addictions to sugar, caffeine, alcohol, or marijuana.

When counseling a woman with a diet lacking essential nutrients, here is the cardinal rule: always begin with praise for whatever is outstanding. In terms of making improvements, base your suggestions on the mother's likes and dislikes. For example, if breakfasts are missing on her report, survey which breakfast foods she enjoys, then point out those with the greatest nutritional value.

Although nausea may be a factor in the first trimester, consider a diet with little variety an indication of inadequate resources. Any woman who has been pregnant will tell you she would never limit herself to just a handful of foods unless she was ill or had no choice. If obtaining food is a problem, refer the mother to public assistance, farmers' market free foods, food banks, and so on. For public assistance programs like Women, Infants and Children (WIC), you may need to write a letter verifying that the mother is pregnant and lacks resources for her baby to grow and develop normally. Every midwife should be knowledgeable regarding social services available in her community. If food stamps are available to the mother, have her dictate a list of everything she likes to eat and then help her formulate meals based on her best choices.

If ethnic or regional dietary preferences appear in the diet report, here's an important tip: do not attempt to replace core foods or ingredients with other, albeit healthier, selections. For example, it would be foolish to suggest that an Asian woman indicating a fondness for white rice substitute brown instead—if you are concerned about her need for whole grains and B vitamins, find a different source. Also work around the less-than-perfect, emotionally based aspects of the mother's diet, that is, her comfort foods. If your recommendations are unrealistic, she may become evasive, and if a complication necessitates another diet report later in pregnancy, she may not be fully truthful.

Before you attempt nutritional counseling, analyze your own three-day diet. You might also contemplate (or journal on) this question I ask my midwifery students: what is your relationship to nourishment? These tasks can help you find compassion for clients struggling with food issues as well as alerting you to any weaknesses in your diet or your commitment to self-care.

Nutrition is the trunk of the tree of health. Almost every complication in the perinatal period can be forestalled or mediated to some degree by good nutrition, so become adept at the work of effective nutritional counseling.

Exercise

Exercise helps pregnant women keep in touch with their ever-changing physical and emotional status while promoting circulation, elimination, and overall good health. But every mother must be cautioned to immediately cease any activity that causes pain or discomfort, regardless of pre-pregnant fitness. If she has exercised compulsively in the past, she is particularly at risk for ignoring distress cries from her body. The goal of prenatal exercise is to achieve harmony and release, not to reach new heights of performance.

That said, new research suggests that vigorous exercise during pregnancy can reduce the risk of diabetes and excess weight gain.[24] You might advise the mother to purchase a heart rate monitor (worn at the wrist) to help her identify and not exceed her maximum heart rate. This varies for every woman depending on her condition, but she will know it as the rate that allows her to work up a sweat without feeling out of breath or exhausted after her workout. Strength training is also recommended, once or twice per week on nonconsecutive days, with eight to ten strength exercises per session.[25]

Stress that moderate vigorous activity should be balanced with rest. Over the course of pregnancy, there will be times when more rest is in order: for example, if the mother is under stress and her baby is in the midst of a growth spurt, her stamina may be reduced and she may crave a nap in the middle of the day (or immediately upon returning home from work). Her appetite may also increase, which could alarm her. Just remind her to listen to and trust her body; it will tell her what to do.

Mothers working long hours need special consideration. It is more difficult for them to be spontaneous: to eat when and what they want, to rest when they should, and to be active when they feel like it. Bending the sharp edges of routine is good, but cutting back on work hours is better. Pregnancy is a precious time of preparation for birth and motherhood, requiring a somewhat flexible schedule if at all possible.

A mother accustomed to high levels of physical activity should continue her routine as long as she is comfortable and taper off gradually if need be. A sudden drop in activity can cause constipation,

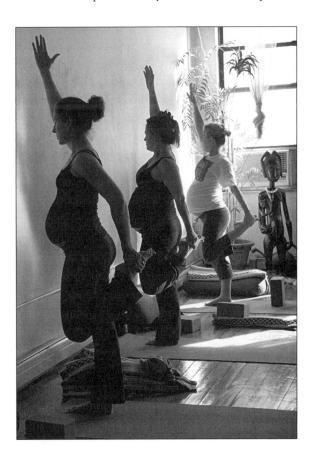

circulatory problems, or nervous irritability. A prenatal exercise group may help alleviate self-consciousness about changing body image. Yoga is my preference for prenatal exercise as it integrates mind and body, movement and rest. At the end of a long day, yoga can dissolve fatigue and boost energy levels for evening. It helps the body recuperate by stimulating the master glands, which keep hormone levels in balance. This creates harmony throughout the system. Many women also feel that yoga fosters their intuition and creativity.

Screening Out

Ideally, **screening out** results from a process of decision making that is shared by both mother and midwife. But sometimes, the midwife must make her own decision. On what basis do you conclude that out-of-hospital birth is not appropriate for a mother or that you are not her most appropriate care provider?

Beyond preexisting medical problems that contraindicate homebirth, other problems, such as abnormal pelvis, extreme obesity, or essential hypertension may have become evident at this visit. Psychological contraindications are more complex. An irresponsible attitude, hostility in response to suggestions for self-care, or an otherwise rigid belief system should give the midwife pause. A poor diet, particularly if the mother is averse to changing it, may indicate deep-seated indifference, passivity, or lack of self-esteem. Excessive use of drugs, alcohol, or cigarettes has similar implications.

If you sense that you won't be comfortable working with the mother, suggest that she consider alternative care. On the other hand, if you feel a connection with her, make room for change. I have worked with mothers who smoked or drank a bit in the early weeks but cleaned themselves up quite nicely after the initial interview. You may want to see what happens at the next visit, which should be scheduled sooner than usual so you can reassess the situation.

For a beginning midwife, the most challenging aspect of screening is determining the relative significance of risk factors. To this end, several state midwifery associations have developed point systems, assigning 5 points to absolute contraindications such as clotting disorders, lung disease, and so on, and 1 to 4 points to less serious concerns like borderline anemia, insufficient exercise, a marginally supportive partner, or less-than-optimal nutrition. Midwives working under these systems agree to consult their peers in any situation where a woman has either a 5 point risk factor or a combination of factors totaling 5 points. Apart from absolute contraindications, risk screening is somewhat subjective, requiring a seasoned ability to make judgment calls best learned from training with an experienced midwife.

Lab Work

If the mother has already had prenatal care elsewhere, initial lab work has probably been performed. Have her make a written request for release of her records, which can be mailed to her or directly to you.

The **complete blood count** (CBC) or prenatal panel is primarily used to determine whether the mother is anemic and, to some extent, what type of anemia she has. Both her **hemoglobin** (HGB) and **hematocrit** (HCT) are critical indicators. HGB is the amount of hemoglobin per red blood cell, and HCT is the percentage of red blood cells per total blood volume. The HGB should be above 11, and the HCT should be 33 or more. Because red blood cells are the oxygen carriers, low HGB or HCT levels mean that mother and baby will suffer some degree of oxygen deprivation. During pregnancy, the mother will be easily fatigued and more prone to infection, and the baby may become growth restricted. If the mother remains anemic at the onset of labor, there are risks of fetal distress, infection, incoordinate or prolonged labor, and postpartum hemorrhage (from "tired uterus"). Even a moderate blood loss can be very serious for an anemic woman; she is predisposed to shock because her blood is poorly oxygenated to begin with. (See the discussion on "Anemia" on page 68 for more information.)

Screening for **syphilis** (VDRL, RPR) is also routine. Syphilis can cause miscarriage, prematurity, neonatal infection, fetal malformation, or death. The desired result on the VDRL/RPR is nonreactive (NR).

Another standard assessment is the **rubella antibody titre**, which indicates whether or not the mother has immunity to German measles. The test is done by a diluting process that detects the presence of antibodies. For example, a rubella titre of 1:48 means that antibodies can be detected even though the sample has been diluted numerous times. It is proof that the mother has had rubella or has been immunized, even if she cannot remember when. An unusually high reading (greater than 1:64) may indicate recent or current infection. Repeat the titre in this case and consult with backup. If the mother's titre is low (less than 1:10), it means she is susceptible to infection and should be immunized after the current pregnancy and at least three months before the next, to minimize her chances of contracting the disease if she becomes pregnant again. Were that to occur, her baby would have a 20 percent chance of heart, vision, or hearing defects.

You must know the mother's **blood type**, too, in case she requires an emergency transfusion. The four blood types are O, A, AB, and B, with an accompanying Rh factor either positive (+) or negative (–).

The Rh factor is an antigen present in red blood cells. Eighty-three percent of women have this factor and are Rh+; 17 percent do not and are Rh–. Here is the concern: if the mother is Rh– and her baby is Rh+, and some of the baby's blood should enter her circulation due to intrauterine trauma, premature separation of the placenta, or placenta previa, she will produce antibodies that can destroy her baby's red blood cells, rendering it severely anemic. This process is called **isoimmunization**. Isoimmunization

is rare with a first baby (as rare as the traumas that can cause it to occur) unless the Rh– mother has had abortions or miscarriages without receiving RhoGAM (an anti-antigen that blocks the development of antibodies). Because of the possibility of undetected miscarriage, every Rh– woman should be screened for antibodies early in pregnancy and again at twenty-four, twenty-eight, thirty-two, and thirty-six weeks. If antibodies are found, the baby will be tracked closely and may need a transfusion while still in utero.

It is standard of care to administer RhoGAM prophylactically at twenty-eight to thirty weeks. This conveys only *passive immunity*, that is, it will not protect subsequent pregnancies. As RhoGAM is commonly formulated with chemicals such as mercury that may be harmful to the fetus, prenatal administration remains somewhat controversial.[26] RhoGAM may also transmit blood-borne diseases, for although blood used to produce it is routinely screened for HIV and hepatitis, viruses as yet unknown may not be killed by current purification treatments.[27] The mother must make her own informed decision. To this end, I highly recommend the book *Anti-D in Midwifery: Panacea or Paradox?* by British midwife Sara Wickham.

Regarding the need for RhoGAM postpartum, you must take a sample of cord blood immediately at birth to determine the baby's Rh factor. RhoGAM must be administered within seventy-two hours to be effective.

Screening for thyroid disease (by blood test) has also become routine, as several studies have shown a correlation between elevated **thyroid stimulating hormone** (TSH) and miscarriage, fetal death, or neonatal death.[28] Normal range is 0.4 to 4.0: higher or lower levels are considered an indication of possible thyroid disease and require consultation with a physician.

Rather than wait until advanced pregnancy to discover signs of diabetes for women at risk, you can request the **HA1c** blood test as part of the prenatal panel (if not already included). HA1c (also known as HbA1c) determines the average amount of glycohemoglobin (blood sugar) over the past two months or so, and thus is considered more accurate than methods measuring current levels only. Normal range is 4 to 6 percent. Yet another reason for this test is that high blood sugar levels in early pregnancy are associated with certain birth defects and miscarriage.[29]

The **PPD** screens for tuberculosis (TB), an infection linked to crowded living conditions among Native American, Asian, Middle Eastern, and military populations. Initial infection is often self-healing, so a woman may be asymptomatic although she remains infected. In this case, her PPD results will be positive, even if her condition is inactive. Women with inactive TB are at no greater risk for active disease in pregnancy, but a mother with active TB may pass the infection to her baby during pregnancy or in the immediate postpartum. She may also infect other family members. Any woman who coughs up blood, has difficulty breathing, and suffers weight loss, fever, or fatigue should be immediately referred to a physician for screening. A mother with an active infection in pregnancy should be treated at once, whereas treatment will generally be postponed if the infection is asymptomatic. If a woman reports a previous positive PPD, *do not repeat the test*, but do consult with a physician regarding additional screening and treatment options.

Urinalysis is also standard in prenatal screening. Besides checking for the usual dipstick items, urinalysis detects the presence of bacteria; values of +4 or more indicate a urinary tract infection (UTI) and mandate cultures to determine what kind of bacteria is involved. Urine cultures are often accompanied by antibiotic sensitivities to assess which medications are most likely to be effective in eliminating the infection. Whenever values are +2 or +3, repeat the urinalysis before considering treatment.

Most women know when they have a bladder infection, but in pregnancy, high levels of progesterone so soften and dilate the urethra that the usual warning signs may go unnoticed. Advise all mothers that even the slightest symptom is cause for immediate screening, and all those with previous history should be screened periodically to rule out insidious infection. Undiagnosed UTI can lead to kidney infection, or **pyelonephritis**, which can complicate pregnancy and lead to premature labor: rule this out by checking for **costovertebral angle tenderness (CVAT)** (see the discussion of backache in "Common Complaints," later in this chapter).

Pap smear is another critical test, checking for irregular cells at the cervix. Often performed with the initial pelvic exam, an early Pap is crucial because hormonal changes in pregnancy may precipitate abnormal cell growth. It should be repeated again at six weeks postpartum. For the **slide method**, the lab supplies slides, cardboard slide holders, and fixative; you must order long-handled, sterile wooden spatulas or cytology sponges to collect your sample. For the **thin-prep method**, you purchase kits containing a small container of solution for preserving cells and a brush for sample collection (after stirring the brush into the solution, you return the entire container to the lab). You will also need a flashlight and speculum. You may prefer to use disposable plastic speculums over the metal version so you won't have to bother with resterilizing; if so, the mother can take her speculum home in case she ever wants to check her cervix in the future.

To prevent lubricating gel from contaminating results, do the Pap prior to pelvic assessment (or at the next visit). With the cervix in view, find the **squamo-columnar junction** (the usual site for abnormality) where the red, columnar cells lining the cervical canal meet the pink, mucosal cells covering the cervix and vagina. If invisible, it is just inside the cervical os; if widely displayed, it is called a **transformation zone**. Take your brush, spatula, or cytology sponge and gently rotate 360 degrees at this juncture. You do not need to scrape as cells come away freely in cervical secretion, but use enough pressure so the mother can feel it. With the slide method, spread your sample on the slide in a lengthwise line, flip your spatula (or sponge), and draw another line next to the first (do not press hard or rub back and forth, as this will destroy the cells). Immediately spray the slide with fixative, air dry, and mark with date and mother's name. For the thin-prep method, stir the brush into the solution.

While checking for abnormal cells, the lab may discover other conditions such as monilia/vaginal yeast, herpes virus, or **human papilloma virus (HPV)**. HPV can manifest as **condyloma accuminata**: visible genital warts or flat lesions that are difficult to see. HPV is now the most prevalent sexually transmitted disease, and evidence indicates it may be contracted without sexual contact. Like herpes, it resides in nerve ganglia in the genital area. There is no cure for this virus, only topical treatment for warts or lesions. Certain genotypes of HPV are known to be precursors to abnormal cell growth, increasing the risk of cervical cancer. Women with these genotypes are advised to have Pap smears every six months. Venereal warts or lesions are usually painless or may not manifest at all, so a woman can have HPV and not know it.

Therefore, while doing the Pap, inspect the cervix carefully for warts or lesions as well as any **unusual discharge or inflammation**. If discharge or inflammation is noted, the mother may have gonorrhea, chlamydia, or other infection. Chlamydia is the second-most common sexually transmitted disease in the United States—four times more common than gonorrhea (although the two often occur together). Women are rarely symptomatic, but their partners (if male) may have discharge or pain and burning with urination. Cultures for gonorrhea and chlamydia should be performed on every woman, taking a sample of secretion from the vagina, the cervix, and the anus.

Gonorrhea infection in the mother can lead to **chorioamnionitis** (infection of the membranes), premature rupture of the membranes, and preterm labor. It can also cause a blinding eye infection in the baby unless antibiotic drops are administered within two hours postpartum. The usual treatment for gonorrhea is a course of ceftriaxone.

Chlamydia can infect the urinary tract and lead to premature labor. With delivery, the baby has a 70 percent chance of infection, which can result in conjunctivitis or life-threatening pneumonia. The usual treatment of tetracycline is contraindicated because it can discolor fetal tooth enamel; erythromycin is nearly as effective and considered safe in pregnancy. For both gonorrhea and chlamydia, the mother's partner must also be treated, and condoms or latex barriers must be used for sexual interaction until additional screens confirm the infection to be fully resolved.

Yet another infection that may be sexually transmitted is **hepatitis B (HBV)**. Screening is done by blood test, which checks for presence and quantity of surface antigens (HbsAG). HBV is transmitted through blood or blood by-products, saliva, vaginal secretions, or semen. This disease is very contagious: women who are HbsAG positive have a high risk of transmitting the disease to their newborns, who, if infected, have a high risk of becoming carriers and transmitting the disease to their own offspring. Therefore, babies born to infected mothers should be immunized within twelve hours after birth. If this is done, breastfeeding is not contraindicated.

Expectant mothers with active HBV infection (signs are nausea, vomiting, upper-right quadrant abdominal pain, chills, and fever) should be hospitalized, and all family members should be screened. In contrast, HBV carriers are generally asymptomatic, with blood work showing long-term core antibodies (indicating infection contracted at birth). A midwife colleague related that upon finding a client to be a carrier, neither her husband nor her other children tested positive, thus no special care was required. Chronic HBV develops in only 15 percent of cases but can lead to life-threatening conditions such as cirrhosis of the liver and hepatocellular carcinoma.

Hepatitis C (HCV) accounts for about 20 percent of viral hepatitis in the United States. The method of transmission is primarily via blood and blood by-products, but HCV is also sexually transmitted. Signs of active infection are similar to those of HBV, but chronic conditions develop in 85 percent of cases. Perinatal transmission is approximately 5 percent (depending on the amount of virus in the mother's bloodstream), but breast milk is not affected. There is no immunization for HCV.

HIV screening is advisable for all women, particularly if they have ever engaged in high-risk behaviors of unprotected sex or needle sharing. In California, state law requires that all women be informed of the availability of, and indications for, HIV screening. Testing can and should be done anonymously, either at a testing site or through the mail. The ELISA test is highly sensitive but has false positive rates of up to 10 percent. Only if a repeat ELISA proves positive will the more specific Western blot antibodies test for HIV be run.

In 2009, the World Health Organization revised its guidelines for HIV-positive pregnant women to recommend antiviral treatment (ARV) beginning at fourteen weeks and continuing through breastfeeding, as studies have shown this to prevent transmission altogether.[30] If the mother is seropositive and remains untreated, she is at risk for premature labor, and her baby has a 25 percent chance of contracting the virus: a 5 to 10 percent risk during pregnancy, a 20 percent risk with labor and birth, and a 5 to 15 percent risk with breastfeeding.[31] With treatment options ever changing, get to know the specialists in your community. Also consult with backup regarding the advisability of comanaging primary care.

As a health worker, you must define your protocol for assisting anyone with a highly infectious and life-threatening disease. Immunization is available for hepatitis B and may someday be available for HIV. In the meantime, even universal precautions (described fully in chapter 4) cannot offer absolute protection—there is always a marginal risk of a needlestick or other inadvertent exposure to infectious body fluids. Identify the standard of care within your midwifery

community, know your limits, and communicate promptly with your clients should the need arise.

Every mother should be offered **genetic screening**. Depending on her ethnicity (and that of the father), she should be advised of any risks to her baby. If parents are of Greek or Italian descent, the fetus is at risk for B-thalassemia; if of Asian or Filipino descent, there is risk for A-thalassemia. Both are life-threatening anemias. If parents are of African descent, the fetus is at risk for sickle-cell anemia. For Ashkenazi Jewish parents, there is risk of both Tay-Sachs and Canavan diseases, which can lead to central nervous system degeneration and death. All northern-European populations are at risk for cystic fibrosis, characterized by lung disease and limited life span.

Alpha-fetoprotein screening (**MsAFP**) is the first line of genetic screening. Offered at fifteen to twenty weeks, this blood test checks for neural tube defects of anencephaly, microcephaly, hydrocephaly, and spina bifida. It also detects up to 20 percent of Down syndrome cases. In many states, perinatal caregivers are required to inform all mothers of the option for AFP screening. Unfortunately, the test has a 20 percent false-positive rate. The **quadruple screen** is much more accurate: combining AFP with levels of unconjugated estriol (uE3), human chorionic gonadotropin (hCG), and inhibin A (a hormone released by the placenta), it has an 81 percent sensitivity with just a 5 percent false-positive rate for Down syndrome.

If the quadruple screen is positive, ultrasound and amniocentesis come next. Ultrasound can detect some but not all anomalies and has a significant rate of false positives, whereas amniocentesis is more accurate. **Amniocentesis** is performed by inserting a needle through the abdomen and into the amniotic sac and then withdrawing a sample of fluid. This cannot be done before fourteen weeks due to insufficient fluid: fourteen to sixteen weeks is optimal. For perspective, the incidence of Down syndrome at age thirty-five is 1 in 365, equal to the risk of miscarriage or infection caused by the procedure. But by age forty, the incidence of Down syndrome increases to 1 in 100.

Chorionic villus sampling is another option. It can be performed at ten to twelve weeks—an obvious advantage over amniocentesis in case some anomaly is found and the mother decides to terminate the pregnancy. However, the procedure carries greater risks of miscarriage and infection because the requisite sample of placental tissue must be obtained through the cervix. And because the chromosomal content of placental tissue does not always reflect that of the fetus, there are a significant number of false positive and false negative findings. More disturbing are indications that the procedure may actually cause fetal anomalies.[32] Chorionic villus sampling is contraindicated for women with a history of cervical incompetence, miscarriage, or premature labor.

Decisions regarding genetic screening are very personal and often agonizingly difficult. Should a woman decide against it, she will undoubtedly be reminded of this repeatedly as friends and family ask if she has had "the test" and whether the baby is all right. Amniocentesis has become increasingly common: in response to fear of litigation, some physicians recommend it for every woman over thirty. For any woman uncertain of her risk status, a session with a genetics counselor can help her make a decision. The midwife should be prepared with updated referrals to specialists who are compassionate and willing to spend plenty of time answering questions.

Glucose testing (apart from the HA1c test in the first trimester) is routine at twenty-four to twenty-eight weeks, although it may be performed sooner, particularly if HA1c results are abnormal. Most common is the **glucose screen**, for which the mother's blood is drawn one hour after she ingests 50 mg glucose (a thick, syrupy drink). If her blood glucose exceeds 140 mg/dl, more testing is recommended. Many midwives find glucose screening unreliable for their clients, most of whom eat very little sugar and are thus less tolerant to the dosage used in testing. The controversy continues as to whether gestational diabetes is not just type 2 unmasked by pregnancy, and thus, whether women with neither historical nor clinical signs are at risk (see chapter 3 for more details).

Another standard screen later in pregnancy is for **group B streptococcus (GBS)**. This common bacterium lurks harmlessly in the vagina of approximately 25 percent of women but may, on rare occasions, have serious consequences for the newborn, such as apnea (cessation of breathing) or spinal meningitis. The rate of newborn infection is one to two per one thousand; of infected babies, 15 to 20 percent die (two to three per ten thousand). However, death rates are significantly higher for premature babies, thus rates for healthy babies at term are less than two per ten thousand.

If a mother chooses to be screened, vaginal/perineal cultures are done at thirty-five weeks (rectal cultures are no longer recommended).[33] If positive, IV antibiotics are advised during labor if it is preterm, if membranes are ruptured for more than eighteen hours, or if the mother develops a fever greater than 100.4 degrees. And here is where the controversy begins. One study, which looked at the rates of blood infections in newborns over a six-year period, found that antibiotic treatment in labor reduced the incidence of newborn GBS but increased the rate of other blood infections.[34] E. coli in particular is on the rise.[35] Some strains of GBS are resistant to all antibiotics: a study of forty-three newborns with various blood infections (including GBS) found that 88 to 91 percent were resistant to the antibiotics their mothers received in labor.[36] Thus some women choose to forego screening, while others want to know their status and try to reduce colonization.

One option for reducing colonization is chlorhexidine (market name Hibiclens) washes.[37] These are only effective for a short time, so they might be used immediately prior to retesting and/or at the onset of labor. Studies have shown them to be as effective as Ampicillin in preventing vertical transmission of GBS, as well as reducing the rate of neonatal E. coli.[38] To do the wash, have the mother use a 30 cc plastic syringe filled with Hibiclens topical solution and insert the syringe while in a standing position only about halfway in the vagina.[39]

Other options that may be effective in maintaining vaginal health and discouraging colonization include the following:

- *Probiotics*: two capsules daily
- *Echinacea*: 700 mg daily
- *Garlic*: 1,000 mg daily
- *EHB by NF Formulas* (antibacterial supplement): follow dosage directions on bottle
- *Tea tree oil suppositories* (cotton ball or small cotton tampon with fifty-fifty blend of tea tree oil and olive oil): twice daily

For more information, see the oft-cited article by Christa Novelli, "Treating Group B Strep: Are Antibiotics Necessary?"[40] For more recent references, another excellent article is Judy Slome Cohaine's "Top 10 Reasons Not to Culture at 36 Weeks," in *Midwifery Today* (Summer 2010).

If a woman comes to her initial visit with no previous lab work and you are unable to do it yourself, send her to a public health facility or women's health center with a full list of requisite tests, including vaginal cultures. Make every effort to acquire these lab skills as soon as possible, though—your clients will greatly appreciate the continuity of care, and you will enjoy the autonomy of practice.

Routine Checkups

The schedule for prenatals is fairly standard: up to twenty-eight weeks, every four weeks; from twenty-eight to thirty-four weeks, every two weeks; from thirty-five weeks on, once weekly. The main reason for the increasing frequency of visits is that complications for mother and baby are more likely to arise as pregnancy progresses. It is also important to have additional personal contact with the mother to foster trust and intimacy as the pregnancy nears completion.

Routine at every visit are a urine dipstick for protein and glucose, blood pressure assessment, fundal height assessment, and, from twenty weeks, fetal auscultation. From twenty-four weeks, the midwife can begin Leopold's maneuvers and assess amniotic fluid volume. Maternal weight may be checked less frequently, but nutrition and exercise should be discussed each time.

At twenty-eight weeks, certain assessments from early pregnancy should be repeated. Ask for another three-day diet log, as needs for protein, calcium, and iron are intensified during the last trimester. Check the HCT/HGB again, for if the mother is anemic, it may take time to find an effective solution. This is also the cutoff point for glucose screening. Otherwise, care during the last trimester should focus on the more personal aspects of helping the mother prepare for labor and the postpartum period.

Throughout the pregnancy, there are many topics for discussion: books and articles the mother has read, videos she has viewed, her experiences in childbirth class, partner and family preparation, postpartum support, sexuality, aspects of newborn care, rest and relaxation, work and play. Take your cues from the mother, but avoid discussing the same subjects over and over. Your task is to expose her and her partner to issues they may not have considered so that you may prepare them for the multifaceted experiences of birth and childrearing.

Don't forget to inquire about the mother's general well-being at every visit, as there are a number of physical complaints that may arise from time to time. Introduce the "Scale from 1 to 10" and ask her to use it to rate her health status, vitality, happiness, degree of readiness for the birth, and so on (with 10 being the highest experience of each). If she rates herself 9 or less, ask her what it would take to make her score a 10. In doing so, you support her in articulating her own health status and identifying what she needs to do or experience to feel her best.

Fetal Development

The **embryonic period** of fetal development includes the first through the seventh weeks of life, postfertilization (or, calculating from the LMP, the third through the ninth week).

The **fetal period** includes all fetal development after the embryonic period and before the time of birth.

Growth and development begin at the moment of fertilization. The pronucleus of the sperm and that of the ovum fuse to form a zygote. Each pronucleus contains only twenty-three chromosomes (the haploid number); when they fuse, the normal forty-six chromosomes (diploid number) are restored.

Also determined at the moment of fertilization is the sex of the individual. The pronuclei are carried in the sex cells, or gametes, of both sexes. The male gamete carries either an X or a Y chromosome. The female gamete carries only an X. An XX combination is female; an XY is male.

Immediately after fertilization, the zygote undergoes cleavage and becomes a morula. As the morula develops and fluid enters the mass, it becomes a blastocyst. When the blastocyst implants in the uterine lining (on the tenth or eleventh day after fertilization), the embryonic period begins.

Development during the embryonic period, dating from the LMP

- The heart starts to beat around the beginning of the sixth week.
- The ears, arms, legs, facial, and neck structures begin to form at the end of the sixth week.
- The brain and eyes begin to develop during the seventh week.
- The nose, mouth, and palate begin to form in the eighth week.
- The neck is established, urogenital development begins, and all other essential structures are present by the end of the ninth week.

- The embryonic period is a critical one in terms of exposure to teratogens, which may cause congenital malformations or death.

Development during the fetal period, dating from the LMP and taken by lunar months

- *Third lunar month (nine to twelve weeks):* The fetus can swallow, make respiratory movements, urinate, and open and shut his or her mouth by the end of the twelfth week.
- *Fourth lunar month (thirteen to sixteen weeks):* Eyelids are fused, body growth accelerates, fingernails develop, reflexes manifest, sex is distinguishable, and the fetus reaches a weight of about 4 ounces (oz.).
- *Fifth lunar month (seventeen to twenty weeks):* Toenails develop, the fetus hiccups, vernix covers the body, and the fetus reaches an average weight of 0.75 lb.
- *Sixth lunar month (twenty-one to twenty-four weeks):* Hair growth is prominent; the fetus is covered with fine, downy hair (lanugo); buds of permanent teeth form; the fetus makes crying and sucking motions; brown fat (source of heat and energy for the newborn) forms, and the fetus reaches an average weight of 1.25 lb.
- *Seventh lunar month (twenty-five to twenty-eight weeks):* Eyes begin to open and shut, the fetus grows longer, and the fetus gains significantly to weigh an average 2.25 lb.
- *Eighth lunar month (twenty-nine to thirty-two weeks):* Fat deposits smooth the body contours, the vernix is thick, breathing motions are rhythmic, and the average weight is 3.75 lb.
- *Ninth lunar month (thirty-three to thirty-six weeks):* The skin is smooth, the baby looks chubbier, and average weight is 5.5 lb.
- *Tenth lunar month (thirty-seven to forty weeks):* The fetus is well proportioned, lanugo disappears, vernix decreases, and weight reaches an average of 7.5 lb.

And always take good notes! For guidelines, refer to the sections on "Medical Records," "Charting," "Informed Choice," and "Client Confidentiality and HIPAA Guidelines" in chapter 8.

Common Complaints

Ligament pains (which are experienced as pelvic sensitivity or groin pain when walking) occur due to stretching of the ligaments that support the uterus as it grows in size and weight. These ligaments run from the base of the uterus to the pelvic bones, making it more or less a floating organ (see illustration, page 48). Periodic rest and good pillow support while sleeping may provide some relief.

Morning sickness is primarily due to elevated estrogen and hCG levels. This low-grade, persistent nausea is called morning sickness because it is most likely to arise when the stomach is empty, although it may also occur in response to evening cooking odors. Mothers widely acknowledge that psychological upsets contribute to morning sickness, thus emotional support and stress reduction are crucial. Also suggest 50 mg vitamin B-6 at bedtime and again at midday. Other remedies include eating simple crackers or plain yogurt upon rising and drinking ginger or raspberry-leaf tea. Many moms report that small meals and nearly continuous eating help, particularly if food choices are high in protein. This makes sense: yet another factor in morning sickness is low blood sugar, mostly from fasting during sleep but potentially recurring throughout the day. If the mother is extremely nauseated, Guatemalan midwife Antonina Sanchez recommends that she "feel the vegetable or fruit that she likes most and eat just that."[41]

If nausea progresses to vomiting, recommend ground ginger capsules with small meals; also maintain daily contact with the mother, at least by phone. Should **hyperemesis gravidarum** develop, the mother is at risk for severe dehydration and should be seen by a physician immediately. Thyroid dysfunction may be a factor: it is estimated that 40 to 70 percent of hyperemetic women have thyroid dysfunction, although it is unclear whether thyroid dysfunction causes hyperemesis gravidarum or the reverse.[42]

Fatigue obviously has a relationship to nutrition, stress and activity levels, and general state of health. But in early pregnancy, fatigue is directly related to physiologic adjustments and hormonal changes and so may serve the positive function of helping the mother rest and tune in to her changing needs. If fatigue is problematic after the first trimester, review the diet. Sometimes mothers need help breaking away from habitual eating patterns: a greater variety of fruit and vegetables can provide the vitamins and minerals needed to boost vitality. Daily exercise and social interaction can also mediate fatigue by stimulating body and mind. Encourage every mother to experiment to find what works best for her. Screen for anemia if fatigue is extreme or persistent.

Indigestion and heartburn result from the displacement of stomach and intestines by the growing uterus, particularly in the last trimester. The best remedy is frequent but small meals, with digestive enzymes (available at health food stores) taken as needed. Because digestion slows naturally in pregnancy to increase the absorption of nutrients, meals should be taken leisurely. The gallbladder functions less efficiently in pregnancy, so reducing fat intake may also help. Advise limiting food in the evening, especially right before lying down.

Skin itchiness (pruritis) occurs in 3 to 14 percent of pregnancies. It may be correlated to liver compromise resulting from liver disease, excessive alcohol or drug use, or prolonged use of pharmaceuticals.[43] Tinctures of dandelion root and yellow dock are excellent liver tonics and may bring relief. Liver-cleansing foods like beets, dark greens, lemon juice, and olive oil should be taken freely, along with foods rich in choline, like egg yolk, wheat germ, and brewer's yeast. For topical application, plain yogurt rubbed into the skin or oatmeal baths (prepackaged by Aveeno) can help.

If the palms of the hands and soles of the feet are particularly itchy, **intrahepatic cholestasis of pregnancy (ICP)** may be the cause, in which bile flow is obstructed either mechanically or metabolically. Although rare in the general population (0.5 percent), it is quite common in women of Chilean, Bolivian, or Scandinavian descent.[44] Consult with a physician backup immediately regarding the advisability of a liver profile.

Minor headaches and other minor pains often respond to relaxing teas such as hops, skullcap, and chamomile. Massage, yoga, and chiropractic care can help. Headache may also result from dehydration, so stress the importance of adequate fluid intake.

If the mother complains of **backache**, see that she is getting sufficient but not overly strenuous exercise and suggest pelvic rocks or hip wiggles (like tail wagging) to keep the lower spine flexible. These movements can be done on hands and knees or while standing, sitting, or driving. She should also use her stomach muscles to maintain good posture; suggest that she periodically hold her stomach taut throughout the day. Make sure she has plenty of pillow support while sleeping: some women swear by egg-carton foam padding for alleviating back pain. If her abdomen is pendulous, she may benefit from an elastic bellyband, which also provides support for the lower back. Again, chiropractic adjustments can help.

If she indicates that her backache is near waist level, rule out kidney infection by checking for **costovertebral angle tenderness (CVAT)**. Do this with the mother in a sitting position, her back fully exposed. Place your hand on one side of her spine at waist level, then make a fist with your other hand and gently strike the hand in place, repeating on the opposite side. If the mother jumps or otherwise indicates pain, note whether her sensitivity was to the left or right and refer her immediately to a backup physician.

Varicose veins of the legs and vulva are caused by high levels of progesterone relaxing smooth muscle and hindering venous return throughout the body, particularly in the extremities. Hereditary factors also play a part. Sitting with crossed legs or standing for long periods exacerbates the problem, but periodically stimulating circulation via exercise or by elevating legs and buttocks can help. Six hundred units of vitamin E per day may also be beneficial. For best absorption, this fat-soluble vitamin should be taken separately from other supplements and with milk, cheese, oils, or other fatty foods.

In the absence of hypertension or proteinuria, **swollen ankles** are a normal result of impaired circulation in pregnancy or excessive periods of standing. The diet should be improved with more protein, fresh vegetables, and plenty of fluids, and moderate exercise should be taken regularly. Elevating the feet and legs helps, too.

Hormones or diet can cause **constipation**, but plenty of fluids and fibrous foods should remedy the problem. Sometimes women mistake thirst for hunger and must learn to distinguish between the two impulses. Regular physical activity is critically important in preventing constipation.

Vaginal infection, particularly **yeast (monilia)**, is common during pregnancy. Characterized by a white, curd-like discharge, yeast is a naturally occurring vaginal organism that tends to overgrow in pregnancy because of increased vaginal alkalinity, which in turn is caused by elevated progesterone levels. Have the mother insert vaginal sponges (boil first to remove mineral deposits) or cotton tampons soaked in acidophilus culture (available in the cold section of health food stores) every three or four hours. Cotton underwear is essential. Yeast infection at term increases the risk of newborn **thrush** (infection of the tongue and mouth that can make nursing difficult).

Bacterial vaginosis (BV) (also known as **gardnerella** or **hemophilus**) is another common vaginal infection. Although ordinarily benign and transient, in pregnancy it can lead to chorioamnionitis, premature rupture of the membranes, and preterm labor. If infected, the mother may detect a fishy odor, particularly after lovemaking. Seldom is there vaginal

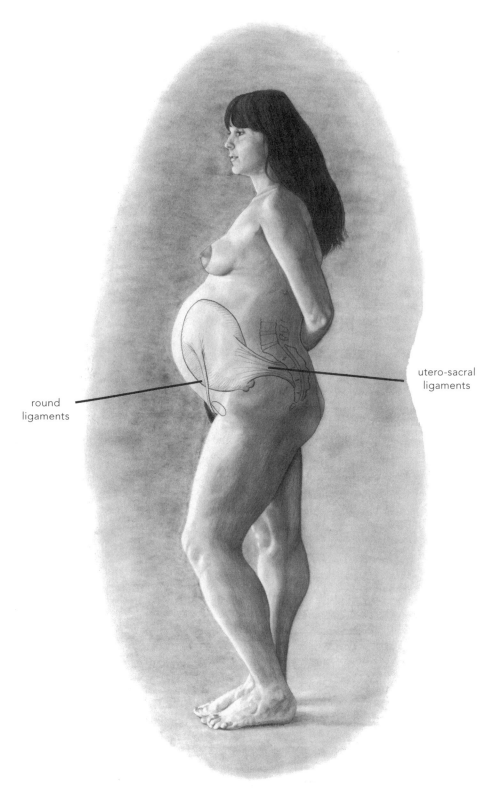

round
ligaments

utero-sacral
ligaments

Supporting Ligaments of the Uterus

irritation or itching. Bacterial vaginosis produces a thin, gray or white discharge that tends to adhere to vaginal walls.

The best way to test for BV without a microscope is by the **whiff test**. Touch a cotton swab saturated with discharge to a bit of KOH solution; if it lets off a potent fishy odor (amine), it's bacterial vaginosis. One remedy is to insert a peeled, unnicked clove of garlic into the vagina, changing three times daily. Follow this with five days of acidophilus treatment, as described for monilia. If this does not work, medical treatment is indicated. (It is also important that the woman abstain from intercourse during treatment and that her partner be checked if symptoms persist.)

Trichomonias infection is characterized by a malodorous, highly irritating, yellow-green frothy discharge. Like BV, it can cause chorioamnionitis, premature rupture of the membranes, and preterm labor. The usual treatment, Flagyl, is contraindicated in pregnancy. As an alternative, the herbal douche formula outlined in the sidebar on page 50 is often effective. It is a bit of trouble to prepare but is gentle and nourishing to vaginal membranes (unlike harsh medicinal formulas). Although douching is generally not recommended during pregnancy, it is safe as long as pressure is kept to a minimum: a hand-held squeeze unit is best, with the water warm, not hot. Insert the nozzle no more than a few inches into the vagina. Garlic suppositories also work for trichomonias, particularly if used in combination with the douche.

Trichomonias is sexually transmitted, thus the mother's partner must also be treated. Men have relatively minor symptoms (such as twingeing with urination or slight discharge), but because the organism can be harbored in both the urethra and prostate, they must take oral medication. Condoms and latex barriers should be used for sexual activity until both partners are cured.

All vaginal infections respond positively to dietary inclusions of dark-green vegetables, seaweeds, high-quality protein, citrus, and plenty of fluids. Unsweetened cranberry juice or concentrate (in capsules) increases vaginal acidity, helpful for most infections (as well as UTIs). With yeast infections, sugar should be completely eliminated as the organism thrives on it; also have the mother cut back on her fruit intake, whether fresh, dried, or juiced. Eating plenty of yogurt with probiotics helps, as does brewer's yeast.

Herpes simplex virus is at epidemic proportions and has thus become a common complaint. Small, painful blisters are the prime symptom of this sexually transmitted viral infection. The initial outbreak is usually severe, like a bad flu. Once the sores disappear, the virus remains in genital nerve ganglia, thus infection may recur repeatedly: there is no cure. Susceptibility is increased during times of severe stress or exhaustion. Some women have outbreaks every few months; others never have subsequent symptoms, or perhaps none for many years. If a mother reports recurring episodes, inquire as to the number, severity, and usual location of lesions, and note this in her chart.

In the event of a recurrence during pregnancy, culture the sores (for a firm diagnosis) and the cervix (to see if the virus is present at this location). With an initial outbreak during the first trimester, immediately consult backup, as herpes can have a devastating effect on the baby's central nervous system.

This is also a concern if lesions are present when labor commences, although studies have shown that women with recurrent episodes develop and pass antibodies to their babies.[45] Still, it is the standard of care that all women with a history of herpes be screened at the onset of labor by speculum exam, to rule out cervical infection. Do this within two hours if the waters release, for although internal procedures are generally contraindicated with **rupture of the membranes (ROM)**, if the mother is infected, the baby may soon be too via **vertical transmission** (virus migrating up into the uterus).

With lesions at the cervix, vaginal birth is prohibited. But birth may proceed vaginally if (1) the outbreak is nonprimary, (2) sores are external, (3) sores are healing, and (4) adhesive surgical film or spray-on bandage is used to prevent contact with the baby.

Treatments for herpes during pregnancy are basically comfort measures. Advise the mother to keep the affected area cool and dry—no nylon underwear, panty hose, or tights. Hot baths tend to aggravate symptoms, whereas applications of lysine ointment, cold milk, zinc oxide, A&D ointment, ice, and calendula cream (marigold extract) are all reputed to be healing and soothing. Dietary changes may also help; one mother reported cutting her usual five-day cycle in half by beginning stress supplements (B-complex) and protein drinks at the first sign of infection. Increased lysine intake is recommended, in supplemental doses of 500 mg daily. Eliminating coffee, black tea, alcohol, and sugar is essential, as is getting plenty of rest. The mother should avoid foods containing arginine (an amino acid that supports the herpes virus), such as nuts and nut products, seeds, and chocolate. Sexual interaction should be discontinued until all sores are completely healed.

Acyclovir (Zovirax) is generally used only for initial outbreaks, or for severe or frequent recurrences.

Douche for Vaginal Infections

One part each of the following:

- *Comfrey root*
- *Yarrow*
- *Mugwort*
- *Rosemary*
- *Peppermint*
- *Alum*

Steep in a nonmetal container using boiled spring water. Allow it to cool. Douche with 1 pint (pt.) strained solution twice daily for two days. On the third and fourth days, douche as usual in the morning, but for yeast infections add one part *acidophilus* in the evening, and for trichomonias, add one part *myrrh* in the evening.

This drug is FDA classified as C-category, that is, risk cannot be ruled out because human studies are lacking or animal studies have shown adverse effects. The newer drugs Valaclovir and Famciclovir are FDA classified as B-category, with no evidence of risk shown in animals but insufficient information available on humans.

Common Fears and Counseling Techniques

Certain fears regarding pregnancy and birth are universal and rooted in survival, such as fear of the unknown, of death, of separation, and of change. These fears serve to alert the mother to the needs of her developing baby as they help prepare her for parenting. Almost every mother wonders if her baby will be normal; most have some fear of labor, wondering if they will be able to tolerate it. Explaining how commonly these fears occur often helps to alleviate them.

Besides these universal fears, there are concerns unique to our times and culture. Working mothers may fear losing career-related identity and being buried in domesticity. Others struggle with changes in primary relationships, fearing losses of intimacy and freedom. Some worry deeply about being able to parent effectively. These concerns are specialized according to the mother's background, her role in society, and the nature of her relationship with her partner. When these fears arise, focus the mother on her own problem-solving capabilities, but sympathize with her distress. (See chapter 3 for specific psychological issues and configurations.)

Validating a mother's hormonally enhanced fears can be trying, so spice the process with humor and relevant personal disclosure. In the midwifery model of care, counseling is an expression of friendship. What are some basic techniques? By receiving impressions and reflecting them back without judgment or distortion, you **mirror the mother's feelings**.

Herbs and Homeopathy in Pregnancy

Shannon Anton, CPM

A partial list of herbs contraindicated during pregnancy includes *goldenseal*, *ephedra*, *cotton root bark*, *blue cohosh*, *pennyroyal*, and *birthroot*. For more information, refer to *The Natural Pregnancy Book*, by Aviva Jill Romm, CPM, MD, or the *Wise Woman Herbal for the Childbearing Year*, by Susun Weed.

As *goldenseal* has become popular, it has also been overused and overharvested. Once abundant and easily wild crafted, it is now endangered in certain areas. To harvest *goldenseal*, you must take the root, thereby eliminating a significant portion of or the entire plant. *Goldenseal* is also extremely strong medicine; overuse taxes the liver and kidneys. There are only a few conditions for which it is a traditional remedy; other potent and more appropriate remedies abound. Do not use it for cold and flu, as you would *echinacea* tincture. There are a few appropriate uses for it postpartum, but do not use it at all during pregnancy. If you must use *goldenseal*, preserve its potency and stretch its volume by tincturing it.

Buying Herbs

Dried herbs should hold a deep color and smell strongly of their substance. Faintly colored herbs with little scent have been stored incorrectly or for too long a time, and their potency is questionable.

Herbal tinctures are composed of either fresh or dried herbs preserved in a liquid form. Herb qualities are extracted using alcohol or glycerin, and then the mixture is strained and stored. Tinctures are taken in drops from an eyedropper or by dropperful. When buying tinctures, try to find out how they have been prepared. Tincture from fresh, wild, or organically grown plants is the best. The company Herb Pharm consistently provides quality tinctures prepared with care and respect for the plants.

Working with dried plant material for tinctures is fine. But consider taking a class from an herbalist for an opportunity to observe herbs as they grow and to learn directly from the herbs about their properties and uses.

Using Homeopathy

Although homeopathy is a rich and exact healing tradition, there are beginners' rules that make it easier to work with these marvelous allies. Homeopathic remedies must be properly stored or they are antidoted (negated). Store homeopathics out of sunlight, protect them from heat and extreme cold, and never keep them near strong aromatic substances like herbs, camphor, peppermint, toothpaste, perfumed products, and so on. Avoid storing them in your medicine cabinet or in your birth bag near your herbal tinctures.

If possible, the mother must avoid eating or drinking for fifteen minutes prior to taking a remedy (in labor, this cannot always be achieved).

The strong potencies listed in this sidebar are not for everyday use; birth is exceptional in its requirements. Potencies of 6x or 30C are applied in most other situations. Unless you are sure of your expertise, never treat issues outside of birth with these stronger potencies.

In critical situations, as when resuscitating an infant or dealing with maternal hemorrhage, dosing and then dosing quickly again is appropriate. Once relief is experienced or a shift is noted, discontinue the remedy. If symptoms return, apply the remedy again.

I urge you to read *Homeopathic Medicines for Pregnancy and Childbirth*, by Richard Moskowitz, MD, to better understand the nature of homeopathic medicines and to further research the following remedies.

Herbs for Pregnancy Support

The most basic and well-known nutritional herbs are also beneficial for pregnancy. Herbal infusions are a simple and delicious way to take herbal nourishment. To make an herbal infusion, use 1 oz. of fresh or dried herb (a good handful) per 1 qt. boiling water (removed from heat).

continued >>

Steep at least four hours in a covered, nonmetal container. You can mix two herbs per 1 qt. water, or double the batch. You may also want to add honey or lemon. If you like, brew *peppermint tea* separately and add it to your infusion for taste.

- *Nettle leaf* provides excellent support for kidneys and is rich in vitamins A, C, D, and K, as well as calcium, potassium, phosphorus, iron, and sulfur. It prevents leg cramps and postpartum hemorrhage, eases postpartum afterpains, nourishes the circulatory system to reduce hemorrhoids, and encourages abundant breast milk.

- *Dandelion leaf* is nature's special gift to nourish and revitalize the liver and also provides great kidney support. It is rich in calcium, potassium, and iron as well as vitamins A, B complex, C, and D. It is also essential in the prevention and treatment of preeclampsia and is a reliable digestive aid.

- *Red raspberry leaf* is the classic uterine toner and pregnancy tonic. It prepares the uterus to function at its best. The leaf can ease morning sickness and gently aid digestion.

- *Red clover leaves and blossoms* greatly nourish the whole reproductive system as well as nourish and balance the endocrine system. They are rich in calcium, magnesium, and trace minerals.

- *Lemon juice and water* safely detoxify the liver during pregnancy (or at any time of stress). It is best to drink it in the early part of the day.

Remedies in Pregnancy

Nausea can be greatly relieved with *ginger tea*. Pour 1 cup boiling water over three to five slices of fresh ginger root. Let steep five minutes and sip slowly. Homeopathic remedies can be extremely effective for easing morning sickness. The remedies are specific to symptoms. Research *pulsitilla, sepia, nux vomica,* and *ipecacuanha*. Additional remedies to consider include *antimonium tartrate, argentum nitricum, petroleum, sulfur,* and *tabacum*. Good references are *Homeopathic Medicine for Women,*

by Trevor Smith, MD, and the already-mentioned *Homeopathic Medicines for Pregnancy and Childbirth*, by Moskowitz.

Anemia is often diagnosed in pregnancy. Herbal and green sources of iron include *dandelion, nettles, kelp,* and *parsley. Yellow dock root* improves absorption. *Floradix Herbs plus Iron*, a concentrated herbal and food compound, is an excellent tonic.

Heartburn responds well to *slippery elm* lozenges, even the worst heartburn. Also try chewing raw almonds, raw papaya, or papaya enzyme tablets.

Sleep difficulties can largely be alleviated by deep relaxation and exercise during the day. A silky eye pillow filled with *flaxseed* and *lavender* has proven to be my own best remedy for sleeplessness. Stronger remedies include half a dropperful of *skullcap tincture* or *valerian tincture*. Or, during the last trimester, try half a dropperful of *hops* tincture. Some women are awakened by anxiety or worry that keeps them from getting back to sleep. *Homeopathic aconite 30C* is very effective to calm and quiet nervous tension and fears. Use this remedy only during anxious episodes.

For **back pain, sciatica**, or **carpal tunnel syndrome**, chiropractic care can be crucial. Joints softened by pregnancy may become misaligned, and if readjusted, other remedies can be more helpful. Even if you are unfamiliar with chiropractic care, don't hesitate to try it in pregnancy.

Saint-John's-wort (hypericum) *oil* is the best remedy I've found for **nerve** or **muscle pain**. Apply it directly over the sore area, as well as a bit above and below. Especially if used before sleeping, *Saint-John's-wort* brings amazing relief. Depending on the severity of pain, use it straight from the bottle or dilute 1 oz. in 6 oz. of almond or olive oil. *Arnica oil* can also be beneficial, though it is *Saint-John's-wort oil* that earned the reputation of "miracle cure" during the Middle Ages. For nerve pain, *Saint-John's-wort tincture* may be taken orally, half a dropperful of tincture every few hours. Homeopathic remedies include *hypericum 30C*, taken every two hours during painful episodes, and topical application of a gel compound, *arniflora*.

Hemorrhoids often respond to *red clover* and *nettle infusion*, which nourishes the circulatory system and can be preventative, especially if taken routinely. Grated raw potato may be used as a compress directly on hemorrhoids, or a thin slice of raw potato may be inserted into the rectum to shrink and relieve painful swelling. The classic standby, *witch hazel extract*, is very effective. Apply directly on hemorrhoids or use compresses. An oral form of the agent active in *witch hazel* can be found in *hamamelis*; take 30C when hemorrhoids flare up.

Constipation requires excellent hydration. Plenty of vegetables and whole foods offer sufficient bulk to avoid constipation. For additional bulk, *psyllium seed* (the main ingredient in Metamucil) can be added to oatmeal or taken in capsules; take lots of water with it. Prune juice is the faithful elixir our grandparents knew and loved; it works great.

Diarrhea can happen for a number of reasons—even pregnant women get the stomach flu. The biggest concern is keeping enough fluid down to prevent dehydration. Often, plain water is abrasive to the system. Add honey or maple syrup to warm or room-temperature water and sip slowly. To stop diarrhea, here are two proven remedies:

- *Rice water*. Cook white rice with a four-to-one ratio of water to rice. Cook only until rice is tender, then pour off excess water and drink it.
- *Tea x3*. Using black tea and boiling water, brew one cup of tea. Save the tea bag, dump the tea. Use the same tea bag and brew a second cup, then dump. Brew a third time and drink.

Both of these remedies are complemented by **polarity therapy**. To practice this, the woman and her partner face each other and fully relax. The partner places one hand on the woman's right shoulder and one hand on her left hip. Waiting until both hands feel even or seem to pulse together, the partner then gives the woman warning that a change is coming and shifts hand positions to hold the woman's left shoulder and right hip. When the energy in both hands feels even again, the partner slowly removes both hands. *Rescue Remedy*, a Bach Flower Remedy, is helpful in any case of physical or physiological upset.

Breech babies may respond to the usual postural exercises for turning a breech baby, but two additional remedies have proven effective. Homeopathic *pulsitilla 30C* taken several times a day can also encourage the breech to rotate. Even more reliable is *moxa* treatment. *Moxa* is a roll of tightly compacted *mugwort*, used in traditional Chinese medicine. When lit, *moxa* looks rather like a cigar. The ash of burning *moxa* is extremely hot, so care must be taken in handling. Place the burning end near the outer, lower corner of the pinky toenail; heat at this "point" facilitates rotation of the breech. Treat the toes on both feet two or three times daily until a change occurs—and don't worry, women know how hot is hot enough! *Moxa* treatment is most effective done on a slant board.

With **preterm labor**, the sooner labor symptoms are addressed, the better your chance of getting them to stop. In times of threatened preterm labor, good hydration is critical. In addition, magnesium supplements have proven invaluable in preventing preterm labor in any woman with predisposing factors, or forestalling it if it occurs. Too much magnesium causes diarrhea; reduce intake as necessary, and space doses throughout the day. Follow this routine until thirty-seven weeks. If preterm labor begins, extra doses of magnesium and plenty of fluids should be taken at once, along with a deep, warm soak in the tub.

Homeopathic *mag phos 30C* is also useful. Using a nonmetal cup, put seven pellets in half a cup of hot (not boiling) water and stir with a nonmetal stick a hundred times. Slowly and continuously sip little sips of this remedy until it is gone. Contractions should slow or stop within an hour. Continue to monitor for preterm labor symptoms: if labor is not slowing or is accelerating, or if cervical change is occurring, consult a physician.

Postdates situations usually respond to the famed *evening primrose oil* remedy; in addition, the cervix may be softened with homeopathic *cimicifuga 30C*, taken once an hour for eight hours. Follow with homeopathic *caulophyllum 30C*, taken as above. If the cervix is already soft, go right to *caulophyllum*. Often, one dose of *caulophyllum 200C* before bed will result in labor during the night.

You can also try **pacing the mother's rhythms**, matching her speed and style of self-expression as a means of making a connection. **Active listening** requires that you use all of yourself—not just your ears, but your heart and soul—to fully receive what the mother is trying to communicate. When the mother has moments of truth or reckoning, give her **positive reinforcement** for her revelations.

Contrary to the medical model's premium on clinical detachment, personal involvement is integral to the midwife/client relationship. By committing yourself to the mother as she works through her problems, you inspire her commitment in return. And by letting your character shine through, strengths and weaknesses alike, you help her find the courage to accept newly revealed truths about herself. When the mother embraces her realizations and begins to make them manifest, the ultimate aim of counseling—**eliciting responsibility**—is achieved.

As midwife healers, giving to our clients nourishes and teaches us. On the other hand, we must at all times respect our clients' privacy and pacing and must consciously avoid projecting personal needs and concerns into the relationship. Working collectively or in partnership with other midwives can keep us from going overboard in this respect and help us maintain the necessary balance between personal involvement and objectivity.

Partner Participation

The mother's partner has his or her own vital role to play in the perinatal experience. Some need time to warm up to playing a significant role, while others are deeply involved from the start. If he or she wants to help catch the baby, provide reading material and visual aids. Explain that sensitivity in the moment is most important and that anyone assisting must follow the mother's lead. Ideally, partner preparation is merely an extension of the couple's intimacy.

Here is Frank's story:

I wanted to share the birth process with my mate and felt that my involvement was necessary and my right as a father. Practicing exercises and massaging Bridget almost every night put me in tune with her body and spirit. By participating in this way, I believed that my mind and body would appreciate the mystical aspects of birth when the time came.

My participation was not limited to prenatal classes, exercises, and reading material. This was our second pregnancy, and once again my goal was to catch the baby and cut the cord. I had performed this mighty ritual during our first birth. That labor was only three hours; Bridget went immediately into hard labor-transition. Even though it was hard to absorb this rapid labor, I still made the catch. Lydia was small, yet perfect to the touch. I caught her and held her close to my joyful, tired body.

I did not catch our second child. His shoulders were stuck and we needed assistance. His birth was twelve hours long, which let Bridget and me absorb ourselves at every stage. We touched, massaged, showered, and supported each other in every way. This made up for not catching Paul.

During this second birth I felt fully in touch with Bridget sexually and spiritually. I noticed that my sensitivity was greater than before, and my love for Bridget and my family grew with every phase of the encounter. Patience, listening, and empathy were at their peak. I felt then that I truly understood both birth and Bridget.

Here is the joint perspective from Watta and her partner, Kenna (herself a midwife):

We both always knew that we wanted to be moms, but somehow each of us had always pictured herself as "the" mom. Learning how to fill the role of nonbiological mother has been a challenge for both of us, but a challenge with great rewards. We have the two most beautiful boys in the world, each one born to a different mother. But they both "belong" to each of us. Here are our stories of learning to be there for each other.

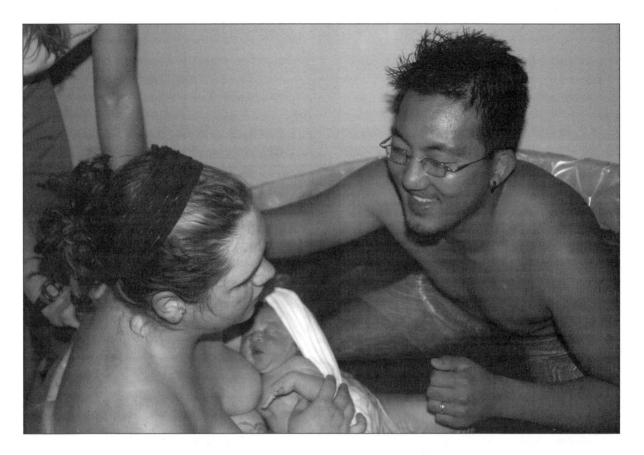

Kenna:

Watta was incredibly beautiful when she was pregnant. I adored rubbing her belly and putting my ear against it to hear the baby's heartbeat. I also struggled a lot with jealousy, as I had wanted to be pregnant for a long time. Our journey to this pregnancy was a difficult one, and many plans had fallen through along the way. I wanted to be there for Watta as a perfectly supportive partner, but trying to suppress my less-than-perfect feelings didn't work very well. It was very hard at times, but in the end, I knew that the most important things held true: I loved Watta, I was completely in love with the baby who was growing in her belly, and together we were a family.

Watching her give birth was one of the great privileges of my life. She was so graceful, even in the midst of all that pain. She was so strong that it made me want to cry. She labored all night with me at her side offering up soft words of encouragement, drinks of Recharge, a bowl to throw up in, and my complete and utter faith that her body knew what to do. Not long after sunrise, she pushed our son Rio out into the water of the birth tub and into my hands. I was, and still am, completely in awe of her.

Watta:

Even though I gave birth first, I wanted Kenna to feel special and as if she was having the first child. As the birth progressed, it was so hard and so long that I got really scared. I was scared for Kenna and I was scared for the baby. I wanted her to have an easy birth, but that's not what she got. I felt really helpless. It was very intense in that I knew what she was going through, but at the same time I didn't know what she was going through.

After twenty-four hours, I was ready for it to be over. I reached a level of exhaustion where, if it wasn't for the midwife, I don't know if I could have kept my faith in the process. It had gone on for so long with no change. Watching her get through it was . . . like she was superhuman, not real in some way. She finally told me to go to sleep. I didn't want to go to sleep until the baby was born; I felt like I needed to be around. But when she told me to go I did—for two hours. That was hard for me, although she did the best part of her work when she was alone.

When we got to the end and the head was coming out, I was right in position to catch the baby. I hadn't planned on that, but the midwife said, "Catch your baby" and took her hands away, so someone had to catch the baby, and it was me! That was such a surprise and such an honor and so great. In that moment of holding the baby, I realized that it was all about Kenna's transformation into motherhood. In the end, the experience was about Kenna and her work.

Here is another account, with comments from the father, Eugene, and the mother, Pamela:

Eugene:
Every man should catch his own baby. I didn't realize that, when my daughter was born eight years ago. We had her at home, I cut the cord, and it was the high point of my life. Yet it would have been even better if I had caught her.

I didn't because I was ignorant. I didn't know how easy it was, and nobody told me that I could or should. But when my son was born, I found out that catching your baby is the next best thing to having it. I urge all fathers to do it, to insist on it.

I enjoyed being down there between Pamela's legs. At my daughter's birth I was at her mother's side and didn't have the intimate perspective. This time I could see what was going on.

Pamela:
I was not sure where I wanted Eugene to be—at my side or at my feet. But as our cycle was near completion, I realized that this was the only time we, the three of us, would be connected in that intense moment of birth. Watching Eugene's concentration, his hands and the message of love that they carried, and seeing my baby's head in the mirror helped me to stay focused. Soon I was feeling those irresistible urges to push and feeling my baby's body moving through the passage. First the head then swoosh the body into the hands of the man I love. A beautiful baby boy was born so right. The connection is made and is never lost.

Eugene:
When Lenny slithered into my hands, I immediately felt bonded to him. I was the first one able to see that he was a boy. That was a special thrill. Though Pamela carried Lenny and gave him up like ripe fruit, I was his first contact with the world as a whole person. In this first, total contact I knew he could feel my protective, loving feelings. And when I gave him to Pamela, completing the cycle, I felt truly satisfied.

Sibling Participation

Children who will be at the birth need preparation, too. Have picture books and videos available for this purpose. Some parents worry that the sights and sounds of birth will be too frightening for small children, but usually these fears are unfounded. Just in case, mothers can play at making "birth noises" with young ones to prepare them. As my midwife (Ann Govan) assured me regarding the presence of my son, then two, at his sister's birth, "They take it like an apple falling off a tree."

Still, it is a good idea to have an adult companion especially for the children, someone who can take them out of the room if they become upset or want to leave for any reason. I recall one mother who wanted her two-year-old at the birth but changed her mind in light of how sensitive her daughter had recently become: crying if anyone around her got hurt and responding intensely to her mother's every mood. With small children, the mother should decide; older children can decide for themselves.

If a child is to be included, the atmosphere at prenatal visits is of utmost importance. Here is one mother's experience of preparing her three-year-old daughter:

From the beginning of our second pregnancy, we wanted to include Lydia in the birth. We felt that this would ease the transition from being an only child and lessen any jealousy that might arise. A homebirth would enable her to comfortably share this joyous family occasion. Although some friends and relatives thought she was too young to participate, our midwife and other friends invited to the birth supported the idea.

Our preparation started with prenatal exams in the home of our midwife, Elizabeth. Lydia accompanied us on all of these visits and, with each one, became more interested in the proceedings. We tried to explain each step to her and encouraged her to take part by imitating Elizabeth. The relaxed atmosphere and obvious enthusiasm of everyone in the room made her more comfortable.

In preparation for the actual birth, we asked a friend who is close to Liddy to look after her during labor and to try to gauge whether she wanted to be in the room while the baby was born. We were happy that she slept through most of my labor because this reduced the chance that she would become bored, plus Frank and I were better able to concentrate on each other and the birth.

Liddy entered the room in the arms of a friend just as I was pushing the baby out. She was very calm, putting to rest our fears that the intensity of pushing might upset her. Even after the birth, much

of my attention went out to Lydia, who seemed a bit shy at first. But a few hours later when the four of us were alone, she warmed up considerably and has continued to show a deep affection for her little brother. We feel that bringing her to prenatals and letting her attend the birth has a lot to do with her present warmth and tolerance.

The Last Six Weeks

The emphasis of caregiving shifts dramatically during this final phase of pregnancy. The birth is imminent, and the baby will soon be here. Parents have last-minute preparations to consider and more questions than before, while the midwife attends more assiduously to assessing the readiness of mother and baby. She carefully palpates the baby for position, size, and growth, and also checks for descent, flexion, and engagement. These additional assessments can be done abdominally or by internal exam.

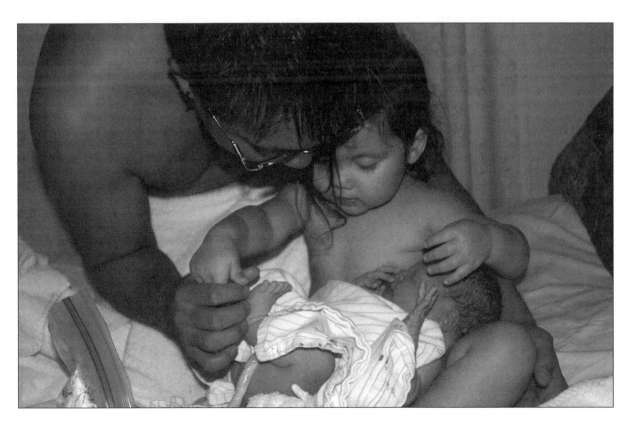

Lack of flexion can be corrected if the head is not too far into the pelvis; in fact, the deflexed head can and should be flexed before it engages. The maneuver is simple—facing the mother's feet, press the **occiput** (back of the baby's head) down into the pelvis while pulling the **sinciput** (forehead) toward you, tucking the baby's chin to its chest (see the illustration "Checking for Engagement and Securing Flexion" on the opposite page).

Internal exams are not mandatory but may indicate to what degree labor is impending. When examining near term, (1) check cervix for dilation and effacement, (2) note station (level of descent) of the baby's head, and (3) note any increase in vaginal lubrication or softening of the musculature. If this is the mother's first full-term pregnancy, the cervix may remain somewhat closed until labor begins, with perhaps 1 cm of dilation, whereas a woman who has given birth before may be 2 or 3 cm dilated at this point.

Effacement, or the softening and shortening of the cervix, depends largely on how much the baby has descended and to what extent it is exerting pressure on lower uterine tissues. If the baby's head is still high and the cervix posterior, it is rare to find much effacement or dilation.

The degree of effacement is recorded in percentage. An uneffaced cervix feels thick, firm, and about an inch long. A cervix 50 percent effaced feels softer, "mushier," with a less distinguishable neck, half an inch or so in length. Sometimes the cervix is almost fully effaced, but the os feels ring-like, with a clearly defined and somewhat rigid edge. This may be due to the presence of scar tissue or may result from extended use of oral contraceptives. The cervix may also efface unevenly if the baby's head comes down at an angle and puts pressure on either the anterior or posterior aspect. It is fairly common to find 60 to 80 percent effacement in the final weeks. Rarely, the cervix is 100 percent effaced at term (paper-thin and smooth against the baby's head) with little or no dilation but great propensity to open precipitously in labor. Some women dilate

to 5 or 6 cm weeks before labor begins; these labors are also apt to be quick.

If you find the os to be rigid and taut, or you suspect the mother may have scar tissue in the cervical canal from previous infection or surgery, have her do self-massage with evening primrose oil (available at most health food stores) beginning at thirty-seven weeks. This will soften and break up any adhesions, preparing the cervix for dilation. This can also be done in early labor, in case it is prolonged. Help the mother find her cervix in case she has never felt it before, and direct her to massage twice daily for several minutes.

The phenomenon of **false labor** occurring in the final weeks of pregnancy is characterized by irregular contractions: instead of increasing in duration and frequency, they eventually just taper off and stop. Little or no dilation takes place because uterine action is incoordinate. The uterus is comprised of three layers: the external, longitudinal layer; the middle, connective layer; and the internal, circular layer. In **incoordinate labor**, only certain long-muscle segments contract, when all must work together in order to pull open the circular muscles of the cervix. Although false labor seldom results in dilation, the term is both discouraging and misleading, as it does facilitate the baby's descent and engagement and may accomplish some effacement.

Descent is the level of the presenting part in relationship to the ischial spines. If the head is 1 cm above spine level, the **station** is termed −1. The head can be as high as −2, −3, or −4 and still be felt internally. If the top of the head is exactly level with the spines, it is at 0 station and considered to be engaged. If the head is 1 or 2 cm below spine level, the respective reading is +1 or +2 station (rarely will the presenting part be lower than +2 before labor begins).

Assessing station can be difficult at first. As when checking the ischial spines with pelvimetry, insert two fingers sideways but *bend only the middle one*, placing it on the spine while extending the index finger to find the presenting part. Your reading will

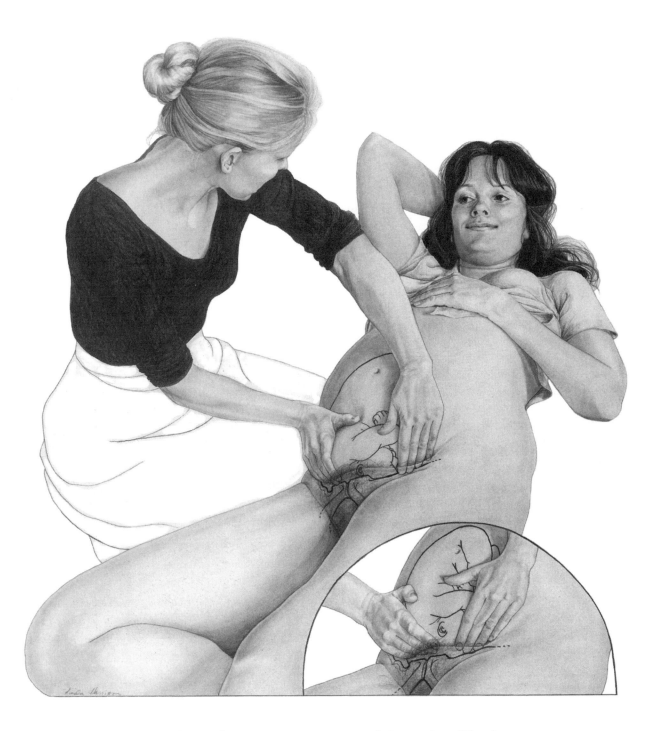

Checking for Engagement and Securing Flexion

be accurate only if you keep both fingers on a horizontal plane. If you must move your index finger up to touch the presenting part, the station is negative. With a positive station, your index finger will be below the spine. If the head is too low for the spine to be felt, your assessment is based on a qualitative sense of how much the head (or butt) fills the pelvis. This skill definitely takes practice.

If you have not done so already, you might want to teach the mother **vaginal awareness practices** to help her avoid vaginal and perineal tears. If she can learn the difference between contracted and relaxed states of her vagina and perineum, she will be able to create either at will. Encourage her to do some exploring when she has privacy and is not hurried, placing her fingers inside and attempting to contract her muscles around them.

One of the best vaginal toners is the **elevator exercise**. In this, the pelvic floor muscles are pulled upward in stages, like an elevator ascending and stopping at each floor. To practice, lift to the first floor and pause for ten seconds, to the second floor and pause for ten seconds, and so on, until reaching the fifth floor. Pause there as long as possible, then release downward floor by floor, with ten seconds' pause at each level, all the way down to the basement, and finally, to the subbasement (from which we give birth). Yet another exercise is the **classic Kegel**, with quick, snapping movements made lower in the vagina, near the vaginal opening. Both these exercises are also helpful postpartum in restoring vaginal tone and speeding tissue healing.

A unique approach to vaginal toning was developed by midwifery educator Verena Schmid. With it, contractions are performed in layers, starting with the internal muscle bands, or **bulbocavernosus muscles**. To activate these, gently draw the pubic bone and coccyx together, and hold. Next, add the **transverse perineal muscle** as you pull the ischial tuberosities (sides of the pelvis) together, and hold. Now draw the entire vaginal canal together by tipping the coccyx forward, and hold. Finally, activate the wide bands of **levator ani muscles** that run between the pubic bone and sacrum as you tip your coccyx back, and hold. Hold all four layers tightly, and then release one by one.[46]

Vaginal massage may be helpful if the muscles are extremely strong or tight. With olive oil for lubrication, the mother places her thumb against the floor of the vagina and moves from side to side in a half circle, with steadily increasing pressure. Deep breathing further facilitates her relaxation and release.

Home Visits

Home visits are obviously a critical part of homebirth preparation. In fact, some midwives provide care exclusively in their clients' homes. A minimum of two home visits is essential: one early in pregnancy to see the mother and her supporters in their own element, and another around thirty-five weeks to be sure that supplies are ready and last-minute concerns are fully addressed. Extra home visits are definitely called for if a mother complains of family problems, reports feeling unsettled in her environment, or her partner hasn't come to prenatal visits for a while, whatever the reason.

The last home visit should include a review of prepared childbirth techniques, especially if the mother and her partner have not taken classes. Children can be included in dinner discussions, then afterward can feel mom's belly and listen to the baby's heartbeat. The entire birth team should be present at this gathering so that roles can be clearly delineated in advance.

Use this visit to appraise the home for order and cleanliness and see that a tabletop or other protected area will be available for laying out supplies. A most critical assessment is for *adequate heat in the birth room*; newborns quickly lose body heat and are almost impossible to resuscitate if cold. Also appraise sleeping arrangements for the baby: beware of the crib or cradle in a separate part of the house. Emphasize

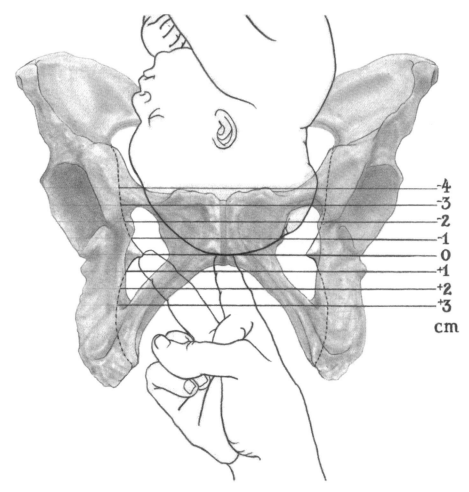

Estimating Station

the importance of skin-to-skin contact in the early weeks, and debunk fears about bringing the baby to bed. You might want to come prepared with handouts or other reading material should your discussion progress to baby care or other postpartum concerns.

This is a perfect time to discuss any unresolved concerns the mother (or her partner) may be harboring with regard to the birth. Because this is a leisurely visit and the mother is in her own environment, she may become more vulnerable than ever before and reveal her deepest fears. However long it takes, consider this time well spent, as the birth may be shorter and smoother because of it. The main purpose of this visit is to affirm her home as the birthplace and

to inspire confidence and intimacy among the entire support team.

If not at this visit, some time in the last few weeks you should broach the subject of debriefing her birth experience once it has occurred. A major challenge to debriefing unhappy outcomes is that, regardless of any feelings of anger or disappointment, women bond with their care providers in the altered state of labor and may thus feel precarious in criticizing them, as if to do so will jeopardize this bond. Reassure her that even if it is difficult for her to be truthful, it is essential for her growth and adjustment in the postpartum period, and her feedback will help you be a better midwife.

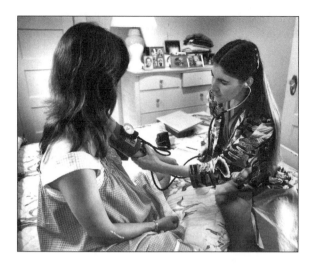

Also let her know that processing her birth can take time. For the first few months, she may experience the "halo effect" of simply being happy that she and the baby are healthy. A year or more may pass before feelings of loss, anger, or trauma may arise; for some women, this might not occur until they become pregnant again or are confronted with another major life challenge. Tell her that it is never too late to contact you for debriefing, and if for some reason she doesn't feel comfortable doing so, she can access the hotline established by Sheila Kitzinger for this purpose: www.sheilakitzinger.com/BirthCrisis.htm.

Preparation for Water Birth

If the mother intends to have a water birth, she will need an ample-sized tub (now widely available for rent). The tub should be scrubbed with iodine and rinsed thoroughly before it is filled with water. It is generally agreed that a mild saline solution can help discourage the growth of microorganisms and keep the birth environment similar to what the baby has known in utero. The mother and her partner should shower before entering the tub. Be aware that it can be difficult to utilize universal precautions when assisting water birth.

Parents' most common concern regarding water birth is for their baby's safety: what if it tries to breathe while still under water? This fear is unfounded, as the baby will not be stimulated to breathe until its body is exposed to air, due to the dive reflex that keeps the glottis closed when the baby is submerged. Still, it is wise to bring the baby out of the water as soon as it is born.

Benefits of water birth include increased relaxation and comfort for the mother, greater intimacy for the couple, and an easier transition for the baby. Water birth can greatly ease a painful or tumultuous labor. German expert Cornelia Enning claims it lowers blood pressure in cases of borderline hypertension and is ideal for breech and posterior babies, as well as for women having a VBAC.[47]

The temperature of the water is very important; it must stay between 86 and 95 degrees Farenheit. Here are some of the physiologic benefits of water birth:

- Neurotransmission of pain is reduced.
- Oxygen uptake via uterine vessels is increased.
- Muscle tone is normalized.
- Glucose metabolism is improved.
- Levels of stress hormones are lowered.
- Placental separation is facilitated.[48]

The mother must be in the water for at least thirty minutes before these effects are fully realized. After two to three hours, benefits as per hormone stimulation diminish.[49] Advise her to stay flexible about being in the water as labor progresses. Never put a cold cloth on her forehead to cool her: if she gets hot, cool the water down or have her come out. If she gets claustrophobic in the tub or feels like she cannot get enough leverage to bear down, she should get out immediately.

Auscultate fetal heart tones using a Doppler with a waterproof probe. If there is fetal distress, meconium, or blood loss during labor, the mother should get out of the water. If she is at risk for postpartum hemorrhage, or factors in the labor lead you

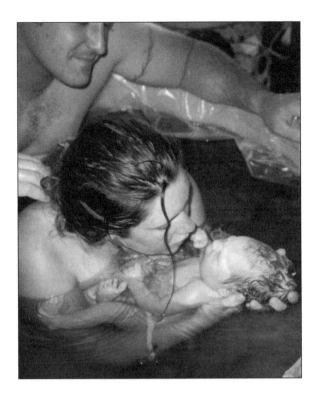

to believe that the baby may be slow to start, have her leave the tub as transition ends.

It is best to avoid touching the baby as it is born. If the mother is undisturbed, she will touch the head herself, and the baby will spiral out (literally pushing itself out with its feet) and turn to face her. It may expel fluid from its lungs (seen jetting into the water), and may reach one arm toward her with the other bent, as if swimming (the asymmetric tonic reflex). Mom and baby will then make eye contact, and she and her partner can lift it and bring it to her chest.

Last-Minute Clients

What about mothers calling for help just weeks before their due date? In general, the last-minute scramble to obtain all the necessary information and develop intimacy in short order will challenge even the most experienced midwife. If the mother has been receiving care and her records are available, your task is less daunting. Without prenatal records, you have no maternal or fetal baselines from which to extrapolate norms during labor. And if her dates are at all uncertain, you have no point of reference regarding the baby's maturity except its current size. You also have little time to assess the mother's needs and expectations of you or to assert your own needs and expectations of her. This increases your liability, and you must decide if the additional effort and risk can be justified.

Your decision to assist must be based on a strong sense of rapport and the conviction that the mother and her supporters are utterly committed to home-birth. If they are coming to you from another midwife's care, explore their motivations to make sure they are not just chasing rainbows. Get right down to it: what do they want from you? Make a home visit as soon as possible and schedule longer or extra appointments. You must still cover all the essential information on emergency care, the mechanics of labor, and birthing techniques. Some last-minute clients expect a major discount; explain that providing care in these short-order circumstances requires a challenging condensation of your services.

Tina, a midwife practicing in rural Hawaii, shared this tale of assisting a true last-minute client. Her account also exemplifies how the midwife's work can overflow into her personal, home, and family life:

> This lady-in-waiting called me two days after her due date—I'd met her before, and I said sure, I'd find time to see her. But I made no promises as I'm wary of last-minute goodies. She had no support, no man, not even a place to call home. She'd seen a doctor three times, but didn't feel comfortable or prepared for the hospital situation.
>
> There she was on my doorstep; I had just returned from one of my huge food-shopping expeditions. So I put the groceries away, made some tea, sat down with the woman, and felt out the situation. She looked pretty tense, had been having contractions all night but didn't want to go to the hospital. She didn't even know if she wanted to keep the child. Very much alone, she felt she had other things to do with

her life besides mothering. But she did have enough incentive to give the baby a good beginning with natural birth and breast milk. She also was willing to give herself some time to feel out motherhood.

It was early afternoon, and I got the feeling that she was definitely in labor and would have her baby that night. But I didn't even know this woman; didn't even know if I liked her! All I knew was that she was confused, and I wanted to help her. She couldn't have her baby at my place—too much traffic with five children. So I told her I'd go to the hospital to ease the doctor confrontation and serve as her support person and coach. She seemed relieved at this decision. She took a walk outside in the banana patch for about an hour and came back a different woman: resigned, courageous, and strong. She began squatting for most of her now regular contractions. I suggested that she lie down and rest in the loft where it was quiet and where Adrian (my one-year-old) was sleeping. The older children came in from playing and we gathered around the table for dinner.

No sooner were the dishes cleared than we heard some serious "Oh Oh Ooh" sounds from the loft. I dropped everything and got ready to examine her, but she was already on her way down the ladder saying she had to go to the bathroom. She came back out to kneel on the living room floor and her water bag broke. "Can I check you?" said I. "No, no, no, oh, oh, oh," said she, "I've got to go to the bathroom again." Then she really began complaining, she said she wasn't comfortable at all, couldn't see any point in all this discomfort, wanted to go to the hospital and get drugged out. She got off the toilet and leaned on the sink, but was still . . . pushing!

Uh, oh . . . what's this? Oh God, quick, wash those hands, catch that baby, plop, flop, she's out, gorgeous! Her mother was stunned but finally uttered something, and the baby gave a cry back. Relief, release! I wrapped the babe in a towel, set another towel on the floor so they could lie down, and waited for the placenta. I opened the bathroom door and there were some little faces eager to greet the baby; the children all heard that first cry. Haydon (nine-and-a-half years old) announced that it happened at two minutes to eight. Chana (eight years old) got a blanket for the baby. Nara (six years old) got my birth

kit so I could clamp the cord, and also a bowl for the placenta. Then I announced bedtime but of course I wasn't heeded; the excitement was too much.

I assisted the mother with baby-holding and bonding and the placenta came out fine. "Now," I thought, "if I can just get them up off this floor and onto a bed in the living room to check for tears . . . hmm, well, she was standing and there was no support." So after a good nursing session I suggested she go to the hospital to be sutured and stay for a few days. She would rest better there and wouldn't have to think about her personal care for a while.

They came to stay with us for several weeks before finally leaving the island. We really fell in love with the baby—it was quite an experience for all of us.

Notes

1. Robert Briffault, *The Mothers* (New York: Atheneum, 1977).

2. Verena Schmid, Midwifery Today conference notes, London, June 2003.

3. Schmid, Midwifery Today conference notes, 2003.

4. Verena Schmid, "Birth Centres in Italy," in *Birth Centers: A Social Model for Maternity Care*, ed. Mavis Kirkham (Oxford, UK: Butterworth-Heinemann, 2003).

5. M. Plaut, M. Schwartz, and S. Lubarsky, "Uterine Rupture Associated with the Use of Misoprostol in the Gravid Patient with a Previous Cesarean Section," *American Journal of Obstetrics and Gynecology* 180 (1999): 1535–42.

6. Ina May Gaskin, *Ina May's Guide to Childbirth* (New York: Bantam Dell, 2003), 300.

7. Catherine Deneux-Tharaux, Ellie Carmona, Marie-Hélène Bouvier-Colle, and Gérard Bréart, "Postpartum Maternal Mortality and Cesarean Delivery," *Obstetrics and Gynecology* 108, no. 3 (September 2006): 541–48.

8. Ina May Gaskin, "Maternal Mortality in the USA: A Fact Sheet," 2011, www.rememberthemothers.net/Fact%20 Sheet%202005.pdf (accessed March 6, 2012).

9. Gaskin, *Ina May's Guide to Childbirth*, 300.

10. Dong Zhang, Mohamed Al-Hendy, Gloria Richard-Davis, Valerie Montgomery-Rice et al., "Green Tea Extract Inhibits Proliferation of Uterine Leiomyoma Cells In Vitro and in Nude Mice," *American Journal of Obstetrics and Gynecology* 202, no. 3 (March 2010): 289.

11. F. M. Cowan and P. Munday, "Guidelines for the Management of Herpes Simplex Virus Infection in Pregnancy," *Sexually Transmitted Infections* 74, no. 2 (1998): 93–94.

12. I. Ofek, J. Goldhar, D. Zafriri, R. Lis, R. Adar, and N. Sharon, "Anti-Escherichia Coli Adhesion Activity of Cranberry and Blueberry Juices," *New England Journal of Medicine* 324 (1991): 1599.

13. Melinda Beck, "Can Mom's Medicine Hurt the Baby? Few Studies Detail Prescription Drugs' Risk to Pregnant, Breast-Feeding Women," *The Wall Street Journal*, March 29, 2011.

14. Peggy McIntosh, "White Privilege: Unpacking the Invisible Knapsack" (in working paper 189, "White Privilege and Male Privilege: A Personal Account of Coming to See Correspondences through Work in Women's Studies," Wellesley, College Center for Research on Women, Wellesley, MA, 1988).

15. R. Mittendorf et al., "The Length of Uncomplicated Human Gestation," *OB/GYN* 75, no. 6 (1990): 929–32.

16. Carol Wood Nichols, "Postdate Pregnancy, Part II: Clinical Implications," *Journal of Nurse Midwifery* 30, no. 5 (1985): 259–68.

17. R. K. Gribble, P. R. Meier, and R. L. Berg, "The Value of Urine Screening for Glucose at Each Prenatal Visit," *Obstetrics and Gynecology* 86, no. 3 (1995): 405–10.

18. B. G. Ewigman, J. P. Crane, D. Fredric, F. D. Frigoletto, M. L. Le Fevre, R. P. Bain, D. McNellis, and the RADIUS study group, "Effect of Prenatal Ultrasound Screening on Perinatal Outcome," *New England Journal of Medicine* 329, no. 12 (September 16, 1993): 821–27.

19. J. P. Newnham, S. F. Evans, C. A. Michael, F. J. Stanley, and L. I. Landau, "Effects of Frequent Ultrasound during Pregnancy: A Randomized Controlled Trial," *Lancet* 342 (1993): 887–91.

20. Eugenius Ang, Vicko Gluncic, Alvaro Duque, Mark E. Schafer, and Pasko Rakic, "Prenatal Exposure to Ultrasound Waves Impacts Neuronal Migration in Mice," *Proceedings of the National Academy of Sciences* 103, no. 34 (August 2006): 12903–10.

21. J. M. Jiminez, J. E. Tyson, and J. S. Reisch, "Clinical Measures of Gestational Age in Normal Pregnancies," *Obstetrics and Gynecology* 61 (1983): 483.

22. Bing-Fang Hwang, Jouni J. K. Jaakkola, and How-Ran Guo, "Water Disinfection By-Products and the Risk of Specific Birth Defects: A Population-Based Cross-Sectional Study in Taiwan," *Environmental Health*, June 2008.

23. U.S. Department of Health and Human Services, U.S. Department of Agriculture Dietary Guidelines 2005.

24. G. S. Zavorsky and L. D. Longo, "Exercise Guidelines in Pregnancy: New Perspectives," *Sports Medicine* 41 (2011): 345–60.

25. G. S. Zavorsky and L. D. Longo, "Adding Strength Training, Exercise Intensity, and Caloric Expenditure to Exercise Guidelines in Pregnancy," *American Journal of Obstetrics and Gynecology* 117 (2011): 1399–1402.

26. Sara Wickham, *Anti-D in Midwifery: Panacea or Paradox?* (Oxford, UK: Butterworth-Heinemann, 2001), 7.

27. Wickham, *Anti-D in Midwifery*, 7.

28. N. Benhadi, W. M. Wiersinga, J. B. Reitsma, T. G. M. Vrijkotte, and G. J.Bonsel, "Higher Maternal TSH Levels in Pregnancy Are Associated with Increased Risk for Miscarriage, Fetal or Neonatal Death," *European Journal of Endocrinology* 160 (2009): 985.

29. T. I. Chang, M. Horal, S. K. Jain, F. Wang, R. Patel, and M. R. Loeken, "Oxidant Regulation of Gene Expression and Neural Tube Development: Insights Gained from Diabetic Pregnancy on Molecular Causes of Neural Tube Defects," *Diabetologia* 46, no. 4 (April 2003): 538–45.

30. WHO, Press Release: "New HIV recommendations to improve health, reduce infections and save lives, " www.who.int/mediacentre/news/releases/2009/world_aids_20091130/en/index.html (accessed March 6, 2012).

31. K. M. De Cock, M. G. Fowler, E. Mercier et al., "Prevention of Mother-to-Child HIV Transmission in Resource-Poor Countries: Translating Research into Policy and Practice," *Journal of the American Medical Association* 238, no. 9 (August 1977): 1175–82.

32. Anne Frye, *Understanding Diagnostic Tests in the Childbearing Year*, 6th ed. (Portland, OR: Labrys Press, 1997), 726.

33. W. E. Jamie, R. K. Edwards, and P. Duff, "Vaginal-Perineal Compared with Vaginal-Rectal Cultures of Identification of Group B Streptococci," *Obstetrics and Gynecology* 104, no. 5 (November 2004): 1058–61.

34. E. M. Levine et al., "Intrapartum Antibiotic Prophylaxis Increases the Incidence of Gram Negative Neonatal Sepsis," *Infectious Disease in Obstetrics and Gynecology* 7, no. 4 (1999): 210–13.

35. M. Dabrowska-Szponar and J. Galinski, "Drug Resistance of Group B Streptococci," *Polski Merkuriusz Lekarski* 10, no. 60 (2001): 442–44.

36. C. V. Towers and G. G. Briggs, "Antepartum Use of Antibiotics and Early-Onset Neonatal Sepsis: The Next Four Years," *American Journal of Obstetrics and Gynecology* 187, no. 2 (August 2002): 495–500. C. J. Baker, M. A. Rench, and P. McInnes, "Immunization of Pregnant Women with Group B Streptococcal Type III Capsular Polysaccharide-Tetanus Toxoid Conjugate Vaccine," *Vaccine* (Netherlands) 21, no. 24 (July 28, 2003): 3468–72.

37. L. G. Burman, P. Christensen, K. Christensen, B. Fryklund, A. M. Helgesson, N. W. Svenningsen, and K. Tullus, "Prevention of Excess Neonatal Morbidity Associated with Group B Streptococci by Vaginal Chlorhexidine Disinfection during Labor," *Lancet* 340, no. 8811 (July 1992): 65–69.

38. F. Facchinetti, F. Piccinini, B. Mordini, and A. Volpe, "Chlorhexidine Vaginal Flushings versus Systemic Ampicillin in the Prevention of Vertical Transmission of "Neonatal Group B Streptococcus, at Term," *Journal of Maternal-Fetal and Neonatal Medicine* 11, no. 2 (February 2002): 84–88.

39. Ronnie Falcao, "Lavage w/Chlorhexidine," www.gentlebirth.org/archives/gbs.html#lavage (accessed March 6, 2012).

40. Christa Novelli, "Treating Group B Strep: Are Antibiotics Necessary?" *Mothering* 121 (November/December 2003).

41. Antonina Sanchez Mendez, Midwifery Today conference notes, Oaxaca, Mexico, October 2003.

42. Timothy J. Caffrey, "Transient Hyperthyroidism of Hyperemesis Gravidarum: A Sheep in Wolf's Clothing,"*Journal of the American Board of Family Medicine* 13, no. 1 (January 2000): 35–38.

43. Frye, *Understanding Diagnostic Tests*, 288.

44. Steven G. Gabbe et al., *Obstetrics: Normal and Problem Pregnancies*, 5th ed. (New York: Churchill Livingstone, 2007), 1112.

45. Dwight Rouse and Jeffrey Stringer, "An Appraisal of Screening for Maternal Type-Specific Herpes Simplex Virus Antibodies to Prevent Neonatal Herpes," *American Journal of Obstetrics and Gynecology* 183, no. 2 (August 2000): 400–06.

46. Schmid, Midwifery Today conference notes, London, 2003.

47. Cornelia Enning, Midwifery Today conference notes, London, 2003.

48. Enning, Midwifery Today conference notes, 2003.

49. Enning, Midwifery Today conference notes, 2003.

For Parents: Self-Care in Pregnancy

Prenatal care is more than the checkups you receive from your practitioner every few weeks—it is the care you give yourself each and every day. Here are some of the main components, with a rating system to help you see how well you are doing. Enter one of the following with each category:

4: You do this automatically, naturally.

3: You do this consistently but with definite effort.

2: You do this occasionally, with some resistance.

1: You just can't seem to do this or haven't thus far.

Nutrition

_____ Eat from the four basic food groups daily.

_____ Take supplements that I know I need.

_____ Drink at least two quarts of water, juice, and so on, per day.

_____ Pay attention to my inner voice of hunger and respond accordingly.

_____ Treat myself to something I know is especially good for the baby and me.

_____ Indulge myself in favorite foods that are also healthful for pure pleasure.

Exercise and Relaxation

_____ Take fresh air and, if possible, sunshine daily.

_____ Do something to work up a sweat each day.

_____ Stretch out my back, legs, shoulders, and neck daily.

_____ Do exercises specific to pregnancy several times a week.

_____ Dance, moving rhythmically and freely with music.

_____ Do vaginal toning/relaxation exercises daily.

_____ Completely let go at least once every day.

_____ Practice progressive relaxation at least twice a week.

_____ Have my partner (or someone else) massage me at least once weekly.

_____ Dress in clothing that allows freedom of movement and is comfortable.

_____ Deliberately release areas where I know I hold tension, several times daily.

_____ Allow myself the necessary comforts to curl up and take it easy before bed.

Emotional Well-Being

_____ Let myself cry whenever I feel like it.

_____ Ask for support, acknowledgment, touch, and sex from my partner (if applicable) whenever I need it.

_____ Vent my frustrations before they become explosive.

_____ Feel free to be loving and tender with my partner (if applicable) day by day.

_____ Feel loving and tender with myself at least once each day.

_____ Give myself time alone and find new ways to enjoy it.

Intellectual Preparation

_____ Read something on pregnancy at least once a week.

_____ Formulate and ask questions of my care provider.

_____ Take stock of my status in pregnancy by reviewing my daily or weekly activities and looking for areas that need improvement.

_____ Discuss technical aspects of pregnancy, birth, and parenting with my partner and/or supporters on a regular basis.

_____ Work on developing my birth plan by noting ideas and preferences as they arise.

_____ Attend information sessions or film series on birth whenever possible.

Social Preparation

_____ Meet with other pregnant women at least once a week.

_____ Talk to mothers of infants or pregnant women in public places.

_____ Observe infant behavior and family interaction whenever possible.

_____ Ask for concrete support from friends and relatives for needs in pregnancy and postpartum.

_____ Think about the changes having a baby will bring and formulate ways to adapt.

_____ Support my partner (if applicable) in talking to other new parents, reading about parenting, or discussing the baby with me.

Mothering Preparation

_____ Connect with the baby physically.

_____ Spend time daily visualizing and sending thoughts to the baby.

_____ Tell the baby it is loved and wanted.

_____ When stressed, explain to the baby and reassure it of your love.

There are several ways to score this exercise. First, add up your score in each section. This will give you a general idea of areas where you are strong and those where you could use improvement. Then tally your overall score, which can be interpreted as follows:

- 124 to 160: Yes, you are enjoying being pregnant and are taking good care of yourself.

- 96 to 123: You are doing well enough but could stand to focus a bit more on the pregnancy. Look carefully at your areas of resistance and see what you can do to discipline or motivate yourself more.

- 40 to 95: Well, perhaps you are very busy with other things, but you definitely need to give your pregnancy some attention. Try combining an activity where you scored low with one where you scored high; for example, if you get outside every day but can't seem to take your vitamins, make vitamin taking a prerequisite to leaving the house.

You'll feel much better if you care for yourself regularly.

CHAPTER 3

Problems in Pregnancy

The challenge in caring for problem pregnancies is to differentiate physical and psychological factors, for they often overlap. We must be wary of oversimplifying physical complications with a psychosomatic view; on the other hand, psychological disequilibrium for an extended period of time can definitely cause physical problems.

Physical problems still in incipient stages call upon the midwife to utilize her insight and expertise to formulate, with the mother's guidance, a remedy as holistic as possible, one combining health-giving physical treatments with self-awareness practices. Safe leeway for finding an effective remedy always depends on close and continued surveillance of the mother's condition. Under these circumstances, prenatal visits should be scheduled more frequently—perhaps as often as every few days with phone contact in the interim. And don't hesitate to consult with another experienced midwife or another expert within your network of health care providers.

Physical Complications

The following section on physical complications will not address every pathological condition of pregnancy but will focus on those pertinent to low-risk women already established as good candidates for homebirth. For more information, consult a medical textbook or your backup physician.

Anemia

Nutritional anemia is common in pregnancy, due to normal physiology. In nonpregnant women, anemia heralds a deficiency either of iron, folic acid, or vitamin B-12. But in pregnancy, a dramatically increased blood volume demands the creation of extra red cells, so until this job is complete, a degree of anemia naturally results.

Creating new blood cells takes more than iron. Adequate protein is necessary as is folic acid, which maintains the integrity of cell membranes. Vitamin C is crucial for healthy cell metabolism, as are zinc, calcium, and many trace minerals. B vitamins are needed to moderate any stress in the system that would otherwise tax cell elimination. In other words, the best way to treat anemia is by dramatically revamping and improving the entire diet, adding more fresh fruit and vegetables, high-quality protein, whole grains, mineral-rich seeds and nuts, and nourishing herbal teas.

Care must be taken with iron supplements, as they are toxic in large quantities. I recommend ferrous peptonate or gluconate, in low doses (25 to 50 mg) spread throughout the day, and no more than 100 mg total. Vitamin C aids absorption, while calcium blocks absorption. Often, no more than a third of supplemental iron is absorbed, with the unused portion irritating the kidneys and intestines and causing indigestion and constipation. This is particularly true of ferrous sulfate. An herbal elixir called Floradix Iron Plus Herbs (or Floradix Floravital Iron Plus Herbs for vegans) is concentrated and easily absorbed by many women. Tincture of yellow dock (12 to 15 drops in water per day) has also been shown to raise the blood platelet count.

If a woman is anemic in early pregnancy, with hematocrit (HCT) at or below 33 or hemoglobin (HGB) at or below 11, suggest overall improvement of the diet as cited above along with 100 mg iron daily taken with 500 mg vitamin C. It takes time to build red blood cells, so repeat the blood work in three to four weeks. Good food sources for iron include prune juice, molasses, pumpkin seeds, sesame seeds, sunflower seeds, beans, raisins, dark greens, and organic beef liver.

Around twenty-eight weeks, HCT/HGB readings often dip with an additional increase in blood volume. Check for this at the onset of the last trimester and, if need be, advise the mother on how to bring the HCT/HGB to optimal levels in time for the birth.

Anemia creates numerous problems for the mother. Fatigue and diminished vitality affect her appetite, her resistance to infection, and her general enjoyment of the pregnancy. She is susceptible to premature labor, but even if she goes to term, labor may be prolonged with incoordinate contractions and clinical exhaustion. As her uterus is less likely to contract well after the birth, she is at risk for postpartum hemorrhage, and with less oxygen-carrying cells in her bloodstream, she may go into shock more rapidly than usual. Anemia in the postpartum period can be devastating, too, as it renders new mothers more susceptible to infection, poor healing, difficulties with establishing a milk supply, and postpartum depression.

The baby of an anemic mother may be growth restricted and without sufficient fat for insulation and stress resistance during the early weeks. As breast milk is low in iron, the baby will normally store enough in the last six weeks of pregnancy for the first six months of life, but if the mother's intake is inadequate, she may have to begin feeding solids before she or the baby are ready. During labor, decreased oxygen levels in the mother's bloodstream can lead to fetal distress, a cesarean, or the need for neonatal resuscitation. For all of these reasons, a woman wanting a homebirth should strive to maintain an HCT of 34 or an HGB of 11.5 throughout most of her pregnancy.

Before treating the mother for anemia, double-check her lab work to rule out folic acid or vitamin B-12 deficiency as the primary cause. How do you identify this? Find the figures for **mean corpuscular volume (MCV)** and **mean corpuscular hemoglobin (MCH)**. The MCV indicates the average size of her red blood cells, while the MCH indicates the average amount of hemoglobin per cell. In iron-deficiency anemia, the MCV is normal but the MCH is lower than usual; this type of anemia is called **microcytic** (small cell) anemia. In B-12 and folic acid anemias, the MCV is elevated but the MCH is normal; these anemias are **macrocytic** or **megaloblastic** (large cell) anemias.

If it appears the mother suffers from a macrocytic or megaloblastic anemia, check levels of folic acid or B-12 on the lab report or, if these are not indicated, order additional testing. In the meantime, reassess the diet. Sources of folic acid include egg yolks, orange juice, melons, strawberries, and dark greens like spinach, chard, kale, and collard greens. Nonetheless, four large servings of the above per day would barely remedy a minor deficiency during pregnancy. So advise the mother to combine food sources with supplemental folic acid, about 2,400 mcg daily.

B-12 is found almost exclusively in dairy foods and animal products and will therefore be lacking in a vegan diet unless a supplement is taken. B-12 deficiency can cause central nervous system damage in the newborn, and, should deficiency persist into childhood, there will be slow, insidious, and irreversible brain damage. Thus all vegan mothers must be sure of their intake. Purported vegetable sources such as fermented soy products, seaweed, shiitake mushrooms, or spirulina actually contain analogs of the vitamin that can block absorption of the active form. Have the mother look for sublingual tablets containing cyanocobalamin or hydroxocobalamin. Soy products or fresh juices fortified with cyanocobalamin or hydroxocobalamin are also good sources. In severe cases, intramuscular injections are the only remedy.

There are certain types of hereditary, microcytic anemias such as **thalassemia** or **sickle cell anemia** that may also render MCV values unusually low. If the MCV is below 80, and the woman is of African, Asian, or Mediterranean descent, consider ordering a hemoglobin electrophoresis (a test for normal hemoglobin).

Problems with Weight Gain

Determining whether weight gain during pregnancy is inadequate or excessive depends partly on pre-pregnant weight. The average weight gain in pregnancy is about a pound per week, although underweight women may gain more and overweight women may gain less. In either case, extensive nutritional counseling may be necessary to assure that adequate nutrients and calories are being taken. As a rule of thumb, the expectant mother should gain at least 10 lb. by twenty weeks and about 1 lb. a week thereafter.

What causes weight gain in pregnancy? There is water retention due to hormones, increased fatty insulation over the belly and backside, increased weight in the breasts, increased blood volume, plus the obvious weight of the enlarged uterus including the amniotic fluid, placenta, and baby. Women lose an average of 15 lb. with the birth or a few days thereafter, with the remaining weight used for sustenance during the first few months postpartum. Making breast milk, getting up several times a night to nurse, and dealing with the stresses of caring for a baby definitely burn up the fat reserves!

If a mother seems to be gaining weight more rapidly than usual, check for a **fetal growth spurt**. It is not unusual to see a gain of 5 lb. in two weeks linked to an increase of 3-plus cm in fundal height. Increased gain may also happen prior to a growth spurt, so wait a few weeks and see if things even out. Double-check the diet to see if the mother has made any deleterious changes and if so, ask why. See if there are foods she is craving that might clue you in to her nutritional needs. Excess sugar intake may signal a need for more protein: recommend low-fat sources like cottage cheese, fish, or chicken breast in place of high-fat sources like ice cream, hard cheese, or cream cheese. Suggest vegetable snacks in place of high-calorie fruits and juices; see which fruits appeal to her and find vegetables with similar vitamin and mineral content. Reiterate the basics, while reminding her to heed her instinctive voice of hunger. Be sensitive to her declarations and try to work positively around her attachment to certain foods.

Mothers with a **history of eating disorders** may require care from a specialist. Anorexic women often have difficulty conceiving and may have problems maintaining a pregnancy. Even when pregnancy is well established, increased appetite combined with changing body image may reactivate eating disorders. Mothers with a history of bulimia are particularly at risk for hyperemesis gravidarium, and those who have been anorexic, for malnutrition. Schedule prenatal visits more often and see the mother in her

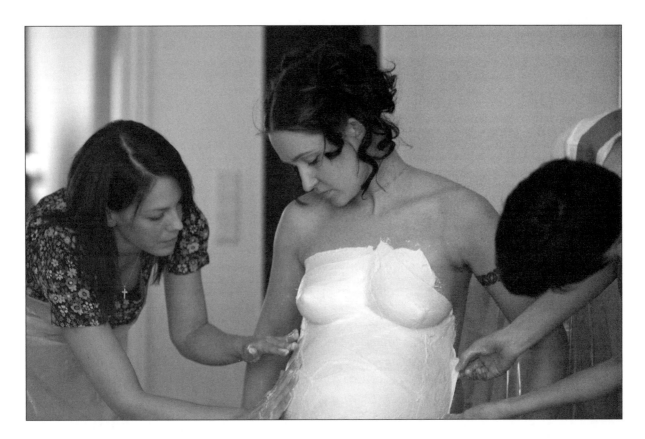

home (where you can share meals together) as often as possible.

In fact, any mother who claims she must "watch her weight" should be taken seriously. If she defines eating as an out-of-control, emotionally based activity, she may never learn to trust her instincts for nourishing herself and her child. She may have strong feelings of guilt associated with eating, linked to years of criticism from family or friends regarding her appearance. Take history in this regard, but avoid dwelling on the negative aspects. Encourage her to bring variety to her diet, honor cravings for treats from time to time, and find some type of physical activity she can embrace. Brisk walking is a good beginning; prenatal exercise classes are ideal.

How about the underweight woman who gains very slowly? She may be somewhat hyperactive, used to running around constantly and more or less "living on air." Help her slow down enough to tune into her pregnant body, particularly if she has nervous symptoms of insomnia, dizziness, or fainting. She may adore fresh juices and raw vegetables, but unless she gets enough calories each day she will not look and feel her best. Thin women often complain of feeling bloated, heavy, or bogged down with more food, especially carbohydrates. If so, suggest smaller meals, with an extra snack at bedtime. Better yet, encourage continuous snacking throughout the day. Explain that the body makes nourishing the baby a priority, so if she is underweight, there may be little left for her own needs. This puts her at risk for anemia, preeclampsia, premature labor, prolonged labor, postpartum hemorrhage, poor recovery, and postpartum depression. With her participation, set a goal for weight gain.

Make sure the mother is not dieting or trying to control her weight to please her partner. See that he or she appreciates the nutritional demands of pregnancy and is fully supportive.

Miscarriage (Abortion)

The proper technical term for miscarriage occurring before twenty weeks is **spontaneous abortion**; beyond this point, it is **fetal demise**. In the vast majority of cases, the cause of spontaneous abortion is abnormal development of the fetus or placenta due to chromosomal anomalies. Less commonly, a mother may miscarry due to viral infection, severe malnutrition, substance abuse, or an antibody effect toward the father's sperm.

Threatened abortion is presumed when the mother has vaginal bleeding in the first half of pregnancy, particularly if combined with cramping or persistent backache. But keep in mind that one in four women experience bleeding in the first trimester, while only half of these actually miscarry.[1] Threatened abortion is signaled with bright red blood loss, either dramatic, or slight and continuous for days or weeks. **Inevitable abortion** occurs if the membranes rupture or if the cervix dilates.

Is there any intervention that can keep a threatened miscarriage from becoming inevitable? Probably not, but certain measures are worth a try. If symptoms are acute, recommend bed rest and complete cessation of all sexual activity. If there is cramping without bleeding, a glass of wine may halt uterine activity and forestall miscarriage. But if it does become inevitable, console the mother as best you can, and focus on helping her safely through the physical aspects of the process.

If she wants to go through her miscarriage at home, be certain she is not anemic and keep close watch for possible hemorrhage. Two cups of blood is the maximum safe blood loss. If the miscarriage extends for more than two days, she is at risk for infection and must take her temperature every four hours. If bleeding or pain persists, she should see a physician to determine whether everything has been shed and the miscarriage is complete. She may also wish to save physical remnants of her pregnancy (insensitively referred to as "products of conception")

to be tested for possible causative factors or to be handled in some ceremonial way.

Occasionally, women have light brown bleeding for many weeks with no distinct episode of resolution. This may be due to **missed abortion**: the fetus has died but is retained in utero. The mother may notice that her breasts have returned to their normal size or that she has lost several pounds. Upon examination, her uterus will be small for dates, with no fetal heart tones. In case of suspected missed abortion, it is important to make a determination with ultrasound as soon as possible. Although rare before twenty weeks, a coagulation disorder known as **disseminated intravascular coagulation** (DIC) may occur in reaction to fetal breakdown, resulting in catastrophic bleeding when the uterus is finally emptied. The incidence of DIC increases exponentially the longer the mother has been pregnant and the longer the fetus is retained after it dies. If a mother with apparent missed abortion reports excess bleeding from the gums, nose, or minor injury sites, she is extremely high risk. Have her seen by a physician immediately.

I've had only one case of missed abortion in my practice. The mother came for her first prenatal at eighteen weeks, reporting light-brown spotting for about a week. She had a history of previous miscarriage, although she had also given birth to a term baby (whose birth I assisted several years earlier). Her uterus felt about right for dates. I couldn't hear the baby with the fetascope but was not concerned as she was not yet twenty weeks. Two weeks later she returned, reporting what she thought was fetal movement but with brown discharge continuous since her last visit. This time I was alarmed at not finding the fetal heart and sent her for an ultrasound. She called to say she had lost the baby and that its development appeared to have ceased at about fifteen weeks. She was screened for DIC and was negative, but she scheduled a therapeutic abortion immediately because she couldn't stand the agony of waiting.

With any type of miscarriage, emotional support is critical at every phase of the process. Studies show that women grieve as deeply with miscarriage as they do with fetal demise, stillbirth, and neonatal death.[2] Feelings of guilt, shame, and anger are common and must be validated. Support groups for women who have miscarried may be found through a local birth resource center or online.

In addition, most women worry about their future prospects for carrying to term. Occasionally, miscarriage becomes habitual (it occurs more than three times), in which case genetic or other factors may be at fault. Refer a woman (or couple) with this problem for consultation with a specialist.

Ectopic Pregnancy

Ectopic pregnancy refers to implantation occurring outside the uterine cavity. Ninety-five percent occur in the fallopian tubes, termed **tubal pregnancy**. Depending on the portion of the tube in which implantation occurs, the fetus may either be expelled into the abdominal cavity as it grows too large, or may cause the tube to rupture somewhere between ten and thirteen weeks. This is a life-threatening complication. With rupture, the mother will lose the baby and is at risk for severe internal hemorrhage, leading to shock or even death. Tubal pregnancy or rupture may be misdiagnosed as pelvic inflammatory disease, severe gastrointestinal upset, or appendicitis, particularly if the woman does not know she is pregnant.

The primary cause of tubal pregnancy is **pelvic inflammatory disease (PID)**, which leaves scar tissue that may partially occlude the tube and cause reduced cilliation or the formation of blind pockets. Ectopic pregnancies have increased fivefold in the last twenty-five years due to the prevalence of sexually transmitted diseases, trauma from intrauterine devices, progesterone-based contraception, and infection following abortion.[3] Prior tubal rupture and reconstructive surgery also predispose a woman to ectopic pregnancy. One of my colleagues whose practice has had more than its share of ectopics does a bimanual exam on any woman with first trimester bleeding to rule out luteal masses.

Symptoms of tubal pregnancy include pelvic pain (consistent and more intense than cramping) and spot bleeding. The pain becomes severe with actual rupture and may be referred to the shoulder area. A definite sign that the mother is experiencing rupture is that the degree of shock far exceeds what would normally be expected for the amount of blood loss. If a mother calls to report symptoms that lead you to suspect tubal pregnancy or rupture, even if per an initial phone consultation, contact backup right away to arrange for admittance to the hospital and have her call an ambulance for transport. Avoid sending her to the emergency room, as the wait may jeopardize her life.

Prior to rupture, treatment of tubal pregnancy involves two options: surgical removal of the pregnancy or the use of methotrexate to dissolve the pregnancy. The latter may seem preferable as it can spare the loss of the tube: it is the only reasonable choice if the other tube is ruptured. But methotrexate is a potent chemotherapy drug, a folic acid antagonist, and teratogen.[4] Every mother in this situation needs to make an informed decision regarding her treatment.

Emotional recovery from ectopic pregnancy is complex. The woman has come close to losing her life while losing a child that may have been long awaited. Her future fertility may be affected. Her partner may struggle as well with multiple shocks of nearly losing her plus the disappointment of losing the baby. Offer counseling and support to both.

Hydatidiform Mole

This extremely rare complication occurs in 1 per 1,500 to 2,000 pregnancies. The hydatidiform ("high-duh-tid-ah-form") mole results from abnormal development of the chorionic villi. These cells ordinarily form the membranes and placenta, but in this case, they develop into a mass of clear, grape-like vesicles that fill the uterus. In 95 percent of cases, an abnormal sperm inactivates the chromosomes of the ovum. This is called a **complete mole**; there is no fetus. In the remaining 5 percent of cases there is fetal tissue present, though chromosomes from sperm and ovum are abnormal in number and the fetus almost never survives. This is called a **partial mole**. Molar pregnancy is more common in women over forty.

Light brown bleeding is the most common symptom, persisting for weeks or months (though rarely past the first trimester). What distinguishes the hydatidiform mole from the other complication correlated to light-brown bleeding—missed abortion—is that the uterus is typically large for dates and feels woody hard or doughy to the touch. The overgrowth of chorionic villi also leads to abnormally high hCG levels; with missed abortion, these levels are subnormal.

Elevated hCG levels tax the liver, giving rise to secondary symptoms of hypertension and proteinuria. Hyperemesis occurs in 25 to 30 percent of cases but tends to develop later than usual in pregnancy, generally in the second trimester. The mole almost always aborts spontaneously but occasionally must be surgically removed. Approximately 20 percent of molar pregnancies progress to invasive cancer, thus follow-up examination and testing are necessary for at least a year.[5] (A former student of mine related that during her training as a nurse-midwife, she took care of a woman who had metastasis to her brain from cancer originating in molar pregnancy.) If you suspect a hydatidiform mole, refer to a physician promptly.

As with ectopic pregnancy, attend to the mother's emotional recovery or any need for additional psychological support.

Bleeding Late in Pregnancy

Occasionally, a mother reports vaginal bleeding a bit heavier than spotting after intercourse in the second or third trimester. The cervix has increased **vascularity** during pregnancy and is often quite **friable**, that is, easily abraded with friction. Or if the mother has a vaginal infection, the mucosa will be irritable and more prone to bleeding during and after sex.

Another possible source of bleeding is a **ruptured cervical polyp**. Polyps are small, tongue-like protrusions at the cervical os, visible by speculum exam. Bleeding from a ruptured polyp is sudden and somewhat dramatic but tends to resolve quickly. If blood loss is significant and persistent in the second or third trimester, it is probably due to placental abruption or placenta previa.

Placental abruption refers to premature separation of the placenta. It may be caused by cord entanglement, physical trauma, or hypertension, but often the cause is unknown. There are several types of abruption. **Marginal abruption** refers to separation at the edge of the placenta only, causing blood to flow from the vagina. **Concealed abruption** refers to separation of the central portion of the placenta while margins remain attached, so bleeding is concealed. **Complete abruption** refers to total separation of the placenta. These are all rare, particularly the last—and fortunately so, because abruption may prove fatal for the baby and sometimes for the mother. If abruption occurs during labor and delivery is imminent, the baby will probably survive and the mother will be fine. But if it occurs late in pregnancy or early in labor, even an emergency cesarean may not be quick enough to save the baby, and depending on the degree of abruption, the mother's life may also be in jeopardy.

Symptoms of abruption vary depending on degree. With complete abruption, vaginal bleeding will be profuse and the mother will go rapidly into shock. With concealed abruption, bleeding is not evident but there is acute, consistent abdominal pain (distinct from uterine contractions in that it is nonrhythmic), with uterus woody hard and exceedingly tender to the touch. With marginal abruption, bright-red bleeding is apparent but abdominal pain may be less intense (and less noticeable in hard labor). In any case, the mother should be rushed to the hospital unless she is about to give birth. Administer oxygen and treat her for shock with feet elevated, head down, and body warmed with blankets.

Repeated episodes of light bleeding or heavy spotting with no abdominal pain may indicate **placenta previa**, that is, placenta implanted low in the uterus. It is believed that the blastocyst seeks unscarred tissue in which to imbed, thus risk factors for this condition tend to be associated with uterine scarring. They include the following:

- Previous uterine surgeries (including more than three D&Cs)
- History of pelvic inflammatory disease (PID)
- Endometritus (uterine infection) with a previous pregnancy
- Multiparity
- Pregnancies with short intervals between

Placenta previa is also correlated to an unusually large placenta; for example, with a multiple pregnancy.

Why does blood loss occur with this condition? In late pregnancy, the lower uterine segment begins to distend and thin as the presenting part of the baby enters the pelvis and presses downward; if the placenta is imbedded in this area, small portions will detach wherever underlying uterine tissues stretch. There are varying degrees of placenta previa: **total previa**, in which the placenta completely covers the cervical os; **partial previa**, in which the os is partially covered; **marginal previa**, in which the edge of the placenta is at the edge of the os; and **low-lying placenta**, in which the placenta is close to the os but does not actually reach it.

Prospects for vaginal birth depend on the degree of previa at the onset of labor. Total and partial previa necessitate cesarean delivery. A marginal previa will inevitably separate as the cervix dilates and, depending on the degree of blood loss, may also require a cesarean. Vaginal delivery is more likely with a low-lying placenta, but maternal blood loss

must be carefully monitored. Placenta previa is also associated with an increased risk of third stage hemorrhage (see page 166) due to poor contractibility of the lower uterine segment.

Placenta previa is often erroneously diagnosed by ultrasound in early pregnancy, but with the exception of complete previa, this condition cannot be determined until the last trimester when the presenting part of the baby distends the lower uterine segment. This makes the placenta appear to migrate upward, when in fact it is the baby's descent that moves it away from the os. Rarely, symptoms may manifest as early as twenty-four weeks. I had one case like this in my practice; I could barely believe the bleeding was due to previa because it occurred so early. The mother was put on bed rest for a number of weeks until an ultrasound showed the placenta to be out of the way, and she had a perfectly normal vaginal birth.

Diagnosis of placenta previa must always be done by ultrasound. As *Williams Obstetrics* admonishes, "Examination of the cervix is never permissible unless the woman is in the operating room with all the preparations for immediate cesarean section, since even the gentlest examination of this sort can cause torrential hemorrhage."[6] Never, ever do a vaginal exam when there is bleeding in late pregnancy! And have the mother suspend all sexual activity until a diagnosis is made.

Gestational Diabetes

This term for decreased glucose tolerance in pregnancy was coined in 1979, when normal blood glucose levels for pregnant women (as distinct from the general population) were first established. These levels remain controversial, as the study on which they were based included women in poor health as well as prediagnosed diabetics.[7] Subsequent studies were also skewed with management protocols such as starvation diets, early induction, and withholding nourishment from the newborn.[8] The data do show a correlation between elevated blood glucose levels in pregnancy and the tendency to develop diabetes later in life, but no correlation to increased risk for the fetus or other prenatal/intrapartal complications.[9] The purported correlation between high glucose levels in pregnancy and stillbirth was merely extrapolated from risks for babies of mothers with type 1 (childhood) or type 2 (adulthood) diabetes.

This might lead us to conclude that screening is pointless, but there is always a chance that a woman with a propensity for diabetes may develop it during pregnancy.

What if a mother is truly diabetic? Elevated blood sugar in early pregnancy is linked to certain birth defects and miscarriage.[10] As pregnancy advances, elevated blood sugar readily crosses the placental barrier to cause a significant rise in the baby, whose pancreas reacts with an overproduction of insulin, leading to an increase in growth, particularly in the chest region (**macrosomia**). Besides complications of prolonged labor and shoulder dystocia associated with this condition, the baby is at risk for respiratory distress because increased levels of insulin can interrupt production of surfactant in the lungs. The diabetic mother has a four times greater chance of developing preeclampsia, ten times greater chance of polyhydramnios, and a high risk of postpartum hemorrhage. The newborn may have severe problems with **hypoglycemia** (low blood sugar) or **hypocalcemia** (low calcium levels) after the birth.

However, with acceptable levels of blood glucose unrealistically low, many women are falsely diagnosed and considered to be high risk. This makes birth at home controversial or, at best, leads to a regimen of additional screening that may negatively affect the mother's experience of pregnancy and her ability to labor with confidence.

It is difficult to estimate the incidence of type 2 diabetes unmasked by pregnancy. Predisposing factors are marked obesity, history of polycystic ovarian syndrome, multiple unexplained pregnancy losses, or previous delivery of a stillborn or macrosomic baby, family history of diabetes, and current symptoms of increased thirst, increased urinary output, recurrent or chronic yeast infections, acetone breath, ketonuria, or persistent glucosuria. Common sense dictates that women with any of these risk factors should receive the HA1c screen in the first trimester, and depending on results, additional screening at twenty-four to twenty-eight weeks. The most common test is the **glucose challenge test (GCT)** for which the mother ingests 50 mg liquid glucose/orange pop, with a blood draw an hour later. As the liquid concoction is somewhat revolting, midwives may use alternatives of apple juice (about three-quarters of a cup, depending on the brand) or eighteen full-sized jellybeans.[11] It is also recommended that the mother carbo-load for three days prior to the test and that it be performed at twenty-four weeks, as insulin resistance increases as pregnancy advances.

If glucose levels exceed 140 mg/dl, the next step in screening is the **oral glucose tolerance test (OGTT)**. For this, the mother should once again carbo-load for three days before the test. She must fast overnight, after which her blood will be drawn to establish baseline glucose levels before she ingests 75 mg glucose. Blood draws are repeated at one and two hours. During this time, she cannot eat but should exercise lightly, which may be challenging as many women suffer nausea, vomiting, bloating, headache, or profuse sweating in response to glucose syrup. Maximum sugar levels in whole blood are (1) fasting, above 90 mg/dl; (2) one hour, above 180 mg/dl; (3) two hours, above 155 mg/dl. Note that both the GCT and the OGTT have extremely high false-positive rates. Although the OGTT is the gold standard in medicine, 75 percent of asymptomatic women with positive results never develop diabetes, rendering the test only 25 percent accurate.[12]

As an alternative to the glucose screen/OGTT, many midwives prefer to check **fasting glucose levels**. This is done first thing in the morning without any special dietary preparation. Using a lancet to prick the mother's finger, blood sugar levels are measured with either a glucosometer or a Visidex testing strip; levels should not exceed 100. If this test is positive, a **two-hour postprandial whole blood test** is the next step. The mother should carbo-load for three days prior to testing; she then fasts for eight hours (overnight) after which a blood sample is drawn for a baseline. Next, she eats a high-carbohydrate meal, such as whole grain pancakes with butter and syrup, eggs or some kind of meat, and a large glass of orange juice, with her blood drawn two hours later. Readings will be more accurate if she exercises lightly after eating. Levels should not exceed 140 mg/dl. If results are borderline, ask about her diet in the days preceding the test and also check to see if she has been under stress, as excess adrenaline blocks insulin. If there is any question, repeat the test in a few days.

Treatment for diabetes in pregnancy depends on the degree. Good nutrition is central: a diet high in protein and complex carbohydrates, with limited simple sugars, is strongly recommended. Regular, aerobic exercise is also encouraged. Monitoring of the baby via nonstress testing and kick-counts should begin no later than thirty-six weeks (for more information, see the section on page 90 on "Postdatism"). In severe cases, insulin therapy is recommended, and the woman will be risked out for homebirth.

If a woman in your practice chooses not to be screened, she will need to sign a waiver indicating her informed decision.

Hypertension

Hypertension (high blood pressure) may manifest in several ways during pregnancy. **Essential hypertension** is a preexisting condition indicated by initial and subsequent readings of 140/90 or more. When readings increase to this level after a normal baseline was established earlier in pregnancy, we call the condition **gestational hypertension**. These two types can be hard to differentiate if a mother begins care in her last trimester and presents with hypertension. In this case, obtain records of previous care, either during the pregnancy or before it. Homebirth is contraindicated for women with essential hypertension and **severe gestational hypertension** (readings of 160/110 or more).

Keep in mind that blood pressure can fluctuate dramatically with emotional upheaval and tension. In *Holistic Midwifery* (vol. 1), Anne Frye cites a study done by Kevin Dalton at Cambridge University, showing fluctuations as great as 40 points systolic and 22 points diastolic in ten-minute intervals.[13] Thus no conclusions should be drawn unless blood pressure is high on at least two occasions a full six hours apart. For greatest accuracy, do repeat readings with the woman on her left side, as this position induces optimal circulation.

Severe gestational hypertension is linked to placental abruption and intrauterine growth restriction, as vasoconstriction affects uterine circulation and the flow of oxygen to the baby. For the same reason,

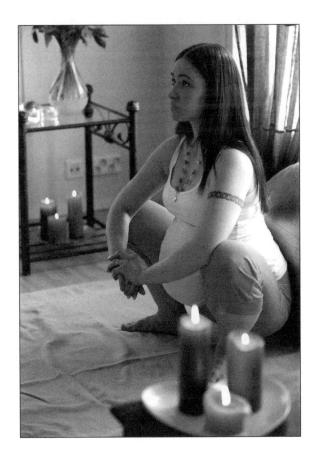

this condition can lead to fetal distress in labor. With readings of 160/110 or more, medical intervention is needed to forestall severe vascular damage. Any woman showing a consistent rise in blood pressure during pregnancy should be screened for elevated **liver enzymes**, **blood urea nitrogen** (**BUN**), and **uric acid**, which could indicate the development of preeclampsia.

Even mothers with a slight elevation in blood pressure persisting for several visits should be treated to prevent the problem from progressing. Here are some suggestions:

1. *Exercise is critical whenever blood pressure is just starting to rise and is appropriate if no more than moderately elevated.* Exercise increases circulation and forces the blood vessels to stretch and dilate, which reduces the pressure inside them. Aerobic activities like brisk walking, hiking, or swimming are most effective. Have the mother start out slowly, depending on what she is used to. One midwife colleague advises all mothers to work up a sweat every day, as a preventive measure. If blood pressure goes above 140/90, rest takes precedence over conditioning. Consult with backup, and in the meantime, the mother should lie on her left side periodically to allow optimal uptake of oxygen.

2. *Deep relaxation goes hand in hand with exercise.* Women with chronically tense circumstances may have little experience of complete release for days at a time, even while sleeping. Relaxation practice helps relieve tension in the voluntary muscles, which in turn reduces tension in the involuntary system. A calm physical state also contributes to emotional stability, which helps prevent overreaction to challenging situations.

3. *No stimulants whatsoever should be ingested or used.* These include coffee, black tea, some carbonated beverages, chocolate, nicotine, and cocaine. The last two stimulants in particular

have been proven to cause vasoconstriction and low birth weight. Strong spices like mustard, black pepper, ginger, and nutmeg should also be avoided.

4. *Good diet and healing herbs help immensely when used in combination with the measures above.* Improper eating and excessive weight gain place undue stress on the system. Encourage the mother to eat plenty of high-quality protein, whole grains, and lots of mineral-rich fresh fruits and vegetables. Watermelon, cucumber, parsley, and onion specifically reduce blood pressure, and garlic is a must. Contrary to popular opinion, salt is a necessary nutrient and should be used according to taste. (See Gail and Tom Brewer's excellent book, *What Every Pregnant Woman Should Know.*)

   Herbs like hops, skullcap, passionflower, hawthorn, and chamomile (listed in order of potency) can be used to induce relaxation. These are perfect for the mother with elevated systolic pressure who mostly needs to calm down. On the other hand, a woman with elevated diastolic pressure can benefit from cayenne pepper, which replicates the effects of aerobic exercise by causing vasodilatation and increased heart rate (take in capsules with meals). Chinese herbs and acupuncture may also be helpful. Ample intake of fluids is critical as are increased amounts of calcium, potassium, and magnesium. A 1996 analysis of 2,500 women showed those who took 1,500 to 2,000 mg of calcium a day to be 70 percent less likely to have hypertension in pregnancy than those who did not.[14] A subsequent study disputed these findings, but other data indicate that calcium does in fact reduce the risk of hypertension in pregnancy.[15]

5. *Counseling may be the first step if you are working with a woman so tense and distracted that she can hardly take responsibility for herself.* Assist her in getting to the roots of her anxiety, which may

help her release tension and find new enjoyment in the pregnancy. If she is enabled to work through whatever is troubling her and can feel good about herself and her situation, attending to messages from her body will not be so difficult.

Here are two contrasting experiences of treating gestational hypertension. With the first, the mother agreed to make immediate changes to her diet and began to exercise daily. Relaxation was difficult, as she had a very active work schedule that couldn't be altered. But she moderated her work activities with a more relaxed attitude and periodic meditation. In a matter of weeks, her blood pressure was down from 150/86 to 120/70. Pride in this accomplishment motivated her to continue her new routine. Toward the end of pregnancy her blood pressure rose again to 136/80 due to extreme stress at work. She began to use relaxant herbs daily, and by her next visit, her blood pressure was back to baseline. Throughout labor, it was steady at 120/70.

In the second case, the mother showed a rise in blood pressure at thirty weeks to 130/86. We offered suggestions on diet, relaxation, and exercise, but she was decidedly indifferent. Her diet was not the best: she ate a lot of red meat and refined foods, and she was 35 lb. overweight when the pregnancy began. Her blood pressure was 140/90 at the next visit, and she grew angry and defiant in response to more ideas of how she might lower it. A few days later, readings of 140/100 prompted us to recommend that she see a physician. At this, she burst into tears, releasing a flood of anger toward her partner for working too much and neglecting her needs. They asked for more time and went home seriously resolved to work on their situation. Two days later, her blood pressure was still 140/100 and continued to rise at the next few exams, so we referred her for hospital birth. She was given intravenous magnesium sulfate (standard treatment for hypertension) during labor and gave birth without further complications.

Occasionally, you will have a mother with a slight rise in blood pressure two or three weeks before term. If she has no other signs of preeclampsia, is well hydrated, and is not unduly stressed, this may be considered normal—the body has its limit in terms of circulatory volume, and the matter will likely resolve as labor begins. Just be sure to attend the birth from the start, and check frequently to see that her blood pressure is stable and within normal range.

During labor, previously normal blood pressure may jump to 140/90 with the most rigorous transition contractions. But a steady rise in the early stages may herald preeclampsia or lead to vascular damage, and the mother should be transported (see chapter 4 for more details).

Preeclampsia

One of the main reasons for routine prenatal care is to screen for preeclampsia: it can occur as early as twenty weeks but is more common after thirty-two weeks. The exact cause of preeclampsia is subject to debate, but this dangerous disease poses a threat to the lives of both mother and baby.

There is ample evidence to suggest that preeclampsia is linked to malnutrition, particularly protein deficiency. In the course of this disease, inadequate albumin (protein) in the blood causes fluid to leak from blood cells, resulting in reduced blood volume, hemoconcentration, and sometimes, generalized edema. Blood flow to the kidneys is thus reduced, which triggers a compensatory rise in blood pressure. Blood flow to the uterus is also reduced, leading to fetal growth restriction (and possible fetal distress in labor). If hypertension becomes severe, vasospasm and irritation of the blood cell walls cause **microthrombi** (tiny clots) to form. The microthrombi stretch the filtering slits in the kidneys so that large protein molecules begin to slip through, leading to proteinuria. Microthrombi can do significant harm to other parts of the body, impairing circulation to the liver (causing epigastric pain, a symptom indicating progression of the disease). Mothers with severe preeclampsia and liver involvement may develop **HELLP syndrome** (**H**emolysis, **E**levated **L**iver enzymes, and **L**ow **P**latelet counts), which increases the risk of adverse outcomes, including DIC as the body exhausts its clotting factors.

Nutritional guidelines for preventing and responding to preeclampsia include a minimum of 80 g protein daily with ample calories, elimination of junk foods, and an emphasis on complex carbohydrates as well as fresh fruits and vegetables. High-fiber foods are recommended, and adequate fluid intake is absolutely crucial.

As for nonnutritional causes, research indicates that a protein made by the placenta, sFlt1, may play a significant role in the disease. This protein, which halts growth, is normally released when the placenta reaches its full size. But evidence shows that with preeclampsia, this protein is produced too soon, stunting placental growth and reducing circulation to the baby. Interestingly enough, pregnant rats injected with sFlt1 develop preeclampsia.[16] These findings may account for the client who eats well, gets plenty of rest, has good support but nonetheless develops the disease.

Newer studies suggest that abnormal development of placental vessels in early pregnancy may be the bottom line. With this, reduced blood flow to the placenta causes overproduction of sFlt1 and endoglin, limiting placental growth and causing damage to the endothelium (thin layer of cells lining the inner surface of blood vessels—see microthrombi, above), resulting in the chain of events we recognize as preeclampsia.[17]

As for early signs of preeclampsia, **hemoconcentration** (due to reduced blood volume) is the first indication, as revealed by an abnormally high hematocrit or one that does not dip as is normal in the latter part of pregnancy. Then comes **hypertension**. **Protein in the urine** may or may not manifest, but labwork will show **elevated liver enzymes, BUN,** and **uric acid. Generalized edema** is no longer considered a cardinal sign but may also occur.

If labs indicate that the mother is ill, she should be risked out for homebirth with her care comanaged with a physician. Visits should take place twice weekly: besides taking her blood pressure, check for proteinuria. Prevent vaginal discharge from affecting results by having the mother take a **clean catch**. She does this by first washing the labia with a cleansing wipe, and then allowing a bit of urine to flow before collecting the sample. Anything over a trace of protein is significant.

Check for generalized edema by observing her hands and face: her features will look coarse; her hands/fingers will be puffy and inflexible. Ankle edema is physiologic and therefore not significant, but edema of the upper shins, breastbone, or sacrum is definitive. Determine the degree of edema by checking for **pitting**: press a fingertip into the skin and see whether or not a depression remains. A 2 mm depression equals +1, 4 mm equals +2, 6 mm equals +3, and 8 mm equals +4. Pitting of +2 or greater is diagnostic.

Hyperreflexia indicates progress to a more serious stage of the disease. Check for hyperreflexia by checking for **clonus**. Have the mother sit in a straight-backed chair, lift and support her calf with one hand, then dorsiflex her foot (bend toes toward her knee). Maintain this hold for a moment and then release. Ordinarily, the foot will fall back to its natural position with no additional movement: if you notice jerking while it is dorsiflexed, or oscillation as it falls, the test is positive. (It is wise to check all reflexes at some point in early pregnancy to establish baselines.)

If your client appears to be preeclamptic, have her immediately rest in bed on her left side while the backup physician is contacted. Tell her to report any of the following indications that her condition has worsened: (1) severe headache, (2) epigastric pain (pain in upper abdomen), (3) visual disturbances, (4) decreased output of urine, (5) extreme nervous irritability, or (6) decrease in fetal movement.

One of my clients became preeclamptic at thirty-seven weeks. I knew it as soon as she walked into my office; her face had that coarse look (due to generalized edema) I had read about in medical texts. At the home visit in early pregnancy, it was clear that her diet was excellent. But just a week before, we had visited her home again and had been served a vegetable dinner with no protein whatsoever. I was concerned and meant to bring it up at this visit, but I was obviously too late. Remarkable in this case was the mother's blood pressure; it never went higher than 120/76. However, her baseline was 98/56, and some experts consider a diastolic rise of more than 15 points or a systolic rise of more than 30 points to be diagnostic. We referred her immediately to backup, and alternated prenatals twice weekly with her physician. Her condition remained borderline: periodic facial edema with blood pressure high (for her), proteinuria from a trace to +2. She took bed rest as much as possible, and we transported as soon as labor was established.

In addition to the aforementioned dangers of preeclampsia, there is a higher than normal incidence of placental abruption (about 8 percent), which can lead to fetal death or jeopardize the mother's life. If preeclampsia progresses to eclampsia, convulsions may threaten the lives of both mother and baby.

Polyhydramnios (Hydramnios)

This is a term referring to excess amniotic fluid. It occurs in less than 1 percent of pregnancies, often in conjunction with multiple pregnancy (8 percent), Rh incompatibility (11 percent), or diabetes (5 to 25 percent). It is also associated with fetal anomalies (18 to 39 percent), particularly with atresia of the esophagus, hydrocephaly, anencephaly, or spina bifida.[18]

Acute polyhydramnios occurs suddenly and dramatically, but this is rare. With the more common form, **chronic polyhydramnios**, there is a slight elevation in fundal height around twenty-eight weeks and larger than usual increments of increase in the weeks that follow. Typically, the baby is difficult to palpate at a time when it should be relatively easy to feel. As a beginner, you may confuse a thick uterine wall with excess fluid: in both cases, heart tones are difficult to hear and the baby is challenging to palpate. Avoid this error by checking for the classic sign of polyhydramnios, **fluid thrill**—place a hand on each side of the uterus, and if a tap from one sends a vibration to the other, the test is positive.

A woman with noticeable polyhydramnios should be seen again in several days regardless of length of gestation. If you find an increase in fluid, send her for an ultrasound to try to determine the cause. Polyhydramnios can lead to premature labor, thus hospital birth is likely unless the condition is borderline. It can also result in serious complications during labor such as uterine dysfunction, placental abruption, and postpartum hemorrhage, all from **overdistension** of the uterus. Fetal malpresentation and cord prolapse are not uncommon.

I recall referring a mother for ultrasound who seemed to have a quite a bit of excess fluid, only to be told that everything was fine. Still, the fundal height was above normal from twenty-eight weeks, reaching 42 cm at term (with head in the pelvis). Early labor was unusual, with spastic and painful incoordinate contractions. We transported, and imagine my frustration when membranes ruptured in a quantity sufficient to bring the entire labor and delivery staff to have a look! At this point, the uterus began to work more efficiently, and labor progressed normally. However, the mother sustained a fairly severe postpartum hemorrhage.

Another mother developed polyhydramnios before I had any idea she was carrying twins. The extra fluid really alarmed me—at twenty-five weeks, her fundus was at 29 cm (a rise of 6 cm in just three weeks, with an accompanying weight gain of 8 lb.). In the next few days, her fundal height increased three more centimeters, she gained three more pounds, and was almost impossible to palpate. I made no mention of twins, but she brought up the possibility. Sure enough, ultrasound showed two babies, plus extra fluid within normal range for multiple pregnancy. Two weeks later she went into labor, and no wonder, with a fundal height of 39 cm at only twenty-eight weeks!

Adequate rest (with feet elevated) can help mediate some of the side effects of polyhydramnios, such as severe ankle edema and varicosities of the legs and vulva. Heartburn remedies, like smaller meals and digestive enzymes, are essential. If you are comanaging the care of a woman with polyhydramnios, check her cervix weekly to look for changes that might portend premature labor.

Oligohydramnios

Oligohydramnios is an abnormally small amount of amniotic fluid. Due to the resulting cord compression, it is associated with intrauterine growth restriction (IUGR), postmaturity syndrome, and fetal distress/hypoxia in labor. It may also occur with fetal anomalies. Although amniotic fluid volume varies considerably from mother to mother, oligohydramnios is readily detected when the fetus is tightly compacted in the uterus and fundal height is lagging. With continuity of care, this will be readily detected.

Studies have shown that amniotic fluid can be increased by adequate hydration: the more fluid the mother drinks, the more amniotic fluid she produces.[19] However, as oligohydramnios rarely occurs in the course of a healthy pregnancy, consider it a sign of something amiss that must quickly be identified (see sections on "Small for Gestational Age and Intrauterine Growth Restriction" on page 87 and "Postdatism" on page 90).

Multiple Pregnancy

Fundal height several centimeters above gestational age should immediately lead you to consider twins. But first, rule out other possible causes of a uterus large for dates (see the section on "Large for Gestational Age" on page 88). Then consider your clinical findings: Have you noticed an abundance of small parts when palpating? Does the baby's head feel small relative to fundal height? Twins are sometimes missed if one is tucked behind the other's body.

Unless a woman has had serial ultrasounds, twins are seldom detected until twenty-eight weeks. Clinical confirmation can be made through the auscultation of two heartbeats. But take care—what appears to be two heartbeats may be just one, audible over a wide range. If you note a 10- to 15-point difference in rhythms with distinct patterns of variability, and you are certain that one is not the mother's heartbeat (check her pulse), you have identified twins. When in doubt, schedule an ultrasound.

There are two types of twin pregnancy. **Identical or monozygotic twins** result from the union of one egg and one sperm, with the fertilized ovum separating into two. **Fraternal or dizygotic twins** represent the union of two eggs and two sperm, that is, two pregnancies occurring simultaneously. Dizygotic twins have separate placentas and separate amniotic sacs, whereas monozygotic twins share a placenta and may also share an amniotic sac, although there are usually two separate sacs. Of all twins, 66 to 75 percent are dizygotic. Monozygotic twins occur at a rate of approximately 1 per 250 births, whereas dizygotic twinning varies dramatically according to maternal race and age. With in vitro fertilization or embryo transfer, the rate of multiple pregnancy is as high as 22 percent.[20]

The use of early ultrasound has shown twinning to be more common than was previously thought. I know of several women who, at about twelve weeks, had such heavy bleeding that they were sure they had lost the pregnancy, only to find they were still pregnant: twins were diagnosed only after one was lost.

It is important to identify twins as soon as suspected, as there are increased risks of anemia and premature birth (upon detection, guidelines for recognizing and reporting signs of premature labor should be immediately provided). Mothers carrying twins need expert nutritional counseling and recommendations for increased rest (feet up for twenty minutes, twice a day). Rarely, with identical twins, **twin-to-twin transfusion syndrome (TTTS)** will cause blood to be shunted from one twin to the other, putting the "donor" baby at risk for growth restriction and other complications.

Risks with twin birth are numerous. Cord prolapse can occur if the first baby is a footling or kneeling breech. The second baby is at even greater risk for this, especially if it remains high in the uterus after the first has been born. It may also become hypoxic, as reduced uterine volume can cause constriction of placental vessels. For the same reason, there is risk of placental abruption. Finally, there is considerable risk of postpartum hemorrhage from an overdistended and tired uterus.

Depending on where you practice and your level of expertise, you may be able to assist the births at home. If not, continue to provide prenatal care in conjunction with a physician. Even if you are no longer the primary provider, you can still provide critical assistance by focusing on the emotional and practical aspects of caring for two babies. And, if the mother is helped to maintain her pregnancy to at least thirty-seven weeks, hospital management may be relatively noninterventive—that is, if vaginal birth is permitted. Increasingly, physicians insist that all twins be delivered by cesarean. Some still assist vaginal twin births, but usually both babies must be vertex. This trend is due to fear of litigation, lack of exposure to vaginal twin births, and lack of training in vaginal breech birth. Beyond the skills and the inclination of the physician, hospital policy may mandate a cesarean. For myself, having witnessed many vaginal twin births before the standard of care changed (a number of them breech, and all spontaneous and uncomplicated), I find it outrageous that women are being funneled into cesarean birth without a choice, regardless of their health status.

If the birth will be in hospital, make sure that the mother and her partner know what to expect from the experience. Even if the birth is to be vaginal, there will be many attendants besides the obstetrician, including the neonatal team. Emphasize the emotional aspects of the birth and the support you will provide before, during, and after.

Breech Presentation and Transverse Lie

It is more than unfortunate that we treat breech birth as a life-threatening complication simply because medical schools have stopped teaching the skills to assist breech vaginally. A fascinating study showed that not only women but also men who were born breech (vaginally) had more than twice the chance of having their first baby born breech, compared with men and women who had been born head first.[21]

The greatest risk with breech birth is **cephalopelvic disproportion (CPD)**. With a vertex presentation, the head has hours to negotiate the pelvis, but with breech, it must be born quickly as exposure of the body and cord to air prompts respiration. In other words, if the body is born but the head gets stuck at the pelvic brim, fetal hypoxia and death will likely result. **Cord prolapse** is another risk, particularly if the baby is footling or kneeling, as there is nothing to prevent the cord from slipping past the body when the water breaks.

What are wise criteria for breech birth at home? The mother should have a normal pelvis with baby sized to fit. The risks diminish if she has previously given birth without difficulty, as previously stretched pelvic joints can speed the process of birthing the head. Many practitioners feel the baby should be either frank breech (legs extended up over the chest) or complete breech (legs crossed over the abdomen, as these presentations provide larger dilating diameters than do the legs or knees. The head should also be well flexed so it can readily negotiate the pelvis. To make certain of these factors, ultrasound must be used.

Even so, complications may arise that require special expertise: an arm impacted behind the head must be deftly and quickly manipulated; a head deflexed with descent must be repositioned without delay. These maneuvers are beyond the scope of this text. Suffice to say, it is unwise to assist breech birth without the assistance of someone experienced in both basic and advanced delivery techniques (as well as neonatal resuscitation).

A new organization in the United Kingdom actively promotes education in breech birth for midwives and obstetricians as well as thorough informed consent for parents. See www.breechbirth.org.uk/index.html for more information (and birth accounts).

Before presenting breech, the baby may be in **transverse lie**. This is common up to twenty-six weeks, at which point the baby usually finds greater comfort in lying longitudinally. If the baby remains transverse after twenty-seven weeks and is high in the uterus, listen for placenta sounds (swishing sounds at the same rate as the mother's pulse) in the lower portion of the mother's abdomen. Do this to rule out placenta previa, which could prevent the baby from presenting either breech or vertex. If the baby remains transverse past thirty weeks, an ultrasound is necessary to locate the placenta precisely.

Sometimes the breech rotates to vertex in the final weeks of pregnancy. Rather than wait and see, have the mother try to turn the baby with **postural tilting** if the baby remains breech beyond thirty weeks. To do this, she must first empty her bladder and then lie with hips elevated about 12 in., either on pillows or an ironing board propped with one end on the couch, three times daily for twenty minutes. Suggest that she do deep relaxation in this position and visualize the baby turning while asking it to do so. If she feels major movement, have her come in right away to be checked.

Other ways she can encourage the baby to turn include the following:

1. Doing somersaults or handstands in a pool

2. Doing elephant walking (on her hands and feet)

3. Placing headphones low on the uterus and playing music (baby may turn toward the sound)

4. Shining a flashlight low in the uterus or between her legs (baby may turn toward the light)

5. Placing a bag of frozen vegetables on the backside of the baby's head (baby may turn away from the cold)

6. Partner talking to baby low on her belly, asking the baby to turn

Another possibility is to use a **rebozo** to turn the baby. This is a long shawl used by midwives in Mexico and Central America for numerous remedial purposes during the childbearing cycle. To rotate a breech, the mother should be on knees and elbows with swayed back (belly sagging toward the floor). Place the center of the rebozo where her buttocks meet her thighs, and then stand at her head with one end in each hand pulled taught. Pull firmly on one end and then the other to establish a brisk, rocking motion for as long as the mother is comfortable. Repeat daily.[22]

If the baby has not rotated after several weeks and is beginning to fill out the uterus, **external version** is another option. This is a tricky maneuver for all but the most experienced midwife, as it requires expert fetal palpation and a highly refined sense of touch. There is also risk of cord entanglement or compression, thus another experienced practitioner must monitor the fetal heart continuously. Start by having the mother drink a beer or glass of wine to promote uterine relaxation, with time to empty her bladder before you begin. Position her in a tilt, and then gently attempt to reposition the baby. Rotate the baby in the direction it is facing, and keep the head well flexed. If any resistance is felt or irregularities in the fetal heart rate are noted, the version should be stopped and the baby returned to its original position. Because of the risks involved in this procedure, informed consent is essential.

Some mothers report massaging their babies into vertex presentation; others report talking the baby into it. But if, despite all efforts, the baby has not rotated by thirty-six weeks, you might ask your backup physician to give version a try. Most physicians wait until thirty-seven weeks to perform external version, for fear of causing premature labor. However, they generally employ a much more forceful technique than do midwives, due to the use of uterine tocolytics (relaxing meds) in conjunction with the procedure. If all attempts at version fail, prepare the mother for hospital birth and, most likely, a cesarean. (Refer also to "Surprise Breech" on page 163.)

Prematurity

Prematurity is defined as birth prior to thirty-seven weeks; after this, the baby is considered to be term. But every week the baby stays in utero as term approaches has benefits, unless the mother has some complication (such as preeclampsia) that would make earlier birth advantageous. According to the March of Dimes, "Babies born after 37 weeks of pregnancy are full-term. However, new research has shown that a baby's brain nearly doubles in weight in the last few weeks of pregnancy."[23]

The greatest danger for the baby born early is that its lungs will not be mature, resulting in **respiratory distress syndrome (RDS)**. Signs include **cyanosis** (blue color), **tachypnea** (rapid respirations), **grunting** (with expiration), **retractions** (skin between the ribs sucks in each time baby inhales), and **nasal flaring**. These are caused by inadequate **surfactant**, a lubricant that permits the alveoli to inflate. However, since the lungs reach maturity at thirty-four weeks, the concern with RDS from this point to thirty-seven weeks springs from the possibility of an inaccurate EDD, which has become increasingly common as ultrasound, rather than menstrual history, is used to establish dates. State regulations may say that a midwife shall not assist births before thirty-seven weeks, but on occasion, if she is confident that a mother's dates are correct based on evaluations of uterine size at twenty weeks

and fetal growth increments as term approaches, she will assist at thirty-six weeks.

Causes of labor prior to this point are vaginal infection or UTI resulting in chorioamnionitis and rupture of the membranes, incompetent cervix, polyhydramnios, multiple pregnancy, uterine anomalies, faulty implantation of the placenta, substance abuse, a short interval between pregnancies, malnutrition, or fetal death. New evidence further suggests there may be a genetic marker for preterm labor, FSHR.[24] Extreme or chronic stress is also a factor: although little acknowledged in the literature, evidence shows that maternal stress may cause up to one-third of premature births by activating the fetal hypothalamic-pituitary-adrenal axis.[25] Along the same lines, there is a link between preterm birth and stressful working conditions or those involving prolonged standing or strenuous physical activity.[26] Mothers with chronic gum disease in the second trimester are at three to eight times greater risk, due to an increase in prostaglandins.[27] Maternal dehydration can also lead to prematurity.[28]

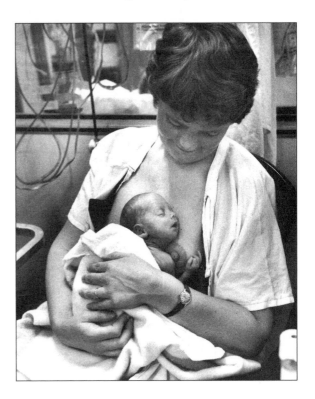

Any mother with a history of miscarriage or previous premature birth is automatically at risk. Make sure she is well hydrated and that her diet is excellent. She should eat fatty fish, like salmon, mackerel, sardines, or trout, once weekly, or take a supplement of fish oil daily, as women who do so have a 1.9 percent prematurity rate compared to 7.1 percent for women who don't.[29] Monitor her carefully from twenty-four weeks on; schedule visits every two weeks and perform a gentle cervical examination each time. Suggest that she reduce her workload, both in and out of the home. Screen at the first sign of vaginal infection and recommend the use of condoms (if appropriate) to reduce risks of STDs and exposure to prostaglandins in seminal fluid that can soften the cervix. If her cervix begins to efface, have her curtail sexual activity, make sure she knows how to distinguish contractions from fetal movement, and see her weekly thereafter. If regular contractions occur or the cervix begins to dilate, immediately contact backup.

Medications commonly used for stopping labor include magnesium sulfate, nifedipine, or terbutaline; these generally do the job but may cause nervous irritability, dizziness, or nausea. They are also quite toxic and should be used no more than several days (especially terbutaline, which if used any longer is associated with risks of maternal heart problems and death).[30] If you find the cervix only minimally changed, contractions are mild, and the mother has no history of alcoholism, suggest she take a couple of stiff drinks. Alcohol inhibits oxytocin and relaxes the uterus. (Before labor-stopping tocolytic drugs were developed, alcohol was given intravenously for premature labor.)

One of my clients began premature labor at thirty-five weeks. Her cervix was 75 percent effaced and about 2 cm dilated (this was her second baby). She took two shots of vodka in grapefruit juice, stayed in bed the entire day, and was fine until the following morning. Her contractions resumed upon arising, so she repeated the previous routine. This went on for a few more days, during which I checked her daily

and in spite of uterine activity, found her cervix to be stable. Contractions then stopped completely. She carried her baby to forty-one weeks and birthed at home, but not without some difficulty: shoulder dystocia, partial separation of the placenta necessitating manual removal, and postpartum hemorrhage made for an interesting trade-off of complications!

Another of my clients carrying twins had a fundal height of 38 cm at thirty weeks, with slight polyhydramnios. She began premature labor and was given Ritodrine, which did little to stop contractions. However, she discovered that postural tilting several times daily definitely stopped uterine activity, probably by taking pressure off her cervix. The obstetrician was so impressed that he called in the staff to observe her innovation. Ritodrine was discontinued, and she carried her babies to term.

If a mother in your care gives birth prematurely, she may have to deal with long periods of separation from her baby and disrupted breastfeeding, although much depends on the gestational age of the baby and hospital policy. Fortunately, a number of intensive care nurseries now incorporate the practice of **kangaroo care** in stabilizing the premature infant. Much as it sounds, kangaroo care involves continuous skin-to-skin contact, with the baby in just a diaper and kept between the mother's breasts with a blanket or a sling. Developed by South American physicians dealing with a growing number of premies and inadequate intensive care facilities, kangaroo care reduced infant mortality from 70 to 30 percent.[31] It has been shown to stabilize newborn heart rates, temperature, and breathing, as well as boosting growth and brain development. Mothers who use kangaroo care report increased confidence, better postpartum recovery, and greater success with breastfeeding. The mother's partner is encouraged to participate, too.

Do all you can to prevent premature labor, but research support organizations for parents with premies. And know that apart from worries about the baby, the mother may grieve the loss of her homebirth dream and may need you to help her process this loss.

Small for Gestational Age and Intrauterine Growth Restriction

With regard to uterine size, causes of **small for gestational age (SGA)** include miscalculated dates, fetus transverse or otherwise low in the pelvis, hereditary tendency to small babies, and **intrauterine growth restriction (IUGR)**. The first three are fairly easy to rule out, but the last is a complication requiring special attention.

Although babies may grow in spurts, fundal height usually increases about 1 cm per week. IUGR is suspected when fundal height has been normal to twenty-four weeks and then begins to fall behind this norm. We can differentiate a baby genetically destined to weigh 6 lb. from one who is growth restricted in that the former will have consistent but slightly less than normal increments of growth, whereas the latter will have decreasing increments of growth. With IUGR, the growth curve flattens out.

The causes of IUGR are numerous, including malnutrition, severe anemia, chronic hypertension, substance abuse, fetal malformation or infection, abnormalities of the placenta and cord, and prolonged pregnancy. Chronic stress and overwork are also implicated: an analysis of studies involving 160,988 women showed that neonates born to women who work at physically demanding jobs weigh less at birth.[32]

Here is an interesting case history. A mother started care at twenty-seven weeks with a fundal height of 23 cm, certain of her dates. Her nutrition was poor and she smoked half a pack of cigarettes daily, but she made a commitment to improve her diet and cut back on smoking. Her baby grew in spurts over the next few weeks and steadily thereafter. Her total weight gain was 20 lb. Ultrasounds at thirty-one and thirty-five weeks determined normal fetal growth, but a baby so small for gestational age that a month was added to the EDD. This seemed arbitrary to say the least, considering that neither the menstrual history nor the couple's sexual history

corroborated this. Nevertheless, if "ultrasound says," we had best believe it!

Her final checkup revealed her cervix to be 1 cm dilated and 60 percent effaced. At thirty-eight weeks by original dates, thirty-four weeks by revised EDD, labor began with ruptured membranes. What to do? Was the baby premature or simply small for gestational age? And what about the impact of earlier IUGR? We estimated the baby to be about 5 lb. and so decided on hospital birth. This was a real disappointment to the parents, who had never accepted the revised dates anyway. After six hours of labor, the mother gave birth to a healthy, vigorous girl of 5.5 lb., estimated at thirty-eight weeks gestational age with no respiratory distress; the lungs were fully mature. There was some indication of fetal compromise in that the placenta was spongy, shredding, and full of calcifications. But the baby showed no other signs of growth restriction; it was neither wizened or emaciated, and had Apgars of 9 and 10.

In retrospect, this birth could have taken place at home. But if the baby is SGA, and care begins late in pregnancy when accuracy of dates is more difficult to determine, hospital birth may be more or less by default. Premature babies face significant risks at birth. On the other hand, complications with a minor degree of IUGR can be managed until a pediatrician sees the baby. These risks include **hypoglycemia** (low blood sugar) and **hypothermia** (difficulty maintaining body temperature), both of which are due to insufficient body fat. These conditions are not immediately life threatening and can be dealt with initially by the midwife, but the baby should be seen by a pediatrician in the first few hours after the birth.

If IUGR is clearly diagnosed and persistent in pregnancy, hospital birth is advisable. Minor degrees of IUGR call for nonstress testing, amniotic fluid volume assessments, and fetal kick-counts beginning at thirty-four weeks (for more on these practices, see the section on "Postdatism" on page 90).

If you are preparing to assist the birth of a minor-degree IUGR baby, have oven-warmed flannel blankets and aluminum outer wrapper ready as insulation. Place the baby skin-to-skin on the mother before wrapping. Keep the head covered, too: use a stockinet cap so that the mother will not have to fuss with the blankets and can focus fully on the baby. Take the baby's axillary temperature several times an hour until you are certain it is stable. Also check the baby's blood sugar with a **dextrostix** (heel prick and test strip). If the level is below 45, contact a pediatrician at once. If it is slightly below normal, have the mother nurse and afterward, give eyedroppers of sterile water and molasses, with a teaspoon of molasses per cup of water (never use honey, due to risk of infant botulism). Repeat the dextrostix every two hours to assess whether feedings are raising the blood sugar level. Be sure to chart each time fluid is given, how much, and how well the baby tolerated it. If the baby vomits, intravenous feeding may be necessary, so contact the pediatrician without delay.

Even a minor degree of IUGR puts the baby at risk for **polycythemia** (excess red blood cells), which predisposes it to severe jaundice. If the baby looks ruddy at birth, do a hematocrit, and if elevated, immediately consult with the pediatrician. Once the baby is fully stable, make certain the parents understand that they must at all times keep it warm and dry and to call immediately if it gets irritable or lethargic. Ask them to report back after seeing the pediatrician, and plan to do postpartum checks for four days minimum.

Large for Gestational Age

Causes of **large for gestational age (LGA)** have already been presented in other sections of this chapter; they include miscalculated dates, hydatidiform mole, gestational diabetes, twins, polyhydramnios, maternal obesity, hereditary tendency to big babies, fetal anomalies, baby high in fundus due to placenta previa or abdominal muscle tone, fibroids (internal or external) displacing the baby upward or positioned atop the fundus, and postmaturity.

Whenever a mother measures large for dates, these possibilities must be ruled out one by one. I recall a woman who came to me at twenty-eight weeks with fundal height of 32 cm, wide abdominal girth (but not overweight), and +4 glucose in her urine. I felt a good-sized head entering her pelvis, butt in the fundus, and small parts everywhere (posterior position, I assumed). She agreed to an immediate glucose screen: it was negative. Next week, no glucosuria but two heartbeats were audible, and an ultrasound confirmed that she had twins!

A big baby is concerning only if the mother's pelvis is not ample. To assuage this fear, **check for engagement**, assessing not only the station of the head but also how well it fits into the pelvis. If the baby is still high, **check for ability to engage** by grasping the head externally and pressing it toward the sacral promontory, then down into the inlet. If the head feels movable and enters the pelvis readily, things are fine so far. Another way to check is to place your hand above the pubic bone with the mom in a semi-sit position, and then have her sit up completely (**Pawlik's maneuver**). If the head bulges into your hand instead of slipping into the pelvis, it will have difficulty clearing the inlet.

I have had only one obvious case of true **cephalopelvic disproportion (CPD)** in my practice. This was a first pregnancy, the mother was certain of her menstrual history but the baby was consistently large for dates. She had a small pelvis with adequate inlet, but android characteristics of close-set ischial spines and a slightly flattened sacrum. She was about 5 ft. 3 in. tall, and the father, 6 ft. tall. I remember feeling alarmed at thirty-seven weeks by the size of the baby's head, particularly in that it overrode the pubic bone and bulged into my hand. Upon discovering this condition of **fetal overlap**, I encouraged her to give birth as soon as she was ready (her cervix

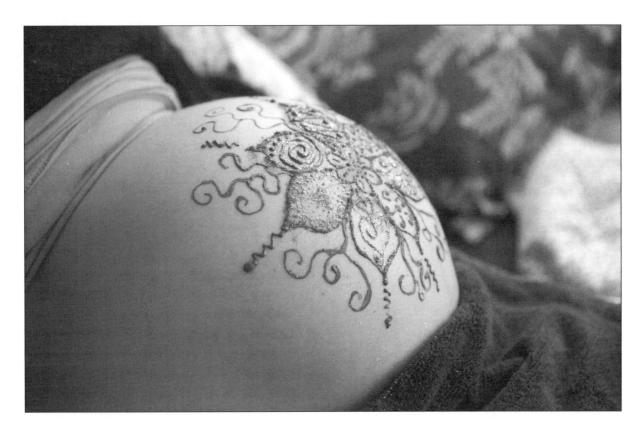

was soft, about 60 percent effaced). She started labor at forty weeks, dilated completely with the help of Pitocin (we transported for arrest at 6 cm), but she pushed for two hours without engaging the head and ended up with a cesarean. Her dates proved correct, as the baby showed no evidence of postmaturity: he simply grew too large for her pelvic dimensions.

If a similar situation arose and dates were certain, I might suggest **natural methods of induction** as early as thirty-seven weeks. Successful induction largely depends on the condition of the cervix: it must be **ripe** (soft and partially effaced) before attempting to stimulate contractions. If the mother's partner is male, sexual intercourse can ripen the cervix via prostaglandins in seminal fluid, with an alternative in cervical massage with evening primrose oil. Lovemaking further stimulates labor via release of oxytocin. The tried-and-true method of castor oil induction is hardly pleasant, but the resulting diarrhea triggers the release of prostaglandins. Have the mother take two tablespoons initially with orange juice, followed by another tablespoon a half hour later, and a final tablespoon in another hour.

Ways to get contractions going include acupuncture techniques, herbal formulas (blue cohosh tincture, a dropperful every few hours), and periodic nipple stimulation. Or have the mother wear one of her partner's shirts (saturated with his or her scent) to get the oxytocin flowing.

LGA births carry certain risks. If the uterus is overdistended, it may not contract efficiently, leading to prolonged labor, arrested progress, or postpartum hemorrhage. If the mother becomes clinically exhausted due to prolonged labor, the baby is at risk for hypoxia and may require resuscitation at birth. There may also be shoulder dystocia. Be prepared for these possibilities.

Postdatism

The current definition of **postdatism** is pregnancy progressing past forty-two weeks. However, it is estimated that up to 19 percent of pregnancies reach this marker.[33] This is hardly surprising, considering the findings of the Mittendorf study (see page 22).

There may be hereditary predisposition for longer-term pregnancy, as with the mother who reports that she was born three weeks late (as were her siblings). Perhaps some babies simply need to gestate longer than others—the fruit on our trees doesn't ripen at exactly the same rate, so why should our babies?

Occasionally, emotional factors may cause a mother to go past her date. If this is to be her last pregnancy, she may be hesitant to let it go. If this is her first baby, she may be wary of the responsibilities of parenting and reluctant to surrender the attention she has enjoyed while pregnant. If she has been obliged or compelled to work to her due date, she may want extra time to enjoy being pregnant and wind down in preparation for labor. Or if her partner has uncertainty about his or her changing role, this too may prolong the pregnancy. When exploring these possibilities, which can be done simply by asking the mother if she feels ready to give birth, make sure she does not feel judged or accused, as this may exacerbate any tension she is already feeling. Encourage her to make her own observations, draw her own conclusions. Such a difficult time, these postdate weeks of waiting!

The risks of postdatism are twofold. If all is well in utero and the fetus continues to grow, cephalopelvic disproportion or shoulder dystocia may result. On the other hand, if the mother ceases to eat and drink sufficiently (perhaps for fear of having a large baby), the fetus may suffer weight loss, cord compression due to oligohydramnios, fetal distress, or even stillbirth. We used to think these risks were linked to placental deterioration, that it was a "timed organ" set to expire with advanced gestation, but research has shown this not to be true. We do know that maternal malnutrition and chronic dehydration can lead to reduced blood volume and oligohydramnios, which in turn can cause cord compression and fetal compromise. This is known as **fetal postmaturity syndrome**.

But when a mother is simply postdates and is well nourished, well hydrated, relaxed, and (based on pelvimetry and estimated fetal weight) has plenty of room to birth her baby, why is there cause for concern? As the classic text, *Human Labor and Birth*, advises:

> While prolongation of pregnancy beyond 42 weeks may have an adverse effect on neonatal outcome in some cases, fetal death is rare. Induction of labor does not improve results. What the latter practice does achieve is an increase in the rate of cesarean section because of failed induction. An uncomplicated postdates pregnancy is not an indication for induction of labor. Early delivery is necessary only when tests of fetal health show that deterioration is taking place.[34]

One assessment that helps determine postdates fetal health is **kick-counts**. Have the mother do this every day for an hour after her largest meal: she should notice about eight to ten movements in this time period.

Another assessment of fetal well-being is **nonstress testing (NST)**, which evaluates fluctuations in the baby's heart rate in response to its own movements. The desired or positive response is moderate acceleration. The NST can be performed in hospital by external monitor, or the midwife can simply listen with her fetascope for twenty minutes and look for heart rate changes with fetal activity. In recent years, the validity of the NST has been called into question as no definitive correlation has been shown between nonreassuring findings and negative outcomes: still, it is standard in postdates screening.

Reduced amniotic fluid volume is much more significant. This can be assessed by serial ultrasound commencing at forty-one weeks or by careful uterine palpation performed week to week by the same care provider. Decreased amniotic fluid volume is concerning, especially in combination with a poor nonstress response (less than a 15 percent margin of error in predicting negative outcomes[35]).

Current medical screening for postdates often combines the above assessments with a few more obtained by ultrasound: **fetal muscle tone** and **breathing movements**. Ultrasound is not essential, though, as these markers can be presumed to be adequate on the basis of normal fetal activity, measured via kick-counts.

Depending on the result of these assessments, consult with backup, leave well enough alone, or, assuming the head is well into the pelvis, recommend natural induction (see page 88, "Large for Gestational Age"). Induction might also be wise if the baby is getting a bit large for the mother's dimensions; check carefully for fetal overlap and beware of the previously engaged head rising up in the pelvis.

For the truly postmature fetus, the most stressful time in labor is the onset. Uterine contractions are much stronger than Braxton-Hicks, thus any degree of compromise will show up almost immediately. Plan to attend the postdates labor from the very beginning, and take heart tones more frequently than usual.

Psychological Issues and Complications

Most emotional upsets in pregnancy spring from hormonal effects: complaints forgotten by the next visit are typically hormone induced. If emotional problems become chronic, ask for more background. You may uncover issues in the mother's relationships, environment, or health unknown to you before.

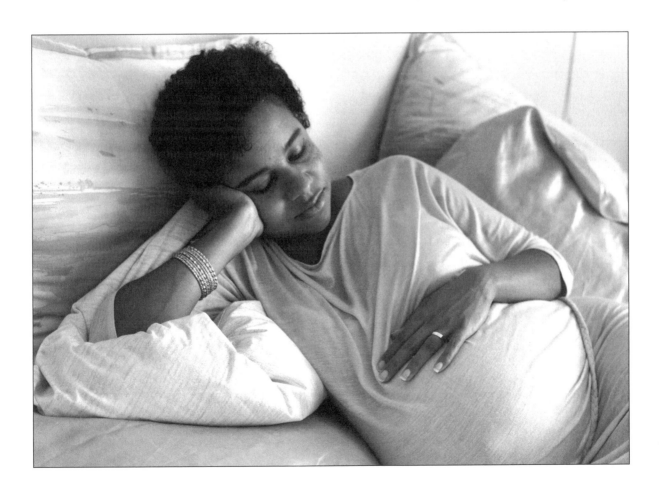

Rarely, a mother becomes increasingly imbalanced as pregnancy progresses, and you may find yourself unable to continue primary care (see "Psychological Screening Out" on page 104).

On the other hand, encourage mothers to use the volatile energy of pregnancy to take personal inventory and forge new modes of self-expression. After many years of practice, I have come to believe that the best way to promote this is to help women see weak or neglected aspects of themselves in a positive light so they will feel good about doing work in these areas. Self-reliance and self-love are the cornerstones of wellness in pregnancy, birth, and parenting.

If some aspect of personality is weak or neglected, another may become overstrong to compensate. For example, a mother extremely physical by nature may be quite distraught over the normal physiological changes of pregnancy; she may not have the emotional resources to cope. If she is highly athletic, she may find the fatigue, nausea, and loss of muscle tone typical in early pregnancy to be extremely frustrating or even frightening. She is at risk for pushing past physical imperatives for rest/relaxation and is therefore vulnerable to stress-related complications, such as premature labor.

I had one such client, a black belt in karate and marathon runner, who broke down and cried at about twelve weeks, "My body just doesn't work anymore!" I explained that her body was actually working very well, making critical adjustments in metabolic rate and circulatory volume. I assured her that her fatigue would abate and that the softening of her muscles and ligaments would make birth and recovery easier. I encouraged her to trust her body's wisdom in adapting to pregnancy and growing a baby. I suggested that she hold on to her strength, but experiment with pacing herself. She then enjoyed her pregnancy. Once in labor, she found dilation challenging but really loved pushing. Afterward, she viewed the entire experience as positive.

In contrast, a more emotionally based woman may savor the changes of early pregnancy, particularly the dreamy quality of her heightened sensitivities. She may drive those around her (particularly her partner) a little crazy with her mood swings and may forget to eat and get regular physical activity. She is at risk for anemia, dehydration, and prolonged labor. Encourage her to acquire factual information, and help her develop a nutrition and exercise plan. She might also keep a journal in which she can make observations on how changes in diet and activity affect her feelings. In labor, the emotionally oriented woman tends to dilate without much trouble but may dislike the intensity of pushing. Help these mothers prepare for the physicality of second stage with activities requiring endurance, such as aerobic dance, hiking, lap swimming, and so on.

The mentally oriented woman usually has a detailed birth plan, based on careful research. She goes by the book on diet and exercise but tends to repress her emotions. If asked how she is feeling, she may answer with just a word or two: "Fine" or "I'm okay." Massage, swimming, or yoga can help the mentally oriented mother find physical and emotional release. Self-contained as she is, it may be difficult to forge a close connection with her until labor. She is at risk for hypertension, postdatism, and postpartum depression.

I had one such client whose mother arrived a few days before her due date. Days and weeks went by, and this woman continued to insist that things with Mom were "just great." The day after her mother left, she went into labor. True to her mental nature, she labored with remarkable control; she didn't want to be touched or assisted by anyone (including her husband). Caring for the baby was her biggest challenge; she kept trying to get him on a schedule!

Few women are as extreme as these examples, but many of us have an aspect of personality noticeably less developed than the others. If you can help a mother identify and activate this latent part, she can find skills for birthing and parenting that otherwise might not have occurred to her.

Another approach to finding balance in pregnancy is that of midwife Verena Schmid, who devised a practice in which mothers experiment with movement to express the core elements of earth, air, fire, and water, discovering what feels easy and what feels challenging.[36] Movement is but one way to do this: as an example, earth is solid, the ground of being, and so a mother might explore her ability to stand firm, be strong, and believe in herself in a variety of situations. Air is intellect, an ability to take the overview, and so a mother might explore her ease at being calm in her truth no matter what. Fire is passion and desire, and so a mother might explore ways of expressing her passion. Water is emotion and feelings of all kinds, and so a mother might explore the depths of letting go.

And yet, beyond any formula lies the Mystery of Birth in which ease or difficulty with dilation, fast or slow pushing, liking one phase of labor and hating another are all in the cards for women and may vary for the same mother from labor to labor. As midwife Janice Kalman says:

> Sometimes birth is energetic, sometimes emotional, sometimes challenging, depending on aspects of relationship, or the mother's physical or psychological state that day. . . . It's always Mr. Toad's wild ride as to how these aspects create the warp and weave of the story of labor. The trick during pregnancy is for the midwife to recognize red flags of fear, anger, anxiety, discord at home or about who will be at the birth, and then, facilitate open communication around these issues and help a woman come to her truth, no matter what the outcome.

That is what counseling in pregnancy is all about—helping women come to their truth, no matter what. Beyond this, certain situations pose special challenges to women in pregnancy. The following sections explore these situations in depth.

Challenges Facing Single Mothers

It has become increasingly common in our society for women to parent alone. Some reach an age when they decide, "It's now or never," even if the relationship with their partner is somewhat tenuous. Women who become pregnant accidentally with men they barely know or with whom they cannot hope to establish a lasting relationship have other adjustments to make. And the mother estranged from but still emotionally attached to her partner has yet another psychological set.

Particularly if the mother is recently separated, pregnancy can be a time of deep apprehension. Alone at night, with the baby kicking and disturbing her sleep, she may wonder how she will ever be able to handle the impending responsibilities on her own. Single mothers sometimes choose homebirth out of fear of being alone and unsupported in the hospital setting: a topic worth exploring to ascertain whether the responsibilities of birthing at home are well understood. And although most single mothers need extra care from the midwife, they must be encouraged to meet other mothers for lasting friendship and long-term support.

How can you help the single mother with this task? See whether she gets out socially. Ask repeatedly about new contacts she has made with other mothers. Encourage her to talk through any concerns she may have about her ability to parent alone, but take care not to assume too much responsibility as confidant. Be on the lookout for signs of depression.

If the mother seems to be keeping the prospect of motherhood veiled, floating through pregnancy with little thought to what lies ahead, initiate a practical discussion of the postpartum period. Ask her how she plans to cope with her own needs in the first few weeks and how prepared she is to care for the baby. Does she have an adequate supply of baby clothes, furniture, and accessories? Has she ever diapered or bathed a baby before? With little time to prepare food or get to the store, how will she feed herself? And if an emergency should arise (whether physical or emotional), whom can she call for help? These are helpful checkpoints for any mother, but for one who is single, they are especially critical.

What about fears concerning the actual birth? Fears of being overwhelmed and losing control are universal, but the single mother is especially vulnerable for lack of an intimate partner. Who will stand by her if she falls apart? Besides you, she should have a woman friend, a female relative, or a doula for support during the birth.

The sexual dimension of birth may also give the single mother pause, at least if she is celibate. Broach the subject with details on the physiology of labor. Discuss the role of vaginal awareness in the final stages of labor, and teach her pelvic floor exercises. Reassure her that masturbation and orgasm are beneficial in pregnancy and help prepare for the birth. Explain the sensations of labor as vividly as you can,

and let her know the benefits of making noise and moving uninhibitedly in response.

This brings up another concern of single mothers: prospects for love after birth. Are women with babies desirable as sexual partners? Let her know that there are plenty of single parents out there looking for companionship. Some single mothers report being pleasantly surprised by a new lover's relief at being spared the pressure to start a family. Enable the single mother to feel confident about her chances for a loving relationship, if this is what she desires.

Difficulties of Working Mothers

As the saying goes, "Every mother is a working mother." But juggling a busy career, household responsibilities, and other children in the home is no small feat, and pregnancy can be the last straw. Particularly if her work is demanding, the mother must

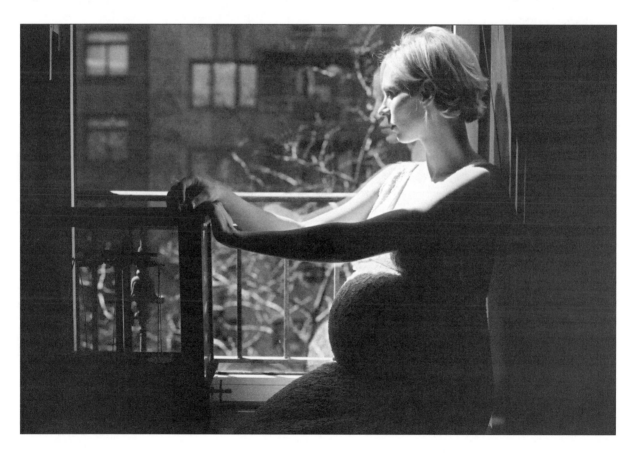

focus on getting sufficient rest and connecting with her baby. Encourage her to be aware of her feelings and pay attention to her body throughout the course of each workday.

Here are some questions for a hard-working mother to help her assess whether her career is negatively affecting her pregnancy:

- Does she have trouble sleeping?
- During her free hours, is she preoccupied with concerns stemming from work?
- How is her sex life?
- Does she make time for deep relaxation every day?
- Does she get exercise on a regular basis?

Her answers to these questions will shed light on how well she is supported, whether or not she is able to unwind, and whether she is making time for the introspection and surrender essential in preparing for labor.

The most common problem for working mothers is chronic stress. This may manifest as insomnia or aches and pains at night and may be mediated by increased vitamins B and C, trace minerals, calcium, and protein. Herbal tinctures of hawthorn, passionflower, or hops can help induce sleep. Chiropractic adjustments also help, and massage can make a big difference. Deep relaxation is essential as is regular aerobic exercise. Any woman dealing with stress needs an excellent diet and a regular means of emotional and physical release.

If income from employment is so important that a mother must continue working even when physical and emotional signals say it is time to quit, suggest that she lie down and relax as soon as she gets home and that she keep weekends completely free. Discuss this plan with her partner and significant others so they will be able to support it fully. Regardless of their situation, I urge all mothers to quit work at least a week or two before the EDD. Particularly if stressed, women who work to term are frequently overdue.

If the mother plans to return to work soon after the birth, stress the importance of taking as much time off as possible to (1) get to know the baby, (2) establish a good milk supply, and (3) develop a new routine at home. None of this can be done without adequate rest and recovery. Recommend that she hire a postpartum doula or line up a woman relative or close friend to assist her full time with everything but baby care. Also help her find a support group: cogent discussion with other new moms can reassure the career woman that she is not alone. Do your best to explain how critical the early weeks are in establishing intimacy and how a few months of undivided attention to the baby make parenting more pleasurable and fulfilling in the long run.

If the mother plans to work and breastfeed, have her contact her local chapter of La Leche League. This magnificent organization offers cost-free phone counseling and referrals to nursing mothers' groups. Without support, a busy mother may unconsciously begin limiting nursing periods, which leads to a reduced milk supply and early weaning.

The "working mothers" category also includes pregnant students who may accumulate tremendous physical tension from sitting still and concentrating over long periods. Help the pregnant student assess her best times for effective, relaxed study, and commit to using these and no others. Also help her take a realistic view of continuing her studies after the birth, for even if she limits in-class hours, she may be so preoccupied with subject matter that she may find it hard to give her baby (and herself) sufficient attention.

Challenges for Adoptive Mothers

Begin by looking closely at any biases you may have regarding mothers who choose to give their babies up for adoption. If you consider adoption to be an evasion of responsibility, you must refer the mother to another care provider. The decision to let go of a baby is a painful one—never an easy choice even in the best of circumstances.

The first homebirth I attended took place in a shed in rural Oregon; I was twenty-one years old and just five months pregnant with my first child. There was no midwife to be found in our community, but the mother had already given birth twice before at home and felt comfortable with the responsibility of birthing on her own. This was in 1971, when humanistic care was virtually nonexistent in hospital.

This experience was remarkable in many ways, especially in that the mother was not keeping the baby but giving it up for adoption to friends who could not have children and would be at the birth. I was stunned by the energy of birth and the mother's strength, but what I recall most vividly was her restraint at the time of delivery. For the hands that caught the baby were the adoptive mother's, and it was she who first took the baby to breast. The women remained friends, and the child continued to have contact with the birth mother.

This account is an example of open private adoption, in contrast to closed agency adoption, where the identity of the birth parents is concealed from the adoptive parent(s) and the child (although in some cases, the birth mother may be permitted to sign a waiver allowing the child to seek her out upon reaching legal adulthood). With agency adoption, a facilitator meets with adoptive and birth parents alike to assess appropriate placement. If your client prefers an agency adoption, advise her to contact the Child Welfare League of America or the Family Service Association. Private adoptions increasingly result from the efforts of an intermediary, such as a lawyer or an independent adoption facilitator, who works for the adoptive parents and charges a substantial fee. It is crucial that the birth mother hire her own legal counsel to protect her rights, and make sure the intermediary is legitimate. Concerned United Parents (800-822-2777) counsels birth parents and provides referrals to local social service agencies.

Suzanne Arms, author of *Adoption: A Handful of Hope*, suggests that both adoptive and birth mothers

need midwives when adoption is planned.[37] Frye observes that for the birth mother, grieving usually begins during pregnancy, and having the baby is a major loss, like a death. Thus the birth mother may want to name the baby, take photos when it is born, snip a lock of hair, take hand- or footprints, or save a baby shirt or blanket from the birth.[38] And unlike my experience in the milk shed, she may want and need to nurse the baby, in order to bond sufficiently to make peace with her decision. She may also ask your assistance in creating a ritual or ceremony with family and friends to formalize her act of letting go.

Adoptive parents have their own anxieties, especially postpartum. Whatever will they do if the birth mother changes her mind? How on earth will they cope, especially if the baby has been theirs for some time? State regulations vary regarding time limits for withdrawal and the number of days after the birth before consents can be signed. Even after papers are signed, there is a probationary period lasting an average of six months, depending on locale. In some states, the biological father must also sign his consent. Know the regulations in your area—if you feel ill equipped to handle the emotional issues, make an appropriate and timely referral.

Issues for Women Who Delay Childbearing

It used to be that any woman having a first baby after age thirty-five was termed an **elderly primigravida** and considered at risk. The main concern was that labor might be complicated by deteriorating health or inhibited by age-induced rigidity of pelvic bones or muscle tissue. But the standard has changed: as increasing numbers of women delay childbearing and maintain their health and fitness through the years, age has proven to be a nonissue.

As for stamina, the older woman who knows herself and clearly wants her baby can manifest phenomenal endurance, more than enough to see her through the longest labor. She has the benefit of life experience and often, a high degree of self-assurance linked to worldly success. With adolescence far behind her, she is less apt to project maturation issues onto her mothering experience than a younger woman might be. She knows how to care for herself, and she knows what works for her.

On the other hand, psychological rigidity may occur with aging. This can cause problems in labor; for example, a mother who thinks she is responding correctly and still feels out of control may get frustrated to the point that her progress is impaired. If she has focused largely on her own development, fine-tuning her likes and dislikes, she may find it hard to surrender established routines to a newborn's needs. And if conception has been by default (the biological clock has run out), disrupted schedules and household chaos in the postpartum period may lead to depression.

You can help by emphasizing that emotional maturity is "gold" when it comes to good parenting. Let her know that the best mothering techniques depend on integrity and forthright communication: attributes she has probably refined over the years. Urge her to form friendships with other mothers, especially if her social circle is composed mostly of childless women and couples. A well-seasoned sense of humor may be her greatest asset; appeal to this with anecdotes that illustrate how levity can mediate the toughest trials of parenthood. A woman of experience is quick to appreciate what it takes the younger, less mature mother much longer to comprehend—that her child is his or her own person, right from the start.

Attitudes have also changed regarding the **grand multipara** (one who has given birth five times or more). Long considered at risk for prolonged labor and postpartum hemorrhage due to lax uterine muscle tone, research shows no risks based on multiparity alone. With close attention to nutrition, exercise, and rest during pregnancy, a mother's physical condition and birth experience can be optimal regardless of age or previous childbearing.

Problems of Estranged Couples

Working with estranged partners is complex and ultimately depends on the mother's assessment of the relationship. She may ask you to help them reconcile their differences or to support her in finding autonomy. Whatever her desires, the latter is always a good idea should reconciliation prove impossible. Help her articulate her core needs and identify those not being met in the relationship. Reaffirm her ability to single-parent if she must, while encouraging her to communicate assertively with her partner.

Estrangement in pregnancy can take a number of forms. Perhaps the couple has been together for a while but has not stabilized, with both parties vacillating on whether to marry or otherwise define their relationship as long term. In this case, be prepared for tearful sessions and a continued repetition of problems. If your counsel starts to repeat itself as well, refer the couple to a specialist who can work with them more intensively.

How best to deal with the estranged partner? Seldom will your assistance be requested; more often than not, he or she simply drops out of the picture. But on a few occasions, I've been beeped in the middle of the night by a drunken and distraught partner wanting to talk: a contact unproductive and more than a little disturbing. If this happens to you, clearly state that you are available during *normal business hours only* and hang up. Take care to be professional in your tone and manner of speaking, as estranged partners can read strange meaning into the midwife's sensitivity and compassion. Refer the couple to counseling and reassert your role as care provider for the mother.

Hopefully, there will come a time well before labor when the couple in distress decides whether they will stay together. If they remain undecided late in pregnancy, it is important to advise them of the difficulties emotional ambivalence can create during the birth. If they cannot work out their differences, suggest that the mother prepare to labor without her partner. Explain that she must feel fully at ease to give birth safely. Contemplation of this fact may make partners decide to reconcile or may cause them to see that it is impossible. If separation seems inevitable, have the mother choose a family member, close friend, or doula as her supporter. As soon as possible, begin to broach the same topics of discussion as you would with a single mother.

Yet another situation is that of the mother with a new love interested in sharing the pregnancy and birth. The newcomer may do well during the birth but may be quite let down postpartum. Passionate, fledgling couples must be briefed on the difficulties of the early weeks, and you must persist through their joking affection to get at the thorniest issues. Have they discussed their respective roles after the birth? How will they deal with sleepless nights, hours of baby-crying, and no time to themselves? Do they understand how emotionally volatile the postpartum period can be and how breastfeeding and lack of privacy may temper sexual activity for quite some time? At some point, see the mother alone to broach the subject of single parenting. Ask her how she would cope if she and her new love grew apart after the birth and whether or not she has any backup plan for physical assistance or financial support. Remind her of her former self-reliance, and suggest she not lose sight of it if the relationship flounders.

Challenges Facing Lesbian Mothers

In the past, lesbian women contemplating motherhood met with ridicule or hostility. Now that same-sex couples are more positively portrayed in the media, these antiquated reactions are falling away. The notion that lesbians are unfit to parent is being replaced with an understanding of how their children may benefit from being carefully prepared for and very much wanted.

Be aware that one or both partners may identify as transsexual, cross-gender, gender-fluid, or gender-queer (a term which signifies gender experiences that do not fit binary concepts and combine gender

identities and sexual orientations). Of course, these terms may also apply to partners in a heterosexual union, and may require some language adjustments on your part. Just make sure you know exactly how the couple wants their relationship presented to the backup physician and medical staff should consultative visits or transport become necessary.

Help with artificial insemination is increasingly available through midwives. Sperm is obtained from sperm banks for 94 percent of inseminations. Otherwise, fresh sperm is secured from known or unknown donors after careful screening for HIV and other diseases. (Sperm banks also screen donors for HIV, which is critical since the virus can survive freezing.) Rarely, the donor may want some knowledge of the child or may wish to co-parent. But the relationship between mother and donor is usually tentative, thus legal contracts are advisable to delineate these agreements and prevent future custody battles. In numerous states, the donor surrenders all claim to the child if insemination is done through a physician.

The actual insemination process often takes many months. The success rate quoted by most sperm banks is only about 19 percent. It takes an average of six to nine months to conceive, and with two inseminations performed each month, the process can be quite costly. Again, this points to the fact that lesbian women desiring motherhood must be thoroughly committed to their decision.

The birth certificate poses a special problem. If the mother indicates that she was artificially inseminated, the state may try to track the father if she later applies for aid. Better to leave the space for father's name blank or write "unknown." With a few exceptions (Vermont, for example), only the birth mother can be registered as legal guardian. In most states, her partner cannot adopt the child. And if anything were to happen to the mother during the birth or postpartum that rendered her disabled or incompetent, her partner would have no authority unless she established power of attorney in advance (in which case she would be treated as next of kin). Excellent books on the subject include *The New Essential Guide to Lesbian Conception, Pregnancy, and Birth* by Stephanie Brill (Alyson Books, 2006), and *The Ultimate Guide to Pregnancy for Lesbians: How to Stay Sane and Care for Yourself from Pre-conception through Birth* by Rachel Pepper (Cleis Press, 2005).

Encourage lesbian mothers to find others in their community for support. Check yourself for homophobia, and if you personally feel you cannot serve lesbian mothers lovingly and well, refer them to midwives who can.

Issues in Family Relationships

The family in Western society has undergone a major transformation: relatives may live at great distances from one another and communicate infrequently. Thus most first-time mothers think little of how family relationships might affect their experience of childbearing and may be surprised to find memories of childhood surfacing as pregnancy progresses. Whether they process these memories or not, many feel the urge to talk with their mothers about birth and baby care.

This desire to reanimate family ties links to the power of bonding, which may remain unconscious until maternal (or paternal) surges turn the wheel and complete the cycle of biological relatedness. Particularly with a first pregnancy, the mother and her partner may express negativity about how they were raised, determined to do better with their child. This process of individuation requires letting go of anger and resentment—reactions of attachment—toward their parents, while culling the best techniques and greatest wisdom from their upbringing.

Help the mother and her partner explore their feelings in this regard while encouraging them to find forgiveness if at all possible. This may require counseling, particularly if there is a history of abuse. Those in their early twenties may confuse bitter memories of adolescence with an otherwise happy childhood: help them to recollect the good times.

The most difficult (and profound) aspect of first-time parenting is reckoning our ideals with our limitations. Stress that parenting is about process, not perfection; about receptivity, not mastery; about flexibility, not control.

Also, the mother and her partner may have opposing ideas about childrearing. One may have preconceptions of what is best, while the other maintains a "wait and see" attitude. Treat any disagreements arising in your presence lightly, as ultimately, time will tell. Just be aware that clients with rigid ideals about parenting may likewise be fanatic in their expectations of birth. Those with unhappy childhood experiences may confide that they do not really like children and wonder how they will ever be able to parent. Those who lack exposure to infants may worry that their enthusiasm is much less than it should be. Unless they are adopting, the hardest thing for prospective parents to grasp is that their baby will be kin, not an abstract infant like the babies of others may seem.

Fear of becoming a parent may be linked to negative role models. If the mother's partner remembers his or her parents as rigid and unfeeling or harried and stressed, he or she may believe (albeit unconsciously) that having a child means behaving this way. Instead of being cause for celebration, pregnancy is viewed as a sobering event concomitant to a loss of personal freedom. This may result in bouts of substance abuse, chronic overwork, fits of depression, or even promiscuity. If the mother reports any such behavior, ask her to bring her partner to the next prenatal, or schedule a home visit when both will be present. Deal tactfully with this polarization by discussing the matter dispassionately, taking a simple, objective look at relevant social patterning. If the issue is not readily resolved, refer the couple to counseling.

For their part, first-time moms often struggle with conflicting role models of self-sacrificing Madonna and self-determined free spirit. Do not let this slip by unattended, or the mother may suffer from postpartum depression.

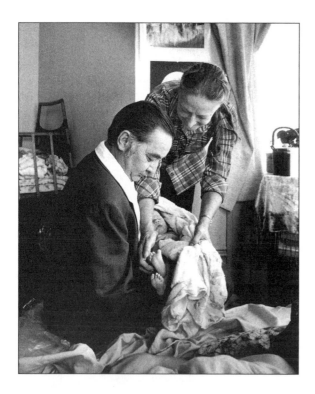

Whatever their situation, partners need to hear it is possible to be a parent and be human at the same time, and that it is infinitely better to express emotions spontaneously than to vent them later as distorted or violent outbursts. Explain that parenting operates on the same principles of honesty and assertiveness as in adult relationships. The more they relax, speak their truth, and trust their instincts, the better they will deal with the expectations of other family members and society at large.

Sexual Problems

Sexual difficulties often stem from mistaken concepts of appropriate masculine or feminine behavior. Polarized gender roles have marked our culture since its inception, and even now, while subscribing to sexual equality, the feminine aspect is underexpressed in our society.

As regards sexual intimacy, most problems spring from an inability to integrate this polarity and effectively communicate needs and desires. Broach

this subject by explaining physical and emotional changes trimester by trimester and how these may impact sexuality, including adaptations appropriate for different phases of pregnancy. This can help a mother more comfortably articulate what she desires from her partner and vice versa. In this respect, discussion with other expectant couples is ideal because all are undergoing similar changes and adjustments.

Both partners should understand that a pregnant woman's desire for sex fluctuates dramatically. At no other time will the emotional aspect have so strong an influence on her response. In turn, her emotions will vary according to the stage of pregnancy through which she is passing. The first trimester can be a honeymoon of all-barriers-down passion and tenderness. Of course, ambivalence toward the pregnancy will temper these feelings. Nausea and fatigue may also interfere.

Once movement is felt, the mother may focus so intently on the baby that she becomes sexually withdrawn. But generally, high levels of estrogen and oxytocin, plus increased pelvic circulation, serve to boost desire in the latter part of pregnancy. This can be a time of balance, ease, and happiness for the mother, and her sexual response usually reflects this. If she complains that her partner is insensitive, suggest she take more initiative or talk to him or her about this when they are not being sexual.

As the birth approaches, the mother may once again withdraw to focus on impending labor. For sex to seem right at this time, she needs to know that her partner is connected to her and the baby, making love to them both. This is a very vulnerable time for the mother, and it is perfectly all right for her to be selective regarding the nature and frequency of her sexual encounters.

But do make sure to explain that birth prompts the same emotional and physical release as does orgasm, and that, barring signs of premature labor or other complications, masturbation is fine during pregnancy, right up to the moment the baby is born (many women report masturbating more than ever before, perhaps several times daily). Even if she is not partnered, encourage the mother to keep her sexual circuits open so she can fully respond to labor's intensity.

If the mother is partnered, make clear that labor is a body-centered experience that will call on her to take the lead. If need be, help her redefine her sexuality as a sharing of her power, rather than her skill in submitting to or pleasing her partner. Encourage her to take sensual pleasure in hot baths, relaxed meals, massage, and so on. Physical practices of yoga or dance may help her get in touch with her rhythms, release tension, and find her own resources for feeling good.

One of my favorite experiences illustrating the sexuality of birth is that of assisting a young couple and their three-year-old daughter on a rare warm and balmy San Francisco afternoon. The mother set up her birth nest in the dining room area, and

I still remember the breeze blowing through white curtains as sunlight filtered through. Labor progressed rapidly but the mother stayed calm, with her daughter tucked comfortably beside her as crowning approached. Her husband sat between her legs, waiting to catch the baby, when suddenly she reached for him passionately, saying, "Kiss me, Jack," which he did as the head slipped out effortlessly. A truly gorgeous and unforgettable moment!

A mother's ease with her sexuality affects not only her labor but also her comfort with her baby, her rate of recuperation, and her commitment to breastfeeding. Help her to explore and celebrate her sexuality as much as possible. For more stories and insight, see my book (coauthored with Debra Pascali-Bonaro), *Orgasmic Birth: Your Guide to a Safe, Satisfying, and Pleasurable Birth Experience.*

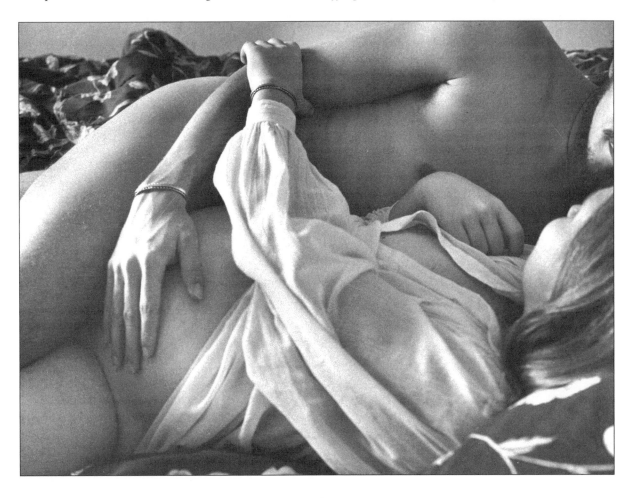

Abuse Issues

Please refer to appendix D, "Mother's Confidential Worksheet." This is meant as a take-home form, but you can also use it as a discussion guide for broaching various abuse and trauma situations the mother may have experienced.

Sexual abuse may be defined as intimate contact in which a child or adolescent is used for the sexual gratification of someone older. The key to differentiating abuse from experimentation is what Anne Frye calls the "power differential": the abuser always has the upper hand.[39] The incidence is estimated to be 33 percent of women, although one study showed that 53 percent of pregnant teens had experienced sexual abuse.[40] Repressed memories of sexual abuse are likely to arise (1) during the perinatal cycle, (2) when a woman gets married or commits to a monogamous relationship, (3) when her own daughter reaches the age when she herself was first molested, or (4) when her perpetrator dies. If the mother responds to relevant questions on the worksheet with some uncertainty but is willing to discuss her experience, ask the following:

1. Have you ever been tricked into an intimate situation you did not desire?

2. Has anyone ever touched you intimately against your will?

3. Have you ever been forced to have sex when you didn't want to?

4. Have you ever been forcibly held down or restrained for sex when clearly indicating you wanted to be free?

Women with a history of sexual abuse often suffer from extreme PMS, chronic pelvic pain, constipation, vaginal infection, pain with intercourse, and eating disorders. There may be history of habitual abortion, hyperemesis gravidarium, or premature labor. An intense reaction to internal exam, speculum exam, breast exam, or even with blood draw is likely. **Vaginismus**, an involuntary contraction of the vaginal muscles if any attempt is made at penetration, is definitely a sign.

Sometimes the abuse survivor develops a dissociative disorder and behaves in a fashion opposite of the above. During exams, she may splay her legs wide or open her labia far apart, but emotionally she is passive, detached, checked out, not there with you. In the extreme, a woman with a history of prolonged sexual abuse may develop multiple personality disorder. Here is a list of characteristics or behaviors common in women who have been sexually abused:

- Describes self as never having been a child
- Is extremely concerned with control
- Is overly willing to expose genitals to others
- Has unexplained pain with intercourse
- Has extreme ideas about sexuality
- Is hypersensitive to touch
- Is repeatedly exploited by others in relationships
- Is deeply estranged from family
- Has a general feeling of being "under it"
- Detaches from self and others
- Says nothing is ever wrong with life, always neutral
- Displays childlike behavior, dress, or appearance
- Has an unkempt personal appearance
- Has chaotic surroundings or habits
- Has overly controlled surroundings and habits
- Shows no personal boundaries
- Has no trust
- Displays anger inappropriate or out of proportion to the situation
- Is unable to appreciate others
- Blindly adores others
- Has fanatic religious or philosophical beliefs
- Jumps into situations or to conclusions
- Has difficulty making decisions[41]

Note that partners who experienced sexual abuse may have many of the symptoms above as well, and if so, may also need assistance in handling the responsibilities of partner support and parenting. Counselor Derek Lainsbury poignantly articulated these issues in his article, "Child Is the Father to the Man" (*Midwifery Today*, Autumn 1999). Reach him at dereklainsbury@hotmail.com.

Experts Penny Simkin and Phyllis Klaus observe that working with sexually abused women can be difficult because they are often needy, controlling, and/or angry.[42] Even if you are doing everything in your power to be of assistance, an imagined slight may snowball into litigation. For these reasons, the mother must receive outside help, as dealing with this problem is beyond the midwife's scope of practice unless she is also a trained therapist. The mother may benefit, too, from group support: Solace for Mothers (www.solaceformothers.org) offers a mothers' forum, a warm line (1866-Solace4), and support for partners in a Family, Friends, and Advocates forum.

With regard to the birth process, certain impacts of sexual abuse are classic. Most survivors have tremendous fear of losing control and cannot bear the thought of grunting, trembling, crying out, involuntary excretions, or feeling helpless in labor. Sensations in second stage may be particularly terrifying, as vaginal distension triggers memories of early violation. Medicated birth and cesarean are common. The survivor may also have great difficulties with breastfeeding, particularly when her baby reaches an age where it begins to fondle the nipple or play at the breast.

A woman who has been raped may express behaviors similar to one who has suffered sexual abuse, depending on how well she has healed from her trauma. She too may be needy and angry and so may have concomitant problems in labor unless she is counseled during pregnancy. As you take her history, be ready to discuss residual fears, embarrassment, or feelings of powerlessness linked to her experience.

On the other hand, women who have done major work to move through traumas of sexual abuse or rape may be quite self-sufficient and responsibly interdependent. And they may have extraordinarily empowering birth experiences. This account from a survivor of childhood sexual abuse serves to illustrate:

> During the birth of my daughter, I felt immense power. I could feel this hard, glorious ball filling my vagina, washing it clean of shame, proving its power and purity. I felt the heat from her head and the stretching of my tissues. I felt burning and stinging. Then I felt a feeling better than any orgasm I had ever had, as her sweet, slippery body left me. I immediately felt I'd do anything to feel that feeling again, that last moment of ecstasy. But by then I was caught in a wave of other ecstasies, the feeling of her warm body against mine, her soft purple skin turning pink in my arms.

Victims of physical abuse/domestic violence require special care. First and foremost, they must be apprised of their legal situation. In many states, health workers are obligated to report claims or evidence of physical abuse to social services, and the abuser will be arrested. Unfortunately, in some states the abuser may be able to post bail the same night, so the mother needs to know where to go to be safe.

Apart from being life threatening, there are serious emotional ramifications of physical abuse. If your pregnant client remains with her abuser, you must make some decisions on how to care for her. Even though her partner may wish to be present at the birth, you must separate her needs from her partner's desires. In many ways, you must treat her as you would an estranged or single mother. She may, with good reason, feel extremely protective of her unborn baby, keeping it inside her as long as possible. The postpartum period is fraught with liabilities for her and the baby, as physically abused women tend toward self-abnegation, frustration, and, unfortunately, child abuse. Get expert consultation, be aware of the resources in your area, and make sure you are safe.

There are numerous other traumas and self-abusive behaviors that may affect the pregnancy, as cited in appendix D. Midwife Mickey Sperlich postulates that mothers with multiple traumas have increased risk for developing post-traumatic stress disorder (PTSD) during the perinatal period. There is evidence that some traumas, such as childhood neglect, are particularly high predictors for PTSD.[43] If you are concerned about your client's level of exposure, know your limits. Refer her to a trusted therapist as you continue to discuss these issues with her.

Psychological Screening Out

Despite her best efforts, a mother may continue to have emotional problems that make you question whether you should assist her birth. Discuss your concerns with your midwifery partner or assistant, who may see signs of improvement you have overlooked. Then again, guard against excessive optimism, and give credence to the emotional aftertaste of working with a troubled mother.

If you decide to assist but the case remains borderline, discuss the situation with backup before the birth is imminent. This will render any complications in labor more comprehensible in the event of transport. Also discuss the case with your peers, not only to benefit from their perspective but also to forestall any rumors in case of an unhappy outcome.

On the other hand, if you have exhausted every resource to improve the mother's situation and still feel it to be unstable, it is wise to excuse yourself from her care and refer her. Provide a list of other potential caregivers, including contacts for hospital birth. Not uncommonly, the mother will be relieved at your decision, and it becomes evident that discomfort with you (or perhaps with the prospect of birthing at home) was part of the problem all along. This amounts to psychological screening out.

Note that the shock of being screened out may prompt her to rally her resources and make long-overdue changes in her health or situation. Thus a mother determined by one midwife to be psychologically at risk may be cared for by another and do just fine. If you agree to receive such a mother into your care, be aware that if she remains emotionally troubled, her chances of developing complications are high and hospital birth may be advisable.

The only way to learn psychological screening out is by experience. I cannot remember a single workshop on this subject where a midwife has not presented a hair-raising case history capped with the final lament, "I knew from the start I shouldn't have worked with her." Those who have borne the consequences via malpractice proceedings will tell you that initial feelings of ambivalence are a warning every midwife should heed.

Once you have made a decision to risk out a mother, hold firm. If you have agreed to support the mother in hospital birth, remember that any last-minute improvements are probably due to increased security with more conventional plans. Do not be tempted to reverse yourself just because things are looking better. This takes the wisdom to let things be. The birth may not be any easier in the hospital than it would have been at home, but at least the legal weight is off your shoulders.

For Parents: Danger Signs in Pregnancy

Report to your midwife immediately if you notice any of the following:

1. *Vaginal bleeding.* In the first trimester, this may indicate threatened, spontaneous, or missed abortion (miscarriage), molar pregnancy, or ectopic pregnancy. In the second or third trimesters, this may indicate placenta previa, placental abruption, ruptured cervical polyp, or other causes; contact your midwife at once.

2. *Initial outbreak of blisters in the perineal or anal area during the first trimester.* This may be herpes virus; contact your midwife at once so a culture can be taken.

3. *Severe pelvic or abdominal pain.* In the first trimester, this may indicate a tubal pregnancy. In the last trimester, this may indicate placental abruption. Both are emergencies; contact your midwife at once.

4. *Persistent and severe midback pain.* This may indicate kidney infection/pyelonephritis; contact your midwife at once.

5. *Swelling of hands and face.* Particularly if your face looks puffy or features look coarse, notify your midwife immediately. This may indicate preeclampsia.

6. *Severe headaches, blurry vision, or epigastric pain (under ribcage).* This may indicate a pre-eclamptic condition becoming critical. Notify your midwife immediately.

7. *Gush of fluid from vagina.* If in the first or second trimester, this may indicate miscarriage. If in your late second or third trimester, this may indicate premature delivery. Contact your midwife at once.

8. *Regular uterine contractions before thirty-seven weeks.* This may indicate impending premature birth. Don't wait to see if they will abate: lie down and call your midwife immediately.

9. *Cessation of fetal movement.* This may indicate fetal demise. The baby should move several times per hour, more right after you have a meal. If fewer movements than this, or fewer movements than usual, report to your midwife at once.

Notes

1. F. G. Cunningham et al., *Williams Obstetrics*, 23rd ed. (New York: McGraw Hill, 2010), 222.

2. Claudia Panuthos and C. Romero, *Ended Beginnings* (Boston, MA: Bergin & Garvey, 1985).

3. Anne Frye, *Holistic Midwifery: A Comprehensive Textbook for Midwives in Homebirth Practice*, vol. 1 (Portland, OR: Labrys Press, 1998), 724.

4. Steven Gabbe et al., *Obstetrics: Normal and Problem Pregnancies*, 5th ed. (New York: Churchill Livingstone, 2007), 194.

5. Anne Frye, *Understanding Diagnostic Tests in the Childbearing Year*, 6th ed. (Portland, OR: Labrys Press, 1997), 319.

6. Cunningham et al., *Williams Obstetrics*, 23rd ed., 771.

7. Henci Goer, *Obstetrical Myths Versus Research Realities: A Guide to the Medical Literature* (Westport, CT: Bergin & Garvey, 1995), 158.

8. Henci Goer, "Gestational Diabetes: The Emperor Has No Clothes," *The Birth Gazette* 12, no. 2 (1966).

9. J. S. Hunter and M. J. N. C. Keirse, "Gestational Diabetes," in *Effective Care in Pregnancy and Birth*, Ian Chalmers et al. (Oxford, UK: Oxford University Press, 1989).

10. T. I. Chang, M. Horal, S. K. Jain, F. Wang, R. Patel, and M. R. Loeken, "Oxidant Regulation of Gene Expression and Neural Tube Development: Insights Gained from Diabetic Pregnancy on Molecular Causes of Neural Tube Defects," *Diabetologia* 46, no. 4 (April 2003): 538–45.

11. K. L. Boyd, E. K. Ross, and S. J. Sherman, "Jelly Beans as an Alternative to a Cola Beverage Containing Fifty Grams of Glucose," *American Journal of Obstetrics and Gynecology* 173, no. 6 (December 1995): 1889–92.

12. Frye, *Understanding Diagnostic Tests*, 319.

13. Kevin Dalton, "Home Telemetry: A Need for Reassessment of PET," report presented at the Royal College of Medicine, London, September 15, 1989.

14. H. C. Bucher, G. H. Guyatt, R. J. Cook, R. Hatala, D. J. Cook, J. D. Lang, and D. Hunt, "Effect of Calcium Supplementation on Pregnancy-Induced Hypertension and Preeclampsia: A Meta-Analysis of Randomized Controlled Trials," *Journal of the American Medical Association* 275, no. 14 (April 10, 1996): 1113–17.

15. G. Hofmeyer, A. N. Atallah, and L. Duly, "Calcium Supplementation during Pregnancy for Preventing Hypertensive Disorders and Related Problems," *Cochrane Library* 4 (2003).

16. S. E. Maynard, J.-Y. Min, J. Merchan, K. H. Lim, J. Li, S. Mondal, T. A. Liebermann, J. P. Morgan, F. W. Selke, I. E. Stillman, F. H. Epstein, V. P. Sukhatme, and S. A. Karumanchi, "Excess Placental Soluble fms-like Tyrosine Kinase 1 (sFlt1) May Contribute to Endothelial Dysfunction, Hypertension, and Proteinuria in Preeclampsia," *Journal of Clinical Investigation* 111, no. 5 (March 2003): 649–58.

17. S. A. Karumanchi, K. H. Lim, and P. August, "Pathogenesis of Preeclampsia," *UpToDate Online*, 2010, www.uptodate.com /contents/pathogenesis-of-preeclampsia (accessed March 6, 2012).

18. Frye, *Holistic Midwifery*, vol. 1, 958.

19. S. Kilpatrick et al., "Maternal Hydration Increases Amniotic Fluid Volume in Women with Normal Amniotic Fluid," *Obstetrics and Gynecology* 81, no. 1 (January 1993): 49–52.

20. Stephen G. Gabbe, Jennifer R. Neibyl, and Joe Leigh Simpson, *Obstetrics: Normal and Problem Pregnancies*, 4th ed. (New York: Churchill Livingstone, 2002), 827.

21. Tone Irene Nordtveit, Kari Klungsoyr Melve, Susanne Albrechtsen, and Rolv Skjaerven, "Maternal and Paternal Contribution to Intergenerational Recurrence of Breech Delivery: Population Based Cohort Study," *British Medical Journal* 10 (March 2008): 1136.

22. Doña Queta Contreras and Doña Irene Sotelo, Midwifery Today conference notes, Oaxaca, Mexico, October 2003.

23. March of Dimes e-Newsletter, June 2011, www.marchofdimes .com/news.

24. J. Plunkett, S. Doniger, G. Orabona, T. Morgan, R. Haataja et al.,"An Evolutionary Genomic Approach to Identify Genes Involved in Human Birth Timing," *PLoS Genetics* 10 (2011): 1371.

25. Charles Lockwood, editorial, *New England Journal of Medicine* 346 (January 24, 2002): 282–84.

26. E. L. Morzurkewich, B. Luke, M. Anvi, and F. M. Wolf, "Working Conditions and Adverse Pregnancy Outcome: A Meta-Analysis," *Obstetrics & Gynecology* 95, no. 4 (April 2000): 623–35.

27. M. Jeffcoat et al., "Periodontal Infection and Preterm Birth: Results of a Prospective Study," *Journal of the American Dental Association* 132 (July 2001): 875–80.

28. H. Minkoff et al., "An Association between the Heat-Humidity Index and Preterm Labor and Delivery," *American Journal of Public Health* 87 (1997): 1205–07.

29. S. J. Olsen and N. J. Secher, "Low Consumption of Seafood in Early Pregnancy as a Risk Factor for Preterm Delivery: Prospective Cohort Study," *British Medical Journal* 324 (February 2002): 447.

30. U.S. Food and Drug Administration. Press release: "FDA Warns Against Certain Uses of Asthma Drug Terbatuline for Preterm Labor," February 17, 2011, www.fda.gov/NewsEvents/ Newsroom/PressAnnouncements/ucm243840.htm (accessed March 6, 2012).

31. S. M. Ludington-Hoe and S. K. Golant, *Kangaroo Care: The Best You Can Do for Your Premature Infant* (New York: Bantam Books, 1993).

32. Morzurkewich et al., "Working Conditions."

33. Gabbe et al., *Obstetrics: Normal and Problem Pregnancies*, 5th ed., 847.

34. H. Oxorn, *Oxorn-Foote Human Labor & Birth*, 5th ed. (Norwalk, CT: Appleton & Lange, 1986), 712.

35. R. D. Eden, L. S. Seifert, A. Winegar, and W. N. Spellacy, "Perinatal Characteristics of Uncomplicated Postdates Pregnancies," *Obstetrics and Gynecology* 69 (1987): 296.

36. Verena Schmid, Midwifery Today conference notes, London, June 2003.

37. Suzanne Arms, MANA conference notes, San Francisco, CA, October 1985.

38. Frye, *Holistic Midwifery*, vol. 1, 936.

39. Frye, *Holistic Midwifery*, vol. 1, 308.

40. T. Hoffman, N. Kellogg, and E. Taylor, "Early Sexual Experiences among Pregnant and Parenting Adolescents," *Adolescence* 34, no. 134 (1999): 293–303.

41. Laura Davis and Ellen Bass, *The Courage to Heal* (New York: Harper & Row, 1998).

42. Penny Simkin and Phyllis Klaus, Midwifery Today conference, audiotape, Eugene, OR, 1996.

43. Mickey Sperlich, "Survivor Moms: Multiple Trauma Exposures and the Development of Post Traumatic Stress Disorder," *Midwifery Today*, Summer 2009.

CHAPTER 4

Assisting at Births

At long last, we have learned enough of the physiology of birth to see that it justifies our trust in the process, a trust that midwives have known since the beginning of time. No longer must we defend a laboring woman's needs for privacy, respect, and nonintervention on a purely psychological basis: these are the biological imperatives of normal birth. Birth works; we just have to get out of the way!

Remember that the birth is the main event: regardless of any prenatal turmoil, we must come to it clear of preconceptions. If we approach open-mindedly, we pay better attention to what is happening in the moment. This quality of freshness will be well appreciated by the mother and her supporters: it is the spark for getting labor off to a good start.

Early Labor

During the last weeks of pregnancy, estrogen levels rise to increase oxytocin receptors in uterine muscle tissue. Estrogen also stimulates the release of prostaglandins, which produce enzymes that digest collagen in the cervix to soften it and initiate labor.

Every woman should know the signs of early labor well before her baby is due. These include **the show** (pink-tinged mucus from the vagina), **regular contractions** (no more than twenty minutes apart), or **spontaneous rupture of the membranes (SROM)** (the waters release). Encourage mothers to call immediately with any of these signs. This gives you a chance to put your personal life in order and prepare to attend, even if the birth does not happen for several days.

If the mother calls to report the show, make sure there is no excess bleeding, which could be related to placental problems. Also let her know that labor may not begin in earnest for several days, so she should go about her normal routine, eating top-quality, non-constipating foods, and getting plenty of rest and sleep. Explain that she doesn't have to do anything to get labor going: what matters most is that she take the best possible care of herself, relax, and let her feelings flow. If she experiences a prelabor burst of energy, reiterate her need for rest and sleep to prepare for the

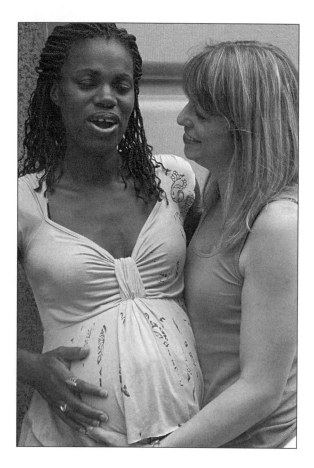

As long as there are no signs of infection, there is no need to get labor going. If she calls at bedtime or the middle of the night, suggest a strong cup of relaxant tea (such as hops or valerian) or a glass of wine (barring history of alcoholism) to get some sleep. Her partner (if applicable) might want to give her a massage, but again, no intercourse, finger-genital, or mouth-genital contact.

Ask her to contact you at once if she notices a green or yellow tinge to her amniotic fluid, indicating that the baby has passed **meconium** (first bowel movement). This is due to relaxation of the anal sphincter caused by a lack of oxygen, or hypoxia. Although this may have been a fleeting occurrence, meconium is suggestive of fetal distress, so you must immediately check fetal heart tones.

If the woman reports a gush of water with no more following, this is a **hind leak**. It is caused by a tear high in the membranes, which releases just enough fluid to allow the baby to settle more deeply in the pelvis so that further flow is prevented. But sometimes a bit of fluid does filter down and is trapped behind the intact membranes still encasing the baby's head; these are the **forewaters**, which feel like an intact but bulging water bag.

Labor beginning with contractions alone is a bit harder to confirm, as rounds of uterine activity can go on for weeks before labor actually starts. Commonly known as **false labor**, this negative term does little more than increase the frustration of stop-and-go contracting, which can be painful and lead to sleep deprivation. Put a positive spin on the situation and explain that although the fibers of the uterus are not yet synchronized to cause dilation to occur, these contractions are toning uterine muscle and are facilitating effacement and fetal descent. We may more accurately term this sort of uterine activity **warm-up labor**.

With warm-up labor, contractions may come every twenty minutes or closer, but they are brief (less than forty seconds) and never form a consistent pattern. If this is the case, suggest a warm bath and

work ahead. Share in her elation, too: this will help her release nervous tension and get into the process.

If the mother calls to report that her waters have released, there are certain precautions she should take to prevent infection, which can occur if bacteria from the vagina enter the sterile uterine environment. She should be meticulous in her toileting, and put nothing in her vagina. If she drinks sufficient fluids at regular intervals, her body will defend itself by increasing the production of amniotic fluid, which flushes the vagina and discourages bacteria from migrating upward. As an additional precaution, she might take one dropperful of echinacea tincture or 250 mg of vitamin C every few hours. And she should check her temperature periodically and note the odor on her pad: it should smell clean and fresh. Ask that she report any changes immediately.

a glass of wine or herbal tincture (see above), which will stop the process if the time is not yet ripe. Sensations similar to warm-up labor may also occur in late pregnancy when the baby is large, unengaged, and then suddenly descends. Known as **lightening** or **dropping**, abrupt stretching of the lower uterine segment can cause cramp-like sensations: the mother may think she is in labor, but her "contractions" are more like twinges, with no particular pattern of dispersal or duration. Have her use the suggestions above and rest up.

Contractions that gradually increase in intensity, coming closer and closer together, characterize **true labor**. Spacing and duration may be erratic at first, but with cervical (menstrual-like) cramping, chances are it's the real thing.

Most women are eager to discuss their first contractions. If labor starts in the morning, ask whether she got enough sleep and then suggest a good breakfast and an outing with her partner or a friend in some natural setting (not the mall). Recommend that she pause when contractions come, leaning against something and releasing her pelvis and hips completely. Remind her to keep eating and drinking and to take a nap in the afternoon if things have not changed (especially if her sleep the night before was limited).

If labor starts in the afternoon, make sure she had a good lunch, and then suggest a hot shower or bath and a nap. In this case, the priority is rest rather than activity, as it is quite likely she will labor well into the night, particularly if this is her first baby. To help her rest, suggest hops tincture in tea or a massage. Remind her that she should plan to have dinner and should call you to check in after she rests.

If labor starts at night, have her follow the guidelines mentioned earlier for getting sleep. Also make sure she had a good dinner and remind her to keep fluids by the bed: she should drink (and urinate) regularly.

This brings up the question of when to go to the birth. With your initial conversation, the mother will probably want to know when you will come to attend her. If she seems to need you at this point, go see her. Otherwise, tell her to call if anything changes. Let her know that you will help her through any rough periods, explaining your willingness to come and go. With a first birth, mothers often call at 2 or 3 cm dilation to report some "really intense" contractions, aware that they are early in the process and worried about how painful it might become. This is an important moment of reckoning with the forces of labor. Explain that as it progresses, her body will release endorphins that will make the pain easier to bear, and as long as she continues to surrender, she will find resources for coping that she may not know she has. You might suggest a hot bath or shower to help her get used to her sensations, or a massage from her partner or another supporter. Remind her that oxytocin is her friend, so anything

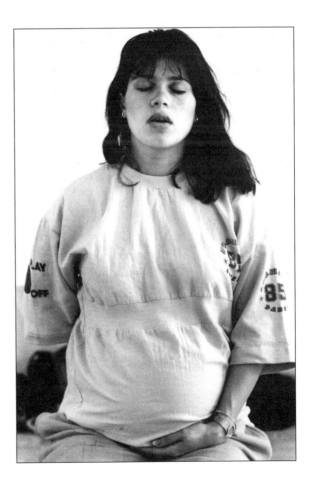

she can do to increase it—lovemaking (as long as membranes are not ruptured), soft lights, intimate atmosphere—will aid and ease the process.

However, there are certain indications to attend the birth immediately. Mothers with psychological issues may need an immediate visit for reassurance and help getting settled. If the baby was high at the last prenatal and the mother reports that her waters have released, immediately go and check fetal heart tones to rule out cord prolapse. If you have any question concerning the baby's ability to handle labor due to intrauterine growth restriction (IUGR) or postdatism, be there from the beginning to monitor fetal response. A report of decreased fetal movement or, as mentioned earlier, meconium-tinged or off-odor waters, necessitates your presence to rule out fetal compromise. And maternal conditions of

borderline hypertension or polyhydramnios should be monitored right from the start. In general, any marginal findings in the last weeks of pregnancy require earlier involvement.

The birth environment also merits attention. It is nearly impossible for a mother to relax and get into her labor if her home is chaotic; beware of loud partying noises in the background. You may need to clear the house of distractions, explaining to well-meaning friends or relatives that it will be a while yet and she needs to concentrate on labor. Send members of the birth team on last-minute food runs, or have them do some cooking or baking (homebirth physician Ric Jones recommends chocolate cake; it fills the house with a wonderful smell and is ideal for the postbirth celebration). The birth room should be neat, well ventilated, and aesthetically pleasing, with fresh flowers or greenery, ample fluids by the bed, massage oil and towels, a heating pad, and so on, laid out and ready for use. Many women use their natural nesting instincts to take care of this in early labor, but those who feel frightened may need help getting organized.

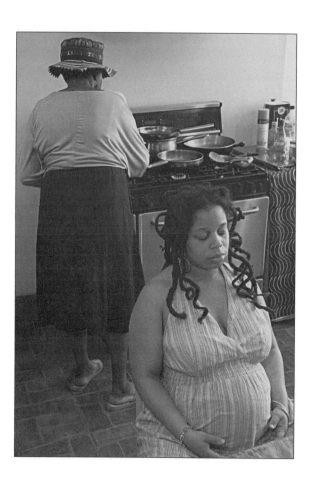

Otherwise, maintain good phone communication and you may be able to guide the mother through early labor without needing to make a visit. This is important if you have a busy practice or are tired from a recent birth. Beginning midwives often struggle with the concept of less than start-to-finish involvement in labor, particularly if they have done doula work, which reaches a peak with the birth of the baby and then eases off. In contrast, the midwife's responsibilities may increase with the birth and peak well after. She may be required to handle a shoulder dystocia, resuscitate a baby, manually remove a placenta, attend to persistent bleeding, or repair a torn perineum. Because the midwife's participation is weighted to the latter part of the birth process, conserving her energy in early labor is essential. But this is only possible if she methodically attends to her clients' needs for support and information prior to the birth, in the context of prenatal caregiving.

When a mother calls to report increasing uterine activity, keep her on the phone for a few contractions. You can usually gauge the intensity of her labor by how long it takes her to recover after contractions end: a lengthy pause before conversation resumes may be indicative of active labor. If she seems to be going deeper with each contraction, or the pause period before she speaks increases, go and attend her regardless of her (or her partner's) evaluation of labor's intensity.

Patterns of early labor vary dramatically. In general, labors that commence with close-set contractions are shorter than those that begin with contractions every twenty minutes. But early labor can become active very suddenly—explain the signs of this to the mother so she knows when to contact you. If she is able to make a smooth transition from early to active labor on her own, she may very well call too late for you to make it to the birth. In general, *contractions a minute long, coming every five minutes, signal the onset of active labor.*

Physical Assessments and Duties in Early Labor

If you attend the mother in early labor, begin your labor record (see appendix F) with notes on how labor started and how it is progressing. Check the mother's urine for ketones (if present, she should eat something), and get baseline blood pressure, pulse, and temperature assessments. Also palpate the baby for position and descent. Do assessments between contractions so as not to disturb the process. On the other hand, take fetal heart tones during and immediately after a contraction to gauge fetal response (more on this in the next few pages). If you have questions about the strength of contractions, palpate the uterus during a contraction to assess intensity. Chart findings immediately.

Vaginal exams are optional in early labor. Despite the curiosity factor, they should be kept to a minimum. Many midwives observe that the physical and emotional impact of vaginal exams contradicts the mother's need to release down and out—and I agree. Still, do not let your commitment to nonintervention prevent you from doing an exam if the mother needs the information to get focused, or if her contractions get weaker and further apart. Particularly as a beginner, you may check more frequently than is necessary until you learn to read signs of progress in the mother's appearance or behavior.

Your goal with vaginal exams in labor is to be as gentle and undisruptive as possible, while quickly obtaining the necessary information. Use sterile gloves with a lubricant (or later, a squirt of Betadine or other antiseptic if the waters have released, labor is active, and you suspect an arrest). Start the exam the moment a contraction ends and the mother agrees. Begin by **checking dilation**, taking care not to stretch the cervix as you assess, and record in centimeters. (If the mother is 6 cm or more, see additional assessments under "Physical Assessments and Duties during Active Labor" later in this chapter.) Then **note the quality of the cervical opening**: is it stretchy and yielding, or tight rimmed? If it feels inflexible and the mother is barely dilated, you can insert six to eight capsules of evening primrose oil high around the cervix, which should soften it in about twelve hours. If labor is well underway and the tight-rimmed cervix seems to be hindering progress, apply pressure to the rim edge: it should break up under your fingers.[1]

Also **note the placement of the cervix**: is it central, anterior, or posterior? Typically posterior when the head is above −2 station, the cervix swings forward as the baby descends. Next, **check for effacement** by estimating the percentage of cervix that has been drawn up into the lower uterine segment (if the cervix is normally an inch long, a finding of half an inch would mean it is 50 percent effaced). Finish by **estimating the station of the head** (see diagram, page 61), noting how evenly it fills the pelvic cavity.

Interpreting your findings depends on how rapidly labor is progressing and how the mother is responding. At this stage, the most crucial assessments are of effacement, dilation, and station. If the mother is losing control at 2 cm, with cervix just 25 percent effaced, she needs a change of scene to rest, relax, and integrate. Or, if it is late at night, contractions are not very strong, and she is dilated just 2 or 3 cm with baby high in the pelvis (–2 or above), sleep is the best idea for everyone involved.

If early labor is prolonged or there is a lull in progress, consider the baby's position. If posterior (back labor), the head may be deflexed and poorly applied to the cervix, and without adequate pressure on the cervix, contractions will be short, irregular, and progress very slow. This situation may self-correct with time; if not, you may be able to manually reposition the head

when the cervix is more dilated. Meanwhile, encourage rest followed by upright and forward-leaning positions to promote descent. (See "Posterior Arrest" on page 152.)

Active Labor

Sometimes you get the feeling that active labor is knocking at the door, but the mother is not ready to get up and answer. Up to 4 or 5 cm dilation, most women have the power to control the ebb and flow of contractions and, unless labor is precipitous, must deliberately let the forces of labor take over. This is the point of realizing that we don't "do" birth, it "does" us! To move into active labor, a woman must give up ideas of how she thought labor would be; in other words, she must surrender.

If contractions are building in intensity and the mother is fighting against them, difficulties occur.

This is often the case when a woman is rocking and moaning with very little dilation. Forced movement during contractions can exacerbate tension and hinder progress; help the mother by showing her how to be still and let her body "melt" while focusing on the rhythm of her breath. Once she lets go and makes this shift, frantic agitation gives way and endorphins are released.

The endorphins are just one ingredient in the "cocktail of hormones" released by the primitive brain to ease and facilitate the birth process.[2] To benefit from this physiologic boost, we must first turn off the neocortex, our thinking and reasoning aspect. And how is this to be done? Consider factors that stimulate the neocortex: speech, bright light, and a sense of being observed (by others, by oneself, or by technology). Laboring women need a quiet, peaceful, private, and intimate environment.

With this, another critical ingredient in the cocktail is released—oxytocin. Perhaps the best way to frame this is to say that an environment suited for love-making is also perfect for giving birth.

Along the same lines is Ina May Gaskin's "Sphincter Law," which reminds us that cervical, vaginal, and rectal sphincters work best in an atmosphere of privacy: for example, in a room with a locking door where interruption is unlikely or impossible. None of our sphincters can be commanded at will to open or relax, and once in the process of opening, they can close down again with fear or self-consciousness.[3]

Thus once the mother has moved to active labor, your role is to do all you can to not disturb her and to make certain that no one else does. If the atmosphere is right and she is still having difficulties, offer help. But rather than ask questions, use gentle touch

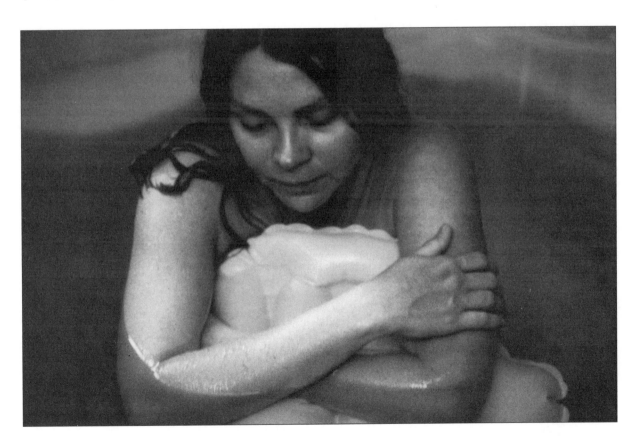

Aseptic Technique and Universal Precautions

Utilization of aseptic technique and universal precautions is crucial to safe midwifery practice. Although these procedures are mentioned throughout the text, this sidebar is meant as a summary and ready reference.

Hand-Washing Techniques

To wash your hands properly, you will need soap, a sink with hot and cold water, a scrub brush with povidone-iodine, and paper towels or a clean hand towel. Proceed as follows:

1. Remove any of your rings with rough surfaces (you may wash under smooth rings). Move your watch several inches up your forearm or remove it.
2. Wet your hands and forearms to the elbows with warm water, taking care not to touch the sink.
3. Add soap to your hands and lather up.
4. Use one hand to wash the other, including the wrist, the forearm, the back of the hand, as well as the fingers and the areas between them.
5. Cleanse under your nails with a nailbrush, fingernail of the other hand, or a nail stick.
6. Repeat for the other hand and arm.
7. Rinse your hands and arms and under the nails, then hold your hands up so water runs down to the elbows.
8. Pat hands and arms dry.
9. Use a dry portion of your towel to turn off the faucet and dispose of the towel appropriately.

These hand-washing techniques should be utilized before and after every examination of mother or baby. If performing a series of exams on different mothers and babies, wash hands between each exam.

Gloving and Ungloving Techniques

1. Wash and dry hands.
2. Peel down the outer wrapper of the glove package.
3. Set inside packet on a clean and dry surface, and open to expose gloves.
4. Pick up a glove at the folded cuff, touching only the inside of the cuff.
5. Pull the glove firmly over hand, being careful not to touch anything with gloved fingers.
6. Put on the second glove, repeating steps 4 and 5, above.
7. Adjust your fingers in the gloves; keep your gloved hands in sight and above your waist.
8. To remove gloves, grasp inside the cuff of one glove, turn inside out and remove, then carefully remove the other glove the same way, taking care not to touch the outside. Dispose of the gloves immediately.

Universal Precautions

The Centers for Disease Control and Prevention (CDC) publish the document *Recommendations for Prevention of HIV Transmission in Health-Care Settings*, which mandates blood and body-fluid precautions with all clients, regardless of bloodborne infection status. The procedures outlined in this document are known as universal precautions. Copies of this document can be obtained from the CDC's National Prevention Information Network at (800) 458-5231.

Here is a summary of universal precautions relevant to midwifery care:

1. Utilize barrier precautions, such as gloves, waterproof gowns or aprons, masks, protective eyewear, and mouthpieces for resuscitation, to prevent exposure of skin and mucous membranes (eyes, nose, and mouth) to blood, amniotic fluid, vaginal secretions, seminal fluid, and breast milk.
2. Make sure to use gloves for blood-collecting procedures, collecting cultures, vaginal exams, assisting delivery, handling of the newborn until he or she is washed and dried, and handling of underpads, clothing, or bed linens wetted with body fluids.

3. If hands or skin are contaminated, they should be washed at once, and a health care provider consulted.

4. All needles and sharp instruments should be disposed of in a puncture-resistant container such as a sharps box—they should never be recapped or otherwise handled after use.

OSHA Guidelines

Midwives in the United States who have employees must meet Occupational Safety and Health Administration (OSHA) regulations to protect employees from health hazards while at work. OSHA provides a list of items you must provide, including gloves of the proper size and in various materials (vinyl for those allergic to latex), masks, eye protection, waterproof aprons, facilities and materials for hand-washing, and first-aid items in case of a needlestick or splatter of body fluids.

Contact your local hazardous waste authority for disposal guidelines and services in your area. Items that must be disposed of according to regulations include sharps needles, tubes with collected blood, disposable products saturated (until dripping) with body fluids, and the placenta (if the mother does not want it). If you are subject to OSHA regulations and fail to comply, you may be fined thousands of dollars. Even if you have no employees, you must still dispose of hazardous items in a manner that will minimize exposure for anyone else who may later handle them, such as garbage collectors or sorters.

and soft words of encouragement. If she is restless, rub her shoulders, her feet, or lower back. Transmit reassurance through your hands; it will ground her and give her focus.

If she complains of nausea, try stimulating the acupressure point known as PC-6, found on the inner wrist. Pressure on this point can also curtail vomiting: apply until she feels better, which may take several minutes. See that she has fresh air and quiet, and have her take small sips of water or tea.

The mother's position can also affect her comfort. Women who labor undisturbed instinctively know what is best, but offer help if indicated. If the baby is low in the pelvis and the mother is experiencing pressure, lying on her side with pillow support or taking a knees-chest position (with butt elevated) may help. If the baby is still high (not engaged), an upright and forward-leaning position will maximize the effects of gravity and evenly distribute pressure on the cervix to keep the contractions coordinate and effective. Walking serves the same purpose. If the baby is really high (−2 or −3 station) and posterior, hands-and-knees with pelvic rocking, or standing and leaning forward with one foot (on the side where the baby's body is lying) on a low stool can encourage rotation. Deep squatting should be avoided, as it closes the inlet.

Positive sensory stimulation via aromatherapy, music, candlelight, or immersion in water can be of great benefit. In fact, once the woman is in active labor, she can get in the tub any time she likes. The water will help relax her voluntary muscles, which in turn will increase blood flow to the uterus and help it work more efficiently. The sense of weightlessness in water can increase her immersion in labor, allowing her to feel it through her entire body rather than just in her cervix or back.

If the mother is partnered, and he or she is eager to get involved but at a loss for what to do, give them privacy so they can find a way to work together. Being in the tub may be enjoyable for both of them, or if they need to be up and active, they might put on some music and dance. Encourage them to be as intimate as they like, and reassure them that if you need to do an assessment—for example, listen to heart tones—you will knock first and wait for their okay.

The above measures work by increasing oxytocin levels. As this happens, the mother's brain waves slow to alpha frequency, as do the brain waves of anyone intimately connecting with her: this is called **entrainment**. Perhaps the easiest way to entrain to a birthing woman is to choose love, running the energy of oxytocin through our bodies and minds. By the same token, we must understand that fear causes the release of adrenaline, not only in us, but also in the mother and others on the birth team. Being calm and loving in attending birth is not sentimental; it is a physiologic necessity!

Sometimes the atmosphere in the birth room becomes stale, and a walk outside is a good idea. Dozing friends and tired birth attendants can be depressing for the laboring woman: those wanting to rest need places to do so away from her. While the mother is up and about, open windows, fluff the bed, light candles, or serve up some food—all good catalysts for stimulating progress.

Physical Assessments and Duties during Active Labor

In terms of physical assessments on the mother, **check her blood pressure** hourly, or every twenty minutes if it was borderline high in pregnancy or is elevated in labor. See that she is well hydrated and urinates hourly. Also encourage her to eat as long as possible, drink fruit juice for a boost of energy, or take an occasional tablespoon of honey to maintain physical and emotional stability.

If labor has been prolonged for any length of time (three hours or so without apparent progress) **do a urinalysis to check for ketones. Ketonuria** indicates that the mother is dipping into her fat reserves for energy. A trace reading is acceptable, but higher levels indicate an electrolyte imbalance and the need for more fluid and calories. Intravenous Ringer's lactate might be given in hospital; at home, replicate

this formula with "labor-aide." Here is the recipe: 1 qt. fluid (water), $1/3$ cup honey, $1/3$ cup lemon juice, $1/2$ teaspoon salt, $1/4$ teaspoon baking soda, and 2 crushed calcium tablets. Better yet, have the mother eat whatever she can; even a piece of toast will help immensely.

Take her pulse every few hours; it should stay within 10 to 15 points of her normal range. If it rises, **check her temperature.** Elevation of both in combination with ketonuria indicates **clinical exhaustion,** threatening to her and the baby in that her blood has become abnormally acidic and less able to carry oxygen. This condition is unusual with homebirth as the mother is free to eat and drink as she desires, but it can become a problem if the mother has been vomiting and is unable to keep anything down. In this case, transport is advisable.

Take fetal heart tones (FHT) every half hour. If anything unusual arises, listen continually until the problem resolves spontaneously or treatment is decided upon. To get a full picture of fetal response, listen through a contraction and for fifteen to thirty seconds after it ends. A slight rise to the peak with a return to baseline by the end is a healthy response, or a **normal acceleration.** Just as our heart rate accelerates with exertion, so should the baby's rate accelerate with the circulatory stress of contractions.

As you must make assessments of increase and decrease quite rapidly, listen in six-second increments and multiply by ten. A baseline above 160 beats per minute (BPM) is termed **tachycardia.** This is cause for concern, as it may indicate fetal infection and/or maternal exhaustion. The baby's baseline must be considered, though: a rise above 160 BPM is serious for a baby with a baseline of 130 BPM, but if the baby's normal rate is 156 BPM, a rise to 170 BPM could be considered within normal range.

Sometimes the heart rate dips and rises dramatically during a contraction, with lows or highs outside normal range, in a pattern we call **variable decelerations (type III).** This is caused by cord

Visual Indication of Dilation

Sacrococcygeal joint

10 cm

7 cm

4 cm

Direction of
purple line

1 cm

Anus

on automatic pilot: the baby's autonomic nervous system cannot adjust its heart rate to the demands of uterine activity. Normal variability is the most important indicator of fetal well-being in labor. You can usually tell if variability is absent without even timing the heartbeat—as one midwife explained, "When the FHT sounds like a metronome, you get an unnatural, creepy sensation." With **late decelerations**, the FHT is normal through the first part of a contraction but *dips down at the peak*, slowly returning to baseline as the contraction ends. This pattern is linked to placental insufficiency and maternal exhaustion; in any case, there is not enough oxygen reaching the baby to see it through a contraction. If the baby is very compromised, the period of deceleration will extend past the end of the contraction: we call this **poor recovery**. If you detect flat baseline or late decelerations during first stage, give the mother oxygen and transport.

As contractions strengthen, it may be difficult to get heart tones throughout, particularly if you are using a fetascope. This is because the uterus contracts so firmly that it obstructs your ability to hear. But you will be able to listen for fifteen to twenty seconds at the beginning and again at the peak when the uterus relaxes, and this is sufficient to identify the baby's response pattern. For example, if you hear the heart rate increase at the beginning of a contraction and then find it at the peak to be noticeably slower, you have detected a late deceleration. Or if you hear it accelerate at the beginning of a contraction and find it at the peak to be slightly higher but gradually returning to baseline, this is a normal acceleration.

At this stage of labor, the midwife's most important task is to pay attention to maternal and fetal well-being while remaining quietly in the background. This does not mean indifference, but it does mean finding the balance between the mother's imperative to make her own way in labor and your need to make responsible assessments and help when help is needed.

entanglement or cord compression, the degree of which varies according to the strength of a contraction and the resulting tension or pressure exerted on the cord. Although not an immediate emergency, fetal distress may ensue if variable decelerations are ignored. The solution is quite simple: have the mother try different positions until she finds one that relieves pressure or traction on the cord and brings the FHT back to normal.

There are several more ominous heart rate patterns: flat baseline with no variability and late decelerations (type II). **Flat baseline** indicates a baby

Also remember that the mother may need to slow down periodically for integration. This is the **plateau phenomenon**, occurring at 4 cm, 7 to 9 cm, or with crowning. *Each of these is a turning point in terms of new sensation.* Four cm marks the challenging shift from control to surrender. At 7 to 9 cm, contractions become so long and overwhelming that new fears arise, which are often compounded by the confusion of bearing-down urges disrupting relaxation. And at crowning, intense stretching of the vagina and perineum marks letting go of baby and pregnancy. Help the mother through a plateau by understanding its nature and giving her freedom to integrate. A plateau of a few hours is fine as long as her condition is good, her morale is high, and the baby is doing well. But if she is holding back or fighting her sensations, encourage emotional release by asking if she is afraid, and if so, what she is afraid of.

As labor intensifies, strictly avoid internal exams. A wonderful technique for estimating dilation, known as the "Purple Line," involves observing the area just above the mother's anus: as she dilates, a dark red/purple line will extend upward and between the cheeks of her buttocks (see "Visual Indication of Dilation" diagram on page 117).[4] Many midwives find this assessment quite reliable. Or, if the mother is upright, you may observe the development of a crease immediately above and parallel to her pubic bone, which will extend fully across her lower abdomen when she is complete.[5] You can also assess descent by palpating the area immediately above the pubic bone: if there is no bulge of head left or you feel shoulders rotating, you can assume the baby is passing through the spines and beginning extension.

Then why do internal exams at all? If the energy of labor feels static (that is, it seems that the mother is dealing with more than a plateau) or your gut tells you it is necessary or the mother insists, do so for additional information. You may be able to identify fetal position and assess degree of flexion in addition to the usual evaluations, which can aid your understanding of the mother's labor pattern and, possibly, allow you to correct a malpresentation so progress can continue.

To **assess position**, the cervix must be dilated to 6 cm or the lower uterine segment must be thin enough to feel the landmarks of the baby's head—**sutures and fontanelles**—through it (see "Fetal Skull" diagram below). Of these, the **sagittal suture** is generally most prominent as it is most subject to molding. As you sweep your fingers across the surface of the head, follow the bony ridge of the suture line and feel for a fontanelle at one end or the other (if the

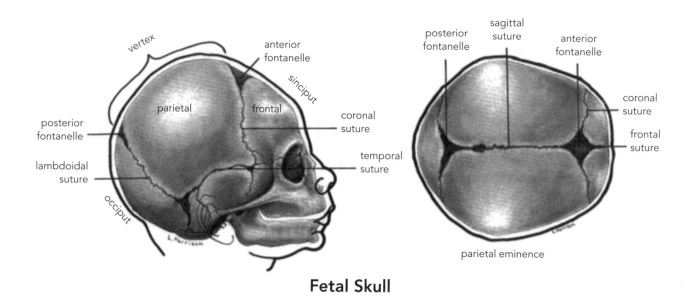

Fetal Skull

Cardinal Spiraling Movements of the Baby during Labor

It is crucial to understand that the baby actively participates in birth; its movements are essential to labor's progress. But we cannot actually see these until the head is emerging, so the movements the baby makes internally have been based more or less on speculation. In *Holistic Midwifery* (vol. 2), Anne Frye presents a compilation of research on this subject, most notably, observations made by x-ray.[6] In light of this, she has revised the standard cardinal movements to the "Cardinal Spiraling Movements of the Baby during Labor" (as follows):

- **Flexion.** Flexion generally occurs as the head enters the pelvic brim. The back curls, too, which helps the head flex as much as possible.

- **Descent.** Descent continues throughout labor due to decreased intrauterine space and pressure exerted by the fundus.

- **Engagement.** As the widest part of the head clears the pelvic inlet and the top reaches the ischial spines, increased pressure on the cervix stimulates labor.

- **Internal rotation of the head.** In response to the oval-shaped musculature of the pelvic floor (not the ischial spines, as was formerly thought), the head rotates to occiput anterior (OA) or occiput posterior (OP), which facilitates passage through the midpelvis.

- **First internal rotation of the body and shoulders.** The shoulders follow the head and enter the pelvis in the transverse diameter.

- **Engagement of the shoulders.** As the head descends through the ischial tuberosities, the shoulders engage in the pelvis.

- **Spinal extension.** As the head moves down, the baby has room to stretch its body so the back becomes less curved.

- **Second internal rotation of the body and shoulders begins.** As the head begins to distend the perineum, the body rotates to the oblique (usually back to whichever side it was on originally) to negotiate the spines and midpelvis.

- **Birth of the head by extension of the lower neck and spine.** Pelvic floor muscles hold the forehead and face back as the head crowns, and extension of the spine further supports flexion. As the head slips past the pubic bone, the perineum retracts around it, and the face is born.

- **Restitution of the head.** The neck untwists as the head realigns with the shoulders.

- **Second internal rotation of the shoulders and chest completed.** The shoulders rotate to the antero-posterior diameter.

- **External rotation of the head.** The head rotates in concert with the shoulders and chest.

- **Birth of the shoulders and delivery.** The anterior shoulder slips under the pubic bone, and then the posterior shoulder is born first, by lateral flexion of the body.

- **Birth of the arms, torso, and legs.** The baby slides out in a spiraling motion. This is especially noticeable in water birth, where warm water may trigger primitive reflexes that cause the baby to actively make a spiraling exit.[7]

baby is term, only one fontanelle can be felt). If the head is flexed, you will feel the **posterior fontanelle**: it is triangular and about the size of a fingernail. The **anterior fontanelle** is diamond shaped and more like a thumbnail; if you feel this, the head is deflexed, which is not uncommon if the baby is posterior. Based on the way the sagittal suture is running and the location of the fontanelles, you can determine the baby's position (in the diagram on the left, the baby is ROT).

Certain situations may prevent you from making this determination, such as a tight forebag, or swelling atop the baby's head known as **caput**. Caput indicates head compression and is associated with extensive molding and possibly, malpresentation: take it as a sign that increased pelvic relaxation is in order. Also note **how the cervix is applied to the head**; it should feel smooth against it. If it is loose like an empty sleeve, the head is either malpresenting or not fitting well into the pelvis (see page 147, "Cephalopelvic Disproportion").

You may not be able to get all this information in one exam. If necessary, check again after the next contraction, using a fresh glove. In terms of dilation, here is a trick of the trade: once the cervix is at 6 cm, we assess dilation not by the size of the opening, *but by how much cervix is left*. The reason for this is simple: the cervix need not dilate to 10 cm to allow the head of a 6 lb. baby to pass through, whereas one weighing 11 lb. will need more than 10 cm space to descend. When we define dilation this way, we focus on how far the mother has to go to be complete. Thus, if you feel 2 cm of cervix before reaching vaginal wall, the mother is dilated to 8 cm; if you feel just 1 cm, she is at 9 cm.

Transition

Labor intensifies sharply as the mother reaches a deeper level of surrender. She is in great concentration and quietude, and her brain waves move to theta frequency: the deepest we can experience in a waking state. Theta is specifically linked to alterations in perception of time, as well as paranormal occurrences. Transition may feel endless when in fact it is of normal length; it is just that contractions are so very intense. This intensity (and that of the theta state) may trigger birth memories in attendants, who may become agitated or may find it hard to stay alert, particularly if labor has been going on for many hours. This is a good time for the mother's main supporter to take a break, and for the midwife and her assistants to spell one another. The mother is usually so immersed in her work that she hardly notices these comings and goings.

To observe women at this time is a privilege; most have a softness about them as their social masks fall away and their deep beauty emerges. The sleepy, faraway place women go between contractions is one of bliss and renewal. Respect this phase of labor for what it is: a peak, out-of-body experience that prepares and rejuvenates the mother for the back-in-the-body, reentry phase of pushing and birthing.

On the other hand, if the baby is pressing on the pelvic floor and prompting an urge to push in conflict with that to relax and finish dilating, the mother may experience transition as a breaking point. Conflicting messages of "Squeeze and bear down" and "No, it hurts, let go and open" can disrupt her concentration. She may become restless and complaining; she may moan, swear, cry out, or lose focus and control. Convey your acceptance, and she may feel easier about expressing awkward or explosive emotions. Watch her body language: her neck shoulders should be loose, and her focus low in her body. She may feel best upright, as maximum pressure on the cervix speeds the last bit of dilation. Or she may choose to stand with contractions, or sit on her heels with knees apart. If she starts to push, don't advise against it. Encourage her to listen to her body and do what it tells her to do.

As for the baby, back-to-back contractions can be very stressful. But with high oxytocin levels, neurotransmitters are calmed and the baby's brain is quieted, protecting it from labor's intensity at this point by deceasing its oxygen needs.[8]

Physical Assessments and Duties in Transition

With a shift in the strength of contractions, **check fetal heart tones** every twenty minutes to see how the baby is adjusting. Remind the mother to drink and urinate. Help her get a sip of tea or water as a contraction ends and before she slips away (bendable straws make this easier). Avoid disrupting her concentration. She may have to lean back slightly for you to obtain clear fetal heart tones with your fetascope, which could disorient her. If you have a Doppler, you may wish to use it now.

The waters often release spontaneously as contractions intensify. What should you do if the water is stained with meconium? This depends on color and consistency: **old meconium** creates yellow-tinged fluid and is evidence of a brief episode of hypoxia earlier in labor or immediately preceding it, whereas **fresh meconium** is particulate, the green/brown fluid (like pea soup) indicating recent or current fetal distress. With fresh meconium, immediately listen to fetal heart tones for several contractions, tracking even the slightest deviation from normal. Unless the baby sounds perfect, with an acceleration response to each and every

contraction, consider transport. Particularly with a first birth, a longer second stage could exacerbate any fetal distress and increase meconium staining.

With the intensity of contractions at this point, continued progress is important. But once again, forgo internal exam—even if the mother says she has to push. Her body is making many adjustments now, she is deep in her primitive brain, and her focus is very much "down and out." If she pushes only at the peak of contractions, or with every other one, she still has some dilating to do.

But if this is a second or subsequent birth, the mother may make a smooth transition to pushing and the baby could come quickly. Prepare by straightening up the room and clearing the floor area (crucial in the event of an emergency). Make sure there are no open flames or lit candles, in case you need to run your oxygen. Remove blankets from the bed and set them aside so they do not get bloodied

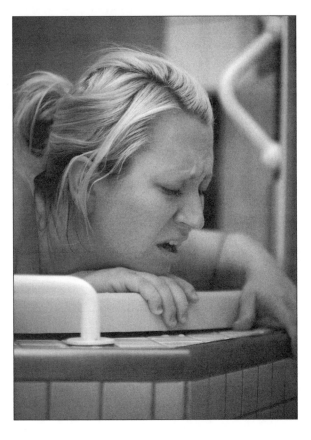
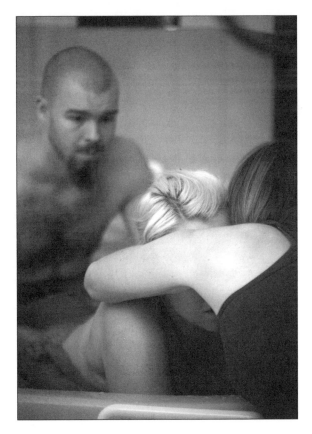

or wet (a good idea even if the birth is to be in the tub, as circumstances may change at the last minute). If you are assisting alone, here is a tip from midwife Tish Demmin: place several strips of masking tape on your pant legs to make notes in case of emergency. This saves you from having to fumble with the chart or worry about getting it dirty.

Scrub up well with Betadine or other soapy antiseptic (see the "Aseptic Technique and Universal Precautions" sidebar for hand-washing techniques). Then set up for the birth: Place your tray of instruments, bulb syringe, DeLee suction device, extra pairs of gloves, and four-by-four sterile pads on a disposable underpad or sterile towel, and if the mother is not birthing in the tub, have a bowl of hot water (with a squirt of Betadine added) ready for perineal compresses. Tear off the tops of the gauze pads so you can reach them without touching the wrapper. Have syringes and medications for controlling hemorrhage (Pitocin and Methergine) readily accessible, and herbal or homeopathic remedies close at hand. Set up your oxygen and resuscitation unit. Also have the mother's supplies (washcloths, baby blankets, and towels) laid out, as well as a bowl for the placenta.

Setting up during transition is a must if labor has moved quickly or the mother's previous births have been precipitous. And one last, critical point—make certain that she urinates before entering second stage. A full bladder can hinder descent and lead to postpartum hemorrhage.

Second Stage

Second stage begins when the cervix is fully dilated. Contractions usually ease from back-to-back to being further apart. If labor has been long or difficult to this point, contractions may stop temporarily, and the mother can take a break or even a nap while her uterus rests and regroups for the work ahead. We call this the **rest-and-be-thankful phase**. This should be encouraged, as stimulating the uterus at

this point can lead to problems later, not the least of which is postpartum hemorrhage.

To best support a mother in second stage, we must understand what is happening physiologically. As pushing urges begin, a surge of adrenaline prompts her to be upright. In following this urge by standing (with her arms around her partner or other assistant) or kneeling and leaning forward, the baby's head swings under the pubic bone and contacts the G-spot. This triggers the opening of the **rhombus of Michaelis**, a kite-shaped area of the lower back with points at the waist, coccyx, and sacroiliac joints, increasing the front-to-back dimensions of the pelvis by several centimeters. As this occurs, the mother will instinctively (1) grab forward for support, (2) spread her knees and let her belly sag, (3) arch her back and wriggle her lower body.[9] This series of movements, termed the **fetus ejection reflex**, brings the baby down.[10] Corroborating this, Sheila Kitzinger relays that Jamaican midwives believe a baby will not be born until the mother "opens her back."[11]

When a mother surrenders to this process, she moves from passive surrender to active participation, often with great excitement. This is the most striking energetic shift in labor as her identity and body

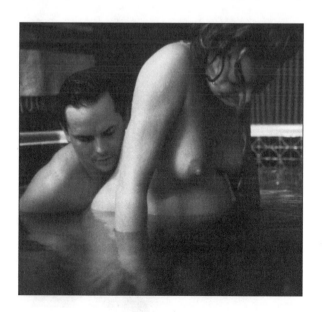

consciousness return anew, accompanied by bursts of energy and enthusiasm. She may even scream or yell as the fetus ejection reflex occurs. (If she struggles or holds back, massage her shoulders to release tension in her chest and throat and encourage her to make sounds. Or if she panics and is shrieking, encourage her to keep breathing: "Breathe the baby out.")

Note the contrast between this and hospital-based conventions of forced, sustained bearing down with prolonged breath-holding, linked to fetal bradycardia and higher rates of episiotomy and neonatal resuscitation.[12] Midwife Jean Sutton relates that in New Zealand hospitals, before forced pushing became the norm, women almost always gave birth side-lying, which at least allowed the back to open.[13] Semi-recumbent or supine positions used in hospital birth today do just the opposite.

If the mother is spontaneous in her pushing, her efforts will vary according to what each contraction demands. She may change position from time to time; bear down hard or not at all; hold her breath involuntarily with a contraction or breathe right through it. Thus she conserves her energy, and the baby gets as much oxygen as possible.

Meanwhile, the baby's adrenaline levels are rising to prepare it for the transition of birth. Head compression intensifies the release of noradrenaline, which helps protect the baby from asphyxia by bringing more blood to its heart, brain, and adrenals as well as the placenta. Endorphin levels rise, too, which offset the potential negative effects of soaring adrenalines. In other words, just as the mother is primed for birth by vaginal stimulation and increased oxytocin, the baby is also stimulated and prepared.

When the head begins to visibly advance with each contraction, the mother may begin to breathe more lightly and rapidly: this helps her ease the head out without tearing. If she is pushing uncontrollably at this point, you might suggest that she breathe the baby out the rest of the way.

Physical Assessments and Duties during Second Stage

Depending on the size of the baby, the mother's dimensions and vaginal muscle tone, and whether this is a first or subsequent birth, second stage can be rather trying for the baby. The greater the head compression, the more likely it is to be compromised. To assess, check the FHT every few contractions, during and immediately after. Once the head is on the pelvic floor, listen with every contraction.

To some extent, **early decelerations (type I)** are normal with head compression, due to stimulation of the vagus nerve. With this pattern, fetal heart tones decelerate as the contraction begins, reach a low point as it peaks, and return to baseline as it ends (in other words, mirror the contraction). Once the head is on the pelvic floor, dips of 10 points are considered normal. Dips of 20 points are not uncommon with perineal dilation, nor are occasional dips to 80 BPM as birth approaches. But persistent dips to 60 BPM or less will soon render the baby hypoxic and so necessitate immediate delivery or transport if the birth is not imminent.

As important as the severity of the dip is recovery as the contraction ends. If recovery is poor, **bradycardia** (FHT consistently below 110 BPM) may result. Mild bradycardia (FHT 109 to 100 BPM) may be acceptable in labor depending on the baby's baseline, but moderate bradycardia (FHT below 100) mandates immediate delivery or transport. With moderate bradycardia or severe early decelerations, give the mother oxygen by mask, 6 liters (L) per minute, as this may improve the baby's condition.

A pattern of early decelerations before the head reaches the pelvic floor is unusual, and may be due to extreme muscle tension linked to a history of sexual abuse (known or unknown). If this is the case, the mother often becomes agitated; if so, let her know she is safe. Suggest an upright position, perhaps standing so she can move freely and feel more in control. Help her with pelvic relaxation techniques, position change, and breathing through contractions. Do not be frightened if she panics; help her move through this.

On the other hand, a prominent sacral vertebra or sharp ischial spine can also cause head compression by reducing the midpelvis. If this is the case, heart tones should return to normal once the head gets past this point. If you suspect disproportion between the baby's head and the mother's pelvis, see page 147, "Cephalopelvic Disproportion," for suggestions.

Variable decelerations may also occur in second stage, indicating **cord nipping**, **pinching**, or **entanglement**. With these conditions, cord sounds (swishing at the same rate as the FHT) may be heard in the vicinity of the baby's torso. If the head is still high, have the mother change position. But if the head is well down, listen constantly and be prepared for cord around the neck.

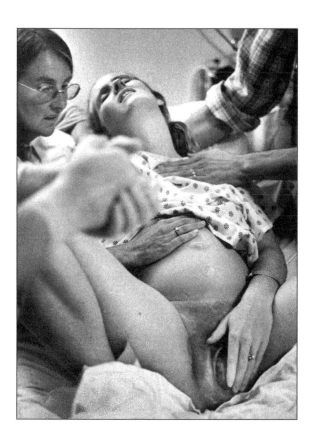

Sometimes the first strong pushes cause the membranes to rupture. If you find the water stained with meconium but heart tones are normal, do not worry. But have your DeLee trap (plastic tubing with a catch compartment) at the ready just in case the baby requires resuscitation (see "Meconium Aspiration" on page 205).

In case of a **prolonged second stage**—more than two hours of urge-to-push contractions—have the mother take ample fluids and tablespoons of honey to boost her energy. If there is no physical impediment to progress and her emotional state is good, be patient. She may become quite tired, though, and so should be encouraged to rest completely between efforts.

If the head is visible but does not advance for a number of contractions, midwife Valerie El Halta suggests the knees-chest position (with butt elevated) to ease pressure on the perineum (it also eases pressure on the head, which may then better accommodate itself to the pelvis). With this, it is not uncommon for the head to suddenly descend to the perineum, and the mother can assume any position she likes for birthing.[14]

At the other end of the spectrum is **precipitous delivery**. Particularly if the mother has given birth several times in short succession, one push may bring the head to the perineum, and the next, the entire baby from head to toe! Far from being the boon it appears, a short, vigorous second stage can cause postpartum hemorrhage. The mother may miss the integration that comes with a longer pushing phase and so may greet her baby in a state of emotional shock. If you anticipate a precipitous delivery, a hands-and-knees or side-lying position may allow second stage to commence more slowly, giving the mother a few moments to assimilate her sensations, and you, a bit more time to prepare for the birth.

Assisting Delivery

The most common birthing positions are hands-and-knees, kneeling with a forward lean, squat/sitting, or standing. The supine position is contrary to the laws of gravity and bad for the baby, due to compression of the maternal vena cava and reduced blood flow to the placenta. Side-lying with one leg raised reduces strain on the perineum (important with a history of deep perineal scarring). Hands-and-knees is particularly good for mothers with big babies or for those who have pushed for a long time with the head low. Squat/sitting (common in water birth) or standing allow the mother to see what is going on and touch or lift the baby up as it is being born.

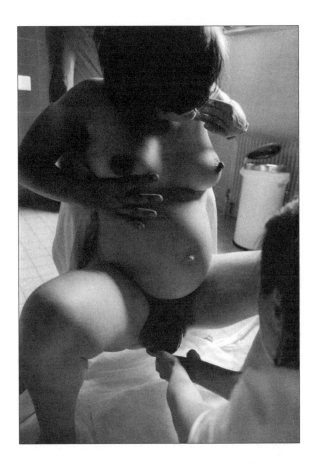

Once the birth is imminent, everyone is in full concentration. No matter how many births a midwife has attended, there is nothing matter-of-fact about witnessing this sacred moment. Every birthing is unique! As a handmaiden to the forces of creation, the midwife's main task is to open and respond with devotion.

One of the hallmarks of midwifery care is trauma-free, tear-free birth. For this, nothing takes the place of the mother's internal awareness in easing her baby out. But if she is struggling with her sensations or involuntarily contracting her outlet muscles, hot compresses to the perineum can help her relax and focus. Hot compresses also stimulate circulation and provide relief from burning at maximum stretch (they are crucial if the perineum blanches at any point). Use sterile gauze pads or clean washcloths soaked in hot water with a squeeze of Betadine or other antiseptic agent. Rarely, pressure of the head on the rectum may cause the mother to pass fecal matter. Wipe with tissue, and if your gauze pad or washcloth becomes contaminated, immediately replace it with another.

It is critical that you continue to assess the FHT. Early decels (decelerations) to 60 BPM or severe bradycardia mean the baby should be born at once. Inform the mother that she must get the baby out quickly and

that you need her full attention and cooperation. Tell her to let go completely and follow your lead on when to push. Sometimes this advice is enough to dissolve the last bit of muscle tension, and the baby births spontaneously with the next contraction.

Otherwise, you may need to do an episiotomy. This is an extreme measure and rarely necessary, but if the mother has tried her best to get the baby out and it is crashing, episiotomy is your only option. As for timing, it should be performed when the perineum is stretched to at least half its capacity with the head not yet crowning. Inform the mother of the situation and obtain her consent. As a contraction ends, position two fingers inside the perineum to protect the head, insert blunt/blunt scissors between them and, as the next contraction brings the head forward, cut straight down about an inch. At this late stage, episiotomy should cause little bleeding, but apply pressure with a gauze pad if necessary. The tissues will be vulnerable to tearing beyond the apex, so give support to the base of the wound. Lidocaine infiltration is optional as the perineum is numb from pressure at this point, but you may wish to infiltrate the area if there is time: see "Suturing Technique" on page 174.

Note that as the baby nears crowning, it may be difficult to get heart tones with a fetascope. Fortunately, this coincides with perineal stretching, which allows you to use the **color of the baby's scalp** as an equally reliable indicator of fetal well-being. As one of my favorite obstetricians said, "I'll hang my hat on pink scalps." Pinkish-blue is good, blue is less favorable, and white-blue is ominous. Rate of venous return when the scalp is gently depressed is also significant. Both these assessments indicate how much oxygen the baby is getting. As long as the baby is doing well, relax and wait for the birth.

Another factor in avoiding tears is **making sure the head is flexed**. If the mother is birthing in an upright position, pelvic floor muscles promote this automatically. But if for some reason the head is not well flexed (anterior fontanelle is at all exposed), apply **counterpressure** to the perineum when crowning begins, holding back the forehead so the smallest possible diameter of the head can pass through. (If the baby is OP, reverse these maneuvers.) Counterpressure is also helpful with a first birth and head crowning rapidly.

If the perineum blanches and a tear appears likely, ask the mother to **push between contractions**: she will feel more relaxed and in control, and your efforts to keep her perineum intact will be more successful without added force from her uterus.

Very rarely, an arrest occurs in the perineal phase. The head appears ready to birth with the next contraction, yet nothing changes for ten, fifteen, even twenty minutes. This may be due to muscle tension associated with sexual abuse, a very big baby, or resistance caused by fear of tearing. In this case, suggest to the mother that she feel her baby's head. This often brings the baby spontaneously. If she doesn't want to touch the baby, arrange a mirror so she can see the head if she wants to. Or have her push between contractions for more control.

As soon as the head is out, do a quick appraisal of color and presence. Note the vitality level of the baby and look for signs of stress: a white-blue head with a clenched mouth usually indicates a baby that needs to be birthed quickly and may need some help getting started. If the mother is in the water, have her get out. Wipe excessive amounts of blood, mucus, or meconium away from the eyes, nose, and mouth. If the baby is gurgling or choking with respiratory efforts, suction with a large rubber ear syringe, squeezing all the air out first. Insert no more than a few inches or you will stimulate the gag reflex at the back of the baby's throat, which can suppress its attempts to breathe.

Suction on the perineum is no longer indicated for meconium; a study of two thousand infants with meconium staining, randomized to be suctioned or not, showed no significant differences in outcome between the two groups, suggesting that meconium aspiration (MAS) occurs not with delivery but with severe distress in utero. But if it appears the baby will need resuscitation (based on color and appearance), suction with a DeLee trap. Be sure that the lid is screwed on tightly so the device will work properly, and then insert the tubing about 4.5 in. into the baby's mouth. Withdraw slowly while sucking sharply and repeatedly (see illustration on "Using the DeLee Mucus Trap"). Tell the mother not to push. If you are still bringing up meconium as you remove the tubing, repeat the procedure.

In this situation, check for **nuchal cord** (umbilical cord around the neck) to rule out one so tightly wrapped that it could be a factor in the baby's compromise. Slip your finger (pad side out) along the back of the baby's neck, and if you find a loop with slack, don't worry. But if the cord is double-looped and very tight, hold the baby's face against the mother's thigh so the body can birth while the head stays stationary: we call this the **somersault maneuver**,

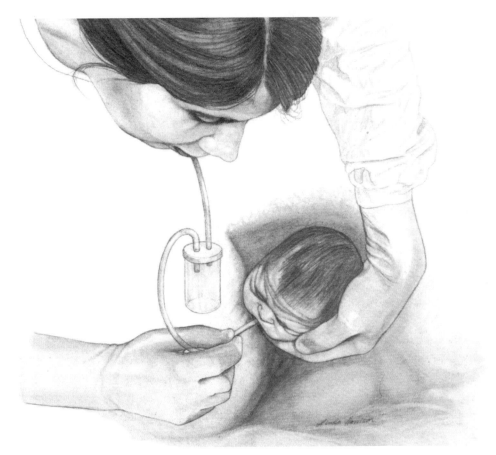

Using the DeLee Mucus Trap

which prevents a tight cord from tightening further. If this does not work, the cord may be entangled around the trunk or legs so that cutting it is your only option. To do this, tell the mother not to push, clamp the cord with two curved hemostats placed 2 or 3 in. apart, cut between them using blunt scissors, and unwind the cord from the neck. As you have cut the baby's oxygen supply, it must be born immediately. Cord cutting on the perineum should be done only in extreme circumstances, as cord blood is vital to newborn stabilization. Researcher David Hutchon explains:

> Clamping the functioning placental circulation results in a dramatic increase in the systemic resistance and an equivalent increase in the afterload of the heart. Even a healthy heart may have difficulty in

recovering from this sudden load. It is uncertain what effect this will have on the homeostatic and regulatory systems of the circulation of the baby. A further effect is hypovolaemia. The pulmonary circulation has to open up at the expense of the rest of the circulation since the blood in the placenta has been blocked off. The hypovolaemia may lead to hypotension and hypoperfusion of vital organs.[15]

Should checking for cord be done routinely? A debate rages on this practice, as it is certainly an intervention and must therefore be justified. Dr. John Stevenson reported that in assisting thousands of births, never once had he cut a nuchal cord, postulating that as the baby descends, so will the uterus, thus the cord will not get any tighter than it is on the perineum.[16] But if the baby is in less than optimal condition (as indicated by heart tones just prior to delivery and/or color of the head at birth), checking makes sense.

If the color of the head is good, there is no need to hurry delivery of the shoulders. In fact, this timeless, sacred moment with baby half in, half out, is a peak experience for the mother. But if the head becomes suffused with blood (turns dark purple), encourage the mother to push the baby out at once (see "Shoulder Dystocia" on page 159).

Who will catch the baby: mother, partner, or midwife? This largely depends on your agreements prior to the birth. If the mother is birthing in water, she will catch her baby if you don't interfere. If she is semireclining or squatting out of water, she can do the same, although she may want some assistance. Take your cues in the moment: if she is not reaching down to catch and her partner is not planning to assist, make your hand into a bowl shape and support the perineum until the top shoulder appears, then lift to a 45-degree angle so the posterior shoulder can birth without causing a tear. Once the shoulders have emerged, encourage the mother to reach down and bring the baby out the rest of the way.

If the mother is birthing hands-and-knees and out of water, you or her partner can reverse the above directions and pass the baby through her legs or help her turn over to receive it. But she may change position at the last minute, lowering her hips so she can birth the baby to the surface beneath her, which she can do by herself.

If the mother is standing or sitting on a birth stool, someone must be beneath her to catch the baby so it doesn't fall. If this is you, make your hand into a bowl shape with fingers toward her pubic bone, palm at perineum. Hold the perineum as the head emerges and until the anterior shoulder appears, then lift the shoulders upward. Have your other hand ready to support the body, but suggest to the mother that she reach down and bring the baby up.

Once the baby is fully exposed to air, cover with three flannel blankets (preferably oven-warmed) to maintain its temperature. The two essentials for

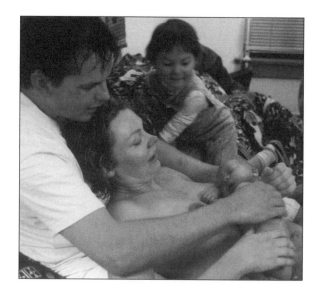

stabilizing the newborn are **warmth** and a **clear airway**, so make certain the baby is breathing well (if so, it will have pinked up nicely). Promptly change the first set of blankets if they are damp. Help the mother get comfortably positioned so that she and the baby can fully relax. See that she is warm and has something sweet to drink, then ease back and give the new family a chance to bond. Keep an eye on the baby's color and responsiveness, and don't forget to do Apgar scores at one and five minutes (see appendix I).

These are the mechanics of spontaneous birthing. But every birth is unique, depending on how passionately the mother has labored, how alert or tired she feels, and how happy she is to be having this baby. For a woman who has really found her way with labor, the moments of giving birth are a time of utter concentration and sensory overload. The pressure of the baby's head on vaginal nerve endings causes an incredible degree of stimulation. And what a release it is as the head is born! Then, as the body surges out, the mother may feel exquisite tracings of her baby's form, followed with waves of relief, ecstasy, and joy. This is orgasmic birth, and it is every woman's birthright.

And yet, as the baby emerges, physical emptiness can come as a shock. It is of the greatest importance that the mother has access to her baby at once, so this shock does not deepen into numbness that can hinder her ability to bond. On the other hand, it may take her some time to bring the baby to breast: women who catch their own babies typically touch and examine before holding the baby close. If the baby is doing well, it is not the midwife's place to touch the baby, let alone put it in the mother's arms. To corroborate, the video *Delivery Self-Attachment* shows several newborns instinctively crawling to the breast and latching onto the nipple without help.[17]

Therapist Raymond Castellino postulates that our rush to put the baby in its mother's arms and get it nursing as soon as possible may come from our own unresolved birth traumas.[18] The mother should be free to receive her baby however she desires.

Third Stage

Once the baby is stable, the mother will want to rest. A drop in adrenaline levels moments after the birth makes it difficult for her to stay upright. Just make sure she is warm enough: if not, adrenaline levels will remain high, which can disrupt placental separation by opposing oxytocin.

The key to a safe and uncomplicated third stage is *watchful observation*. Many a bonding period has been disrupted by an overzealous birth attendant intent on getting the placenta out as soon as possible. Then again, many a hemorrhage has been precipitated by an unattentive attendant missing signs of placental separation. Watchful observation means exactly that: the midwife's participation is indicated by key signs and signals rather than by rote.

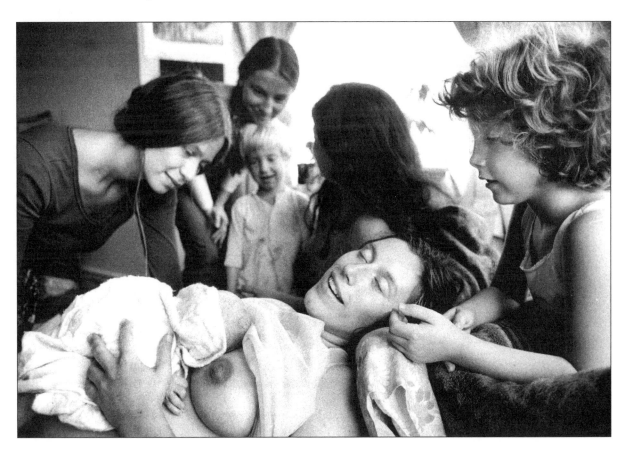

Herbs and Homeopathy during Labor
Shannon Anton, CPM

Most labors do not require the assistance or intervention of herbal or homeopathic allies. However, these remedies used appropriately can make a difference in challenging circumstances, primarily to preserve the precious energy of the laboring woman.

Early Labor

If early labor is intense like transition, with contractions three minutes apart (and especially if the woman is shivering), try homeopathic *cimicifuga 200C*. Labor may seem to diminish but is finding a more effective pattern. This support helps preserve the woman's vital forces. If not yet regular but unrelenting and not given to rest, promote regular contractions with homeopathic *caulophyllum 200C*.

If labor is on again, off again in nature, and especially if the woman is more whiny and clingy than usual or needs a lot of validation that what she feels is emotionally normal, try homeopathic *pulsitilla 200C*.

Active Labor

If the labor is one in which the woman appears to be scrambling away from herself and her contractions, try homeopathic *sepia 200C*. If the cervix is 100 percent effaced, about 3 cm dilated, the os feels like a loop of thread, and labor appears very active or transitional, prepare for the birth as if it was imminent and give homeopathic *gelsimium 200C*. Frequently, the cervix eases open to complete dilation. If the woman is not yet fully dilated but feels an urge to push, give *arnica 200C* to prevent cervical swelling.

If there is a strong urge to push at only 6 to 7 cm dilation, or there is a cervical lip, try homeopathic *sepia 200C* and *arnica 200C*, followed by *sepia 200C* every ten to fifteen minutes. I rely on these remedies absolutely and find them to be among the best-kept secrets of homeopathy for labor.

If dehydration or exhaustion occurs, consider homeopathic *China officinalis* or *Carbo Veg* (Carbo vegitabilis), or *ustilago 200C*. In addition, an enema of warm water and honey or a dose of *royal jelly* taken orally can greatly revive for the short term. Another good remedy is *Essence of Chicken*.

Second Stage

If contractions come less and less often during second stage, give homeopathic *caulophyllum 200C* to keep labor going and prevent postpartum hemorrhage. Each dose should have a noticeable effect. Repeat as necessary to establish a regular pattern of contractions. Homeopathic *aconite* is invaluable for helping women release fear or anxiety in labor. However, not all women benefit from crying or talking out their feelings; some are more internal in their process of release. *Aconite 200C* supports quietude and letting go.

Homeopathic *arnica* is excellent when pain in labor seems out of proportion to the strength of contractions. *Arnica* can also render contractions more regular and effective. If the cervix is unyielding or swollen, *arnica 200C* can alleviate irritation and reduce swelling. I give *arnica 200C* to most mothers in my practice as soon as they feel bearing-down urges in second stage, dosing again as soon as possible after the baby is born. I rarely see swelling of the perineum postpartum. I suggest that my clients continue to take *arnica 30C* for the first few days postpartum for soreness and body fatigue.

The Immediate Postpartum

I rely on two herbs during third stage: *angelica* and *shepherd's purse*. I carry both in tincture form and keep them next to my Pitocin. I find these herbs sufficient to handle most blood loss following birth. In case of sudden, torrential hemorrhage, I give an IM injection of Pitocin as well as the appropriate herb. In some instances, I am sure it was the herb that stopped the bleeding as the Pitocin would not yet have had time to enter the mother's circulation. Nonetheless, with any dramatic blood loss, I give both.

Angelica tincture helps bring the placenta when the wait is prolonged. I give a dropperful under the tongue with a swig of water following. Remind yourself (and the mother) that *angelica* brings the placenta "like an angel." Use also for partial separation of the placenta.

Shepherd's purse tincture is best used after the placenta is out and you are certain it is complete. Because it promotes clotting so expertly, *shepherd's purse* can cause clots to form immediately as the placenta separates, which may lead to uterine distension and additional blood loss. If you are not sure the placenta is complete, use *angelica* to bring on more contractions.

If you are confronted with a vaginal tear that has ruptured a small vessel, apply direct pressure to the tear and give a dropperful of *trillium/birthroot tincture*. *Trillium* constricts small blood vessels and works perfectly in this application. You may find it unnecessary to tie off the vessel with suture.

NEWBORN RESUSCITATION

While CPR and oxygen are essential, homeopathy is always appropriate and sometimes critical in newborn resuscitation. Ifeoma Ikenze, pediatrician and homeopath, taught me most of these applications. In my experience, their potency has been lifesaving. I keep these remedies near my drug box, with red labels to make them easily identifiable. To give a remedy to a newborn, tuck one pellet in the cheek of the baby's mouth. A dose is assimilated by contact with the mucous membranes. In critical situations, repeat the dose in a minute or two. I have never heard of a baby aspirating a homeopathic remedy, even with use of a bag mask unit.

- *Respiratory arrest.* If there are minimal or no respiratory attempts, and the baby looks bluish or feels slightly cold, give *Carbo Veg 1M*.

- *Circulatory collapse.* If the baby is pale as a ghost, floppy, cold, or weak, give *camphora 1M*.

- *Weak heart rate.* If the baby appears lifeless and pale, with no respirations, give *arsenicum 1M*.

- *Mucus or wet lungs.* If the baby is gray-blue, choking or gurgling, if suction does not clear mucus, or if the lungs sound moist and sticky, give *antimonium 200C*. Dose and repeat, along with percussion. Consider blow-by oxygen or steam from the shower. *Aconitum 1M* is for the baby that is struggling and warm, perhaps crying inconsolably as if from a great fright, with rapid heart rate and respirations, and color red, not blue. This baby appears to be shocked by the abruptness of birth and may have difficulty integrating all the stimuli. Another solution is *Rescue Remedy*, given orally or on the soles of the baby's feet. *Arnica 200C* is a wonderful remedy for extreme molding or caput. If the mother chooses not to give vitamin K, homeopathic *arnica* is appropriate.

MATERNAL DIFFICULTY WITH URINATION

A new mother may have difficulty urinating immediately after birth. It's important to make sure she is able to empty her bladder, as a distended bladder can interfere with her uterus staying contracted. Her bladder may also be injured if it becomes too distended. Homeopathic *arnica 200C* can help reduce swelling of the urethra. Also try turning off the lights, dribbling water in the sink, having her put her hands or feet in warm water, or putting a few drops of *peppermint oil* in the toilet before she tries to urinate. Give her privacy but make sure she has support should she become faint. Keep in mind that *peppermint oil* will antidote any homeopathic remedies she has taken. This is usually fine, but if using homeopathic *arnica*, dose again after she's settled back into bed.

FAINTING IN THE IMMEDIATE POSTPARTUM

Giving birth causes incredible changes in a woman's body. Getting to her feet, or even sitting upright, can cause dizziness and fainting. If so, place her in shock position and try this old, reliable, but strange remedy: *burnt hair*. Take a lock of hair from her partner or closest relative present. Burn the hair to cinders and place the crunchy bits under her tongue. Believe it or not, this will stabilize her dramatically: in response to a perceived burn injury, her nervous system will constrict peripheral circulation and send blood flow to vital organs. She may also benefit from a *pinch of the placenta* under the tongue or at the gum line. You may want to try a dose of *Rescue Remedy*. Or, using a soft bristled brush, stroke from her feet to her knees, then from her knees to her hips. *Strong black tea* will also helps normalize circulation.

The umbilical cord should be left alone until it has stopped pulsing. If there is a true knot, loosen it for maximum blood flow. Cord blood stimulates lung function and provides critical perfusion in the baby's brain and other vital organs during its transition to breathing. If this is to be a **lotus birth**, the cord will not be cut at all: placenta and baby will be kept together until the cord dries and detaches. Many midwives feel that keeping the cord intact at least until the placenta has birthed prompts the mother to remember that her work is not yet completed.

If for some reason **the cord is to be cut** before the placenta is birthed, make certain it has stopped pulsing completely by checking the base where it joins the baby. Place one clamp about 4 in. from the mother's vagina, with 4 in. between it and the second clamp. Have her, her partner, or other family member cut between the clamps.

Meanwhile, **watch for signs of placental separation**. If the cord has been cut, keep an eye on the clamp nearest the mother; it will move downward as the placenta detaches, and the cord will appear to lengthen. Also watch for the characteristic gush-flow of placental separation. Rarely, the placenta separates only in the center, with no blood evident at the outlet because margins remain attached. The uterus will increase in size and become boggy, and if the mother continues to bleed, she may go into shock. To rule out concealed separation, rest a hand on the fundus as soon as the baby is out, and recheck often until the placenta delivers. This is known as **guarding the uterus**. Do not massage or prod, as this can result in partial separation and hemorrhage. In other words, no "fundus fiddling": *keep your hand still.*

While teaching a workshop to midwives in London, I encountered an interesting interpretation of physiologic third stage management. Several participants complained that in spite of doing "everything right" (i.e., hands off the woman while waiting for the placenta), several mothers had gone into shock from concealed bleeding. This happened because they were taught that guarding the uterus was too invasive. I

say we let common sense be our guide: guarding the uterus can be done with great subtlety, and the information provided by this procedure can be lifesaving.

Assisting Placental Delivery

The placenta usually delivers twenty to thirty minutes after the birth, although it may take an hour or more. Nine times out of ten, it separates all at once. Typically, the mother shifts her attention from the baby to you, with a look that tells you she is feeling something new. This is an opportune time for her to squat, as delivery of the placenta is best with the mother upright and hunkered down, positioning internal organs in such a way that they compress the fundus and discourage the formation of clots. If the mother is exhausted and does not feel like moving, you can assist her. Encourage her to focus on getting the placenta out.

Standard of care in hospital is to use **controlled cord traction** to remove the placenta. But beware: if the placenta is not separated and you pull on the cord, you run the risk of inverting the uterus (that is, turning it inside out), which could kill the mother. If you wish to use cord traction to assist the placenta out, you must *first make sure it is fully separated* by donning a clean glove and gently following the cord to the cervical os. Only if the placenta is lying behind the cervical opening (or in the vagina) may you use controlled cord traction to remove it.

To perform controlled cord traction, hold the uterus in place by pressing the edge of your nondominant hand in above the pubic bone and up toward the mother's head. As you apply traction to the cord with the other hand, guide the placenta along the L-shaped curve of the birth canal—first down and then out. Do this when the uterus is contracted and with the mother's pushing efforts.

When separation occurs, the membranes may remain adherent until the placenta drops through the cervix and its weight detaches them completely.

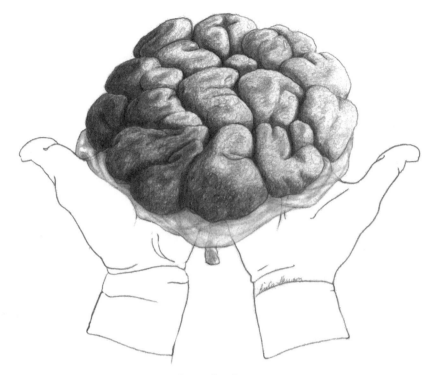

Cotyledons

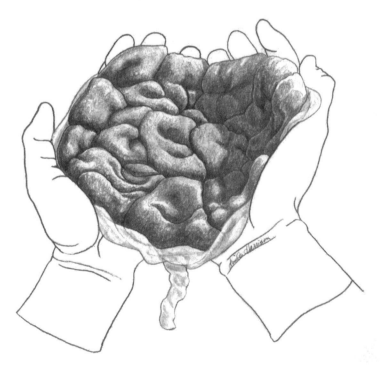

Placenta: Maternal Side

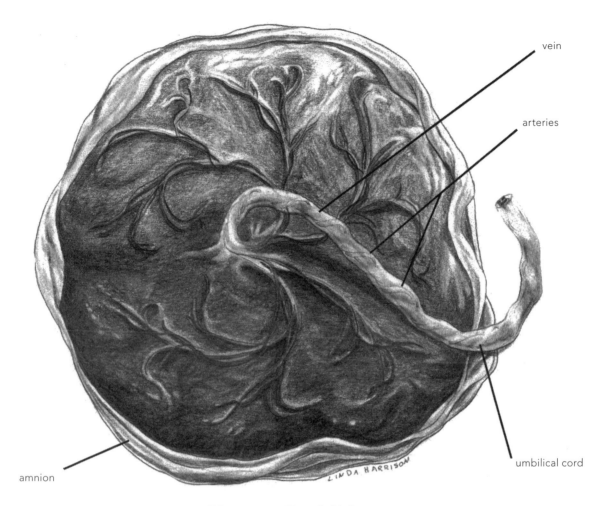

vein

arteries

umbilical cord

amnion

LINDA HARRISON

Placenta: Fetal Side

If the placenta is born but the membranes are lagging (rare if the mother squats), coax them out by holding the placenta with both hands and moving it in a give-and-take motion. Or twist the placenta around repeatedly so that the membranes form a rope, then coax outward. Should the mother happen to be standing when the placenta comes, support it as it delivers, for the membranes may shred or tear if they are not yet separated and the placenta is allowed to fall any distance.

The placenta may deliver either fetal or maternal side first. If the fetal side presents, we call this separation by the **Shultz mechanism**. This correlates to fundal implantation of the placenta with

separation beginning at the center. If the maternal side presents, we call this separation by the **Duncan mechanism**. This correlates to low implantation of the placenta with separation starting at the edges. Students often remember these terms as **shiny Shultz** (glossy membranes) and **dirty Duncan** (meaty maternal side).

As soon as the placenta is out, check immediately to be certain the uterus is well contracted. If not, or if the mother was lying back as she birthed her placenta, give the fundus a few quick squeezes to expel any clots that may have formed. Continue in your watchful observation, keeping an eye out for bleeding and feeling the uterus periodically for firmness. If the uterus feels soft or asymmetrical in shape, or excess bleeding is noted, rub up a good contraction and encourage the mother to nurse the baby. You might also give her several droppers of shepherd's purse and blue cohosh tinctures.

Slow trickle bleeding must be watched very carefully. *Make sure the mother's bladder is not distended*, as this can interfere with the uterus clamping down. Another cause of trickle bleeding is **sequestered clots** (once a clot forms, it will distend the uterus so more bleeding occurs and the clot will get bigger and bigger: more on handling this on page 169, "Fourth stage hemorrhage"). Yet another possibility is **retained placental fragments**: examine the placenta thoroughly to be sure it is complete. You can do this right at the bedside, while you keep watch on the mother.

First examine the **maternal side of the placenta**, which is composed of numerous lobes called **cotyledons**. Start by pulling away any clots, and then hold the placenta in your hands so that it opens convexly, exposing the rents between cotyledons clearly. Next, cup it together and see if the edges of the rents match up and join evenly. Check the edges of the placenta to make sure they blend cleanly into membrane and nothing appears to have been torn away.

Turn the placenta over to **check the fetal side**. If the cord has been cut, **note how many vessels are present**: there should be three holes (two arteries and a vein) visible at the end. If there are only two, the baby may have anomalies not immediately apparent and the pediatrician should be notified. The bluish-white substance in which the vessels are suspended is called **Wharton's jelly**. The amount of this varies, but it should be present at the juncture of the cord and the placenta. If the vessels are suspended in membrane alone, you have discovered a relatively rare **velamentous cord insertion**. Next, note where the cord joins the placenta: **central insertion** (at the center) or **marginal insertion** (at the edge).

Also check for vessels running from the edge of the placenta into the membranes, leading to a separate miniplacenta we call a **succenturiate lobe**. If vessels are found to terminate with a hole in the membranes, the lobe is retained and will cause postpartum hemorrhage. It must be removed manually, either by you or at the hospital (see "Third stage hemorrhage" on page 166 for more on this procedure).

A full bladder, sequestered clots, or retained placental fragments must be dealt with before blood loss can be controlled. Neither uterine massage nor oxytocic drugs/herbs will make a lasting difference with these obstacles in the way. This brings us to the cardinal rule for handling postpartum hemorrhage: *determine the cause of bleeding before taking action.* Should blood begin to flow steadily or in spurts, it is time to resort to emergency measures (see "Fourth stage hemorrhage" on page 169).

If this is a lotus birth, you will need to **preserve the placenta** until the cord separates from the baby. Some midwives suggest sprinkling the placenta with salt, but this tends to make it sticky and difficult to handle; Anne Frye advises rubbing powdered rosemary thoroughly into the maternal surface. The placenta can then be wrapped in an underpad and its own receiving blanket, or bundled in with the baby. Another option, suggested by midwife Gloria Lemay, is to use a thermal lunch bag with zipper closing, placing an ice pack in the bottom, then the placenta, then another ice pack on top with bag zipped up to the corner where cord comes out (keep several alternate ice packs in the freezer).

If the cord has already been cut, use a disposable clamp and recut several inches from the baby's navel. Get the baby and mother warm, cozy, and cleaned up. See that the mother is comfortable: this is so important. If she has slouched down in her pillows, help her into a sitting position with support under each elbow to allow her to cradle the baby more easily. Bring her something to drink, like juice at room temperature or tea with honey to boost her energy. Once she is relaxed and alert, she will nurse and bond more readily, which will help keep her uterus well contracted.

Checking for Tears

Once the placenta is out, and the mother is bonding with her baby, ask her permission to **check for tears**. Discard bloodied underpads beneath her and replace with several fresh ones. If necessary, gently wash her perineum with warm water. Arrange good lighting—a high-intensity lamp works well—then open some sterile gauze, put on sterile gloves, use the gauze to part the labia, and see what you can see. Check for any abrasions, obvious tears around the urethra and perineum, or internal muscle splits at the floor of the vagina (see "Assessment and Repair of Lacerations and Episiotomy" on page 173 for further instructions).

If the mother needs repair, it need not be done immediately. As the new family relaxes and draws closer together, give them privacy, go to the kitchen for a break, and have something to eat or drink. Tell the mother to call out if she feels herself bleeding or feels at all weak or dizzy. Check her uterus and blood flow every ten to fifteen minutes, and bring her more juice and food. As her band of supporters begins to disperse and she is ready to get up, perhaps to go to the bathroom, make sure someone stays with her. Then attend to cleaning up, changing the bed linens, straightening the room, and so on.

Newborn Exam

Because of blood-borne disease risks, wear gloves for the newborn exam unless the baby has been bathed and is free of maternal secretions. Before

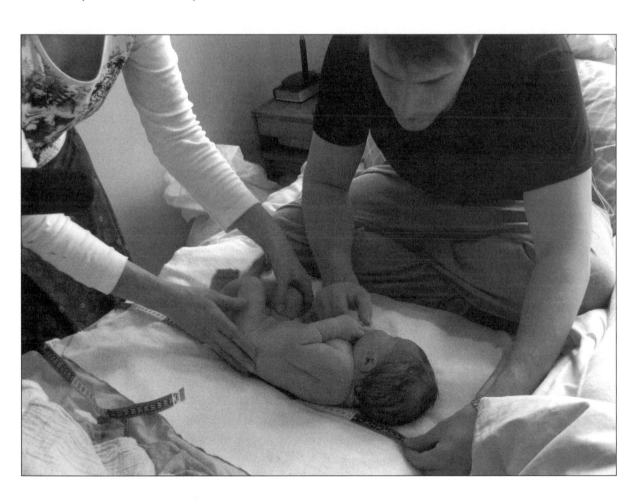

you begin, be sure the mother is ready: she should have had a chance to bond with and nurse the baby at least once. Do the exam on her bed, so she and her partner (or other supporter) can watch. The baby will be more relaxed if the room is warm. If the room is at all cool, place a heating pad on low setting under a towel or several receiving blankets to create a cozy exam surface. Unwrap the baby gradually, exposing just the area to be examined. Explain each step as you move along. You will be checking the baby from head to toe: first the front side, then the back. (See "Newborn Examination" in appendix I.)

Begin by **checking the baby's heartbeat**. Listen closely for anything unusual (such as arrhythmia) and then time it carefully. The heart rate often drops a bit after birth: normal newborn rate is about 110 to 150 BPM. Next, note the **baby's general condition and activity level** with a brief description; for example, "pink, vigorous, strong cry" or "good color and muscle tone, quiet." Any impact the birth may have had on the baby should be noted here, such as trauma during labor or need for resuscitation.

Then **check the skin**. Note the color; a bright-red tone is associated with prematurity and a condition known as **polycythemia** (excess red cells). This finding necessitates a hematocrit and may require referral to a pediatrician, depending on results. Premature babies typically have **lanugo**, or a fine covering of hair, on various areas of the body: make note of amount and location. Also note the amount and location of **vernix**, a creamy white coating more common in babies born early (if present, massage into the baby's skin or it may cause inflammation, particularly in the skin folds). **Desquamation** (peeling skin) is associated with IUGR and postmaturity and is no cause for alarm in and of itself, but it may alert you to more serious problems associated with these conditions (such as dehydration or hypoglycemia). A yellow tinge to the skin indicates **jaundice**, which is abnormal at this stage and should be referred to a pediatrician immediately, as should **circumoral**

cyanosis, a blue ring around the mouth linked to heart, circulatory, or intercranial pathology. Babies of Russian, Mediterranean, African-American, or Hispanic parentage may have **Mongolian spots**, dark-blue splotches at the base of the spine, which are normal and usually vanish in time (you can wait until checking the baby's back to look for these). Also note any **birthmarks** or **hairy moles**.

It is important to **check the head** carefully for **extreme molding**, **bruising**, or **swelling**. All of these indicate some degree of trauma during labor or birth. Normal molding causes the head to assume an elongated shape but usually diminishes within a few hours. **Caput**, or generalized swelling on top of the head, may result from extreme molding. **Cephalhematoma** appears as an abnormal, lump-like swelling confined to a particular area of the head (it does not cross suture lines) and is associated with internal bleeding between the scalp and the skull. Cephalhematoma, bruising, or extreme molding are signs of significant trauma, necessitating administration of vitamin K. A pediatrician should see the baby as soon as possible.

Check the eyes for red spots, **hemorrhages of the sclera** due to pressure in the birth canal. Also look for evidence of **jaundice**: the whites of the eyes should be white, not yellow. Check to see if the **pupils are equal in size and reactivity** when exposed to light. Check for **tracking** by moving your finger back and forth close to the baby's face. Check the **shape** and **spacing of the eyes**, noting any irregularities. With the mother's consent, **instill medication**: erythromycin ointment is standard and effective against both gonorrhea and chlamydia. (Note that this procedure is legally mandated in the United States. The prevalence of chlamydia and its typically asymptomatic presentation in women argue for the routine use of eye prophylaxis, but the mother has the right to refuse. If she declines, she must sign a waiver.)

Next **check the ears, nose**, and **throat (ENT)**. **Check the ears for normal shape** and **reactivity to sound**. Also **note ear placement**: the top of the ear should be level with the corner of the baby's eye. Low-lying ears are associated with kidney problems or other anomalies: if you discover this, have the baby seen immediately. If the baby has not been bathed, you must reglove before **checking the lips and palate** to prevent maternal secretions from entering the baby's mouth. Use your little finger and feel all around the roof of the mouth and back to the throat, making certain the palate is intact. In so doing, you will **stimulate the sucking reflex**: note its strength in the reflexes category. Also **check the frenulum** (under the tongue) for normal length.

Checking the thorax for retractions is usually done right at the time of birth. A positive finding indicates respiratory distress, which should have long since been dealt with. But if the baby had meconium or thick mucus at birth, make sure that there is no lung damage or obstruction. Observe how the chest and stomach move when the baby breathes: ribs and belly should inflate and deflate together. If the skin pulls tight between the ribs, or the chest and the abdomen move in a seesaw fashion, the baby has retractions and should be seen by a pediatrician at once.

Next **check the abdomen**. Occasionally, you will discover an **umbilical hernia**, appearing as a bulge at the base of the cord stump. Contrary to popular belief, this is not caused by a particular method of handling or tying the cord but is a congenital defect that can be remedied by surgery when the child is about two years old. Also **feel the belly for masses or swelling**; all should feel smooth and even (it is easier to do this if you flex the baby's knees toward the abdomen with one hand while checking with the other). Lastly, listen with a stethoscope for the **presence of bowel sounds**.

Check femoral pulses by lightly placing fingertips (both index fingers) in the left and right groin areas. You should feel pulsing on each side, and the pulses should match (charted as symmetrical). If not, the baby may have a congenital heart problem: contact the pediatrician immediately. (If you have

trouble performing this evaluation, you may be compressing the vessels so much that you can't feel the pulse. Try using a lighter touch.)

Check genitals carefully to be sure that all essential parts and openings are present. Girls frequently have **vaginal mucus**, which may be blood tinged due to high hormone levels. Boys should be **checked to see that both testes are descended**. Do this by placing your finger at the top of one side of the scrotum to close off the inguinal canal, feel carefully for the testicle, and repeat on the other side. If the scrotum is edematous and difficult to palpate, shine a flashlight against it to visualize the testicles. This is particularly important if the baby was breech, as **torsion of the scrotum** may cause testicles to be lost unless the problem is detected within several hours of the birth.

Several reflexes have usually been demonstrated by now: sucking with palate check and swallowing with breastfeeding. To verify the **palmar (or grasp) reflex**, have the baby grab your little fingers: you should be able to lift its back slightly off the bed. Next, hold the baby to face you, support both back and head, and tip it slowly backward to activate the **Moro (or startle) reflex**: the arms and hands should extend evenly. Also check **Babinski's reflex** by stroking a foot from bottom to top with your thumb: the toes should fan out. Then place your thumb at the base of the toes: they should curl as you activate the **plantar reflex**. You can also check the **stepping reflex** by holding the baby in a standing position: it should take a few steps forward. The presence of normal reflexes indicates neurological health and maturity.

Now turn the baby over and **closely examine the spine**. Note **Mongolian spots** and record with other findings regarding the skin. **Check for straightness and complete fusion**, looking for any **sinuses** (openings), especially in the sacral area. Even the tiniest opening indicates a condition called **spina bifida**, which can lead to major infections like meningitis: report immediately to the pediatrician. If the opening is large and there is a protrusion through it, the condition is more severe. Cover with sterile gauze soaked in warm saline, notify the pediatrician, and transport.

Then **check the lungs**, listening through the baby's back. Position your stethoscope near each shoulder, and then at midback on either side of the spine. Count respirations and chart. The lungs should sound clear, with air resonating as if in a hollow chamber with no rattling or scratchy noises. This is particularly important if there was meconium: if so, and the baby's lungs sound obstructed, try percussion and steam (see "Meconium Aspiration" in chapter 6), or contact the pediatrician immediately.

Check the anus by observation: it is not necessary to insert a thermometer to check for patency. Even if the baby has not passed meconium, it will often have a plug visible at the opening: this is also proof of patency.

Of great interest to parents are the baby's weight and measurements. **Measure the head circumference** at the widest point, from occiput to frontal bone, and record in centimeters (the average is 34 to 37 cm). Then **measure the chest** across the nipple line: the difference between head and chest should be no more than a few centimeters. If the head is much larger, there may be an abnormal amount of fluid in the brain, which should be checked immediately by a pediatrician. If the chest measurement is the same or larger than that of the head, and the baby is over 9 lbs., the mother may have had some degree of glucose intolerance and the baby should be checked for hypoglycemia.

Measure the baby's length by setting the tape alongside its body with top edge level with the tip of the head, then stretch the leg out and measure at the heel. Chart in both centimeters and inches. To **weigh the baby**, use either a standard baby scale or the more convenient hanging type in which the baby is temporarily suspended in a stork-style bundle. Don't forget to subtract the weight of the blankets. Chart in both pounds and grams.

Finish by **checking the extremities**. Begin by **counting fingers and toes**, **noting uniform length**, and **checking for webbing**. Note symmetry of muscle tone in the arms (largely accomplished already by checking the Moro reflex). This is crucial if there was shoulder dystocia, which could cause injury to the clavicles or nerve damage known as **Erb's palsy**. **Check each clavicle** by palpating from the sternum to the shoulder: if there is a fracture, you will note an unmistakable crinkling sensation called **crepitus**. Administer vitamin K and contact the pediatrician.

Finally, **check the hips** by doing the "click test." Rotate the legs firmly in their sockets while your fingers rest on the hip joints and feel for clicks that might indicate dislocation. Then flex the knees to the abdomen, and as you press them gently, feel once more for any clicking or unnatural movement of bone slipping out of the socket. If you find anything unusual, turn the baby over again and **check hip creases from the backside**. These should be symmetrical; if not, contact the pediatrician.

Wrap the baby in dry blankets. If it is content, this may be a good time for the mother's partner or other supporter to hold it while she takes a shower or stretches her legs a bit.

Postpartum Watch

Your postpartum watch should last at least two hours, or until the mother's blood pressure, pulse, temperature, and lochia flow are within normal range for at least an hour. She should urinate before you go and have something to eat and drink. Make sure she has nursed successfully and understands that even though her milk will not come in for a few days, colostrum is sufficient for the baby's needs until then. Go over your postpartum instructions carefully (see appendix K), making sure that everything is clear and that the mother understands normal and abnormal newborn behavior. Leave copies of the "Birth Record" (appendix H) and "Newborn

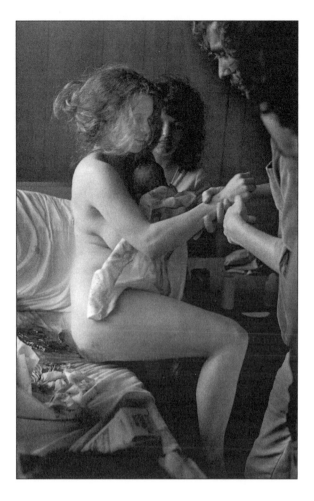

Notes

1. Anne Frye, *Holistic Midwifery*, vol. 2 (Portland, OR: Labrys Press, 2004).
2. Michel Odent, "The Dehumanization of Birth," lecture, California Association of Midwives Conference, Santa Rosa, CA, 2003.
3. Ina May Gaskin, *Ina May's Guide to Childbirth* (New York: Bantam Books, 2003), 170.
4. D. L. Byrne and D. K. Edmunds, "Clinical Methods for Evaluating Progress in the First Stage of Labour," *Lancet* 335, no. 8681 (1997): 122.
5. Frye, *Holistic Midwifery*, vol. 2.
6. Kyle Steele and Carl Javert, "The Mechanism of Labor for Transverse Positions of the Vertex," *Surgery, Gynecology and Obstetrics* 74, no. 4 (October 1942): 477.
7. Frye, *Holistic Midwifery*, vol. 2.
8. Roman Tyzio, Rosa Cossart, Ilgam Khalilov, Alfonso Represa, Yehezkel Ben-Ari, and Rustem Khazipov, "Switch in GABA Signaling in the Fetal Brain during Delivery," *Science* 13 (July 2007): 194.
9. Jean Sutton, "Birth without Active Pushing: A Physiological Second Stage of Labor," in *Midwifery: Best Practice*, ed. Sara Wickham (London: Elsevier Science Limited, 2003), 91.
10. Michel Odent, "The Fetus Ejection Reflex," *Birth* 14, no. 2 (1987): 104–05.
11. Sheila Kitzinger, *Ourselves As Mothers* (New York: Bantam Books, 1993).
12. Roberto Caldeyro-Barcia, "The Influence of Maternal Bearing-Down Efforts during Second Stage on Fetal Well-Being." *Birth and the Family Journal* 6, no. 1 (March 1979): 17–21.
13. Sutton, "Birth without Active Pushing," 90.
14. Gloria Lemay, "Pushing for First-Time Moms," *Midwifery Today* 55 (Autumn 2000): 9–11.
15. David Hutchon, "A View on Why Immediate Cord Clamping Must Cease in Routine Obstetric Delivery," *The Obstetrician & Gynaecologist* 10 (April 2008): 112–16.
16. John Stevenson, "Lessons from a Homebirth Practice," *The Birthkit* 39: Autumn 2003.
17. L. Righard and Kittie Frantz, "Delivery Self Attachment" (video), Geddes Productions: Sunland, CA, 1995, based on the study by M. Alade and L. Righard, "Effect of Delivery Room Routines on Success of First Breast-Feed," *Lancet* 336 (1990): 1105–07.
18. Raymond Castellino, private conversation, April 2004.

Examination" (appendix I) for the pediatrician. Encourage her to call anytime, about anything, at any hour. If she seems at all uncomfortable with you leaving, wait a little longer.

You should also be sure that you are in stable condition before going. Particularly after a long or complicated birth, you may be absolutely exhausted and should rest and relax with your assistant or midwifery partner before attempting to drive. A midwife from my area had the great misfortune of falling asleep at the wheel on her way home from a birth: her car hit a tree, and she sustained major injuries. Those first few hours after the birth fly by: make a habit of getting something to drink or eat immediately so you are ready to go when it is time.

CHAPTER 5

Complications in Labor

Complications arising in labor present the midwife with challenges and tests. Prenatal problems are not so pressing as there is usually time to consider, consult, and reevaluate from visit to visit. But in labor, decisions must be made both carefully and quickly.

Close and vigilant attention is key to detecting complications at their inception. When complications develop, keep an overview of the situation as you pinpoint the area on which to focus a remedy. Sensitivity and objectivity must be combined to determine whether treatment is proving effective. Never forget that nearly all interventions have side effects, which must be tracked throughout labor and the postpartum period. Nonetheless, commitment to the principle of nonintervention cannot be used to excuse hesitation in complicated circumstances. There is a delicate balance between the mother's right to give birth undisturbed, to proceed at her own pace and find her own way, and the midwife's responsibility to use her knowledge and skill so that stamina and safety are maintained to the end.

Maternal emotions must always be factored in. Sometimes emotional problems portend physical danger, yet there is still safe leeway for turning the tide and getting labor back on course again. By the same token, emotional breakthroughs can render progress that is nothing short of miraculous.

The art of handling complications may be approached as follows:

1. Determine the possible causes of the complication and rule them out one by one to reach a diagnosis.

2. Test your diagnosis through further observation plus discussion with the mother and perhaps a midwife colleague.

3. Modify your diagnosis if need be, formulate a remedy with the mother's input (if time permits), and implement it.

4. Follow up with close and careful checks on vital signs and progress to determine effectiveness and results.

5. Watch carefully for any side effects and reevaluate as indicated.

It helps tremendously if the entire birthing team is intent on working together. If the mother seems noncommittal despite your best efforts to address the problem, perhaps the birth is not meant to happen at home. Waiting in limbo is dissipating, particularly when the forces of labor are struggling to move ahead. If the mother concurs that transport is a good idea, it should occur as quickly as possible.

Sometimes a mother requests transport, not from fear or desperation but because she senses that something is wrong. Never try to dissuade her from her instincts in this regard.

Transport is a complication in itself, especially if labor has been long and everyone is tired. The mother may need help getting dressed, packing a bag, making child care arrangements (if necessary), and notifying key friends or relatives. Her partner (if applicable) may be moved to tears out of frustration, sadness for the loss of their homebirth dream, or from sheer exhaustion. Meanwhile, you must contact the obstetrician and hospital to arrange for admission. Trying to be clear headed and articulate while stressed or suffering from sleep deprivation may be quite a challenge. Have your chart in order so questions from hospital personnel can be kept to a minimum when you arrive (update in the car if necessary). A one-page transport summary sheet is also helpful (see "Transport Record from Home Delivery" in appendix G).

When life-threatening emergencies arise, the focus is on survival, with little or no time for integration. But in the majority of transport situations, you have opportunity to give reassurance, support, and hope to the mother and her partner on the way to the hospital. This is definitely one of the greatest services a midwife can render.

Prolonged Labor and Maternal Exhaustion

To address this subject, we must first consider these questions:

1. How do we define prolonged labor?
2. What is the difference between a labor that is simply long and one that is prolonged?
3. And how is length relevant to labor's normalcy?

Concern with labor's length began in hospital, where a prompt turnover of beds was of practical and financial concern. Next came practitioner impatience: doctors with overbusy schedules or better things to do than wait around for women to give birth wanted to define how long was too long. And then physician Emanuel Friedman developed the **Friedman Curve**, which, *based on averages*, defined normal length and progress for first and subsequent labors. According to his research, first labors averaged 6.4 hours in the early phase, 4.6 hours in the active phase, and 1.1 hours in second stage: with subsequent pregnancies, these figures are cut by 50 percent. Dilation averaged 1 cm per hour for first labors and 2 cm per hour for subsequent births.[1]

Needless to say, Friedman's work has been widely misinterpreted and misused. For example, a mother birthing in the hospital and working through a perfectly normal plateau phase, or experiencing a lull in progress due to lack of sleep or nourishment, or whose large or posterior baby needs extra time to descend, will likely be diagnosed with "failure to progress." Many unnecessary cesareans are performed on this basis, even though several studies show average labor lengths double those of Friedman's.[2]

From the midwife's point of view, labor is prolonged when clinical exhaustion threatens. With a commitment to a minimum of vaginal exams, it is critical to stay alert and aware, watching for contractions that are monotonous in rhythm, labor energy that feels static instead of dynamic, or a mother who

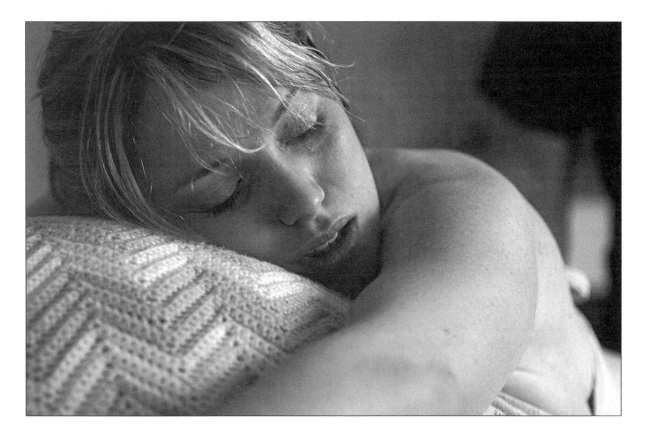

is stressed and disconnected rather than passionately engaged. The concern is less a matter of labor's length than of energy-sapping arrests in the process.

Arrests in labor can have a number of causes, both physical and emotional. Often the two are interwoven, and you must sort through numerous factors to get to the central issue. For example, if you are assisting a mother with a large, unengaged posterior baby, it is not uncommon to see an arrest of progress at 6 cm due to head deflexion impeding descent and resulting in inadequate cervical stimulation. The mother may also be fearful of labor or may become frustrated and impatient as time goes by, but in this case, no amount of counseling or encouragement can override fetal malpresentation as the principal cause of arrest.

In the normal course of labor, a long early phase is no cause for concern if the mother is handling contractions well and continues to eat, rest, and sleep.

This may sound simple, but all too often mothers become so reactive to early contractions that this critical balance is lost. If the mother is not sleeping, recommend hops tincture or a glass of wine. Women birthing in hospital get little or no advice in this respect and typically arrive at the labor ward utterly exhausted and only a few centimeters dilated.

In general, early labor should not interfere with normal life. If the mother is well rested, encourage her to go for a walk, to a movie, or to visit friends. If she is only a few centimeters dilated and is panting, groaning, and plugging away, she needs help winding down so she can conserve energy for the hard work ahead.

Occasionally, you may have the confusing case of a mother who appears to be in active labor, with contractions coming every five minutes, lasting up to a minute. But after a few hours, contractions taper off, and internal exam reveals her to be only 2 or

3 cm dilated. Women who are strongly athletic or highly intellectual by nature tend to this pattern, based on the inability (at least at this juncture) to let go and cross into the active phase. Uterine inertia often results, with a meal and some sleep the best solution. Labor will soon start up again—and dilation may take place quite quickly.

I attended a birth like this early in my practice: for twelve hours (mostly at night) the mother walked, was in and out of the shower, drank labor-promoting teas, and so on. Then labor stopped completely, and it felt odd (but liberating) to be sitting around the following afternoon, sharing a glass of champagne (we went ahead and opened it) and relaxing together. My partner and I decided to go home but after six hours were called back to find the mother dilated to 7 cm, handling labor beautifully and birthing shortly thereafter. When we asked her what had happened, she replied, "Well, after you left we got in bed and talked a lot, fell asleep, and then it just started up again really strong."

Up to 5 cm dilation, contractions may come and go, and the plateau from early to active labor may last for quite some time. Just remember that *a plateau is not an arrest.* Arrests occur only when a woman is at least 6 cm dilated: from this point, the uterus is hard at work and tends to persist regardless of maternal tension. If the mother resists the forces of labor in the active phase, she may become **clinically exhausted** long before her uterus takes a break. This condition is also known as **ketoacidosis**: the affected mother's blood becomes abnormally acidic and less able to carry oxygen. Unless this condition is reversed, fetal distress will result. Clinical exhaustion is diagnosed with a combination of **ketonuria**, **elevated temperature**, and **elevated pulse**.

If signs of clinical exhaustion manifest, remedial measures of nutrition and hydration should be implemented immediately (see the recipe for "labor-aide," in section "Physical Assessments and Duties during Active Labor" on page 116). The baby must also be monitored more closely for signs of distress,

unless labor has tapered off and the mother is resting. This brings us to the cardinal rule: *if labor slows down or stops, do not stimulate it*! Diminishing contractions indicate a uterus that is fatigued; for it to rebound, the mother must be encouraged to eat, drink, and rest. If the uterus is forced to contract while trying to recover its strength, prolonged second stage, fetal distress, and postpartum hemorrhage will likely result.

Have the mother eat some toast, yogurt, or anything that appeals to her. Then give her a glass of wine, shot of brandy, or dropperful of hops tincture in juice or tea to help her rest. Typically, women are not able to sleep at this stage of labor but can rest deeply even if light contractions persist.

When an arrest occurs, treating the symptoms will not rectify the situation: you must determine the cause. Another reason arrest typically occurs at 6 cm is that the cervix can dilate this far without pressure from the presenting part, but from this point on, the head (or butt) dilates the cervix the rest of the way. *The presenting part must press on the cervix uniformly for labor to intensify*. Rule out any impediments to this with a thorough internal exam. Check the position and attitude of the head very carefully. If posterior, it may be deflexed, increasing its circumference and resulting in asymmetric cervical pressure. If this is the case, or if the baby is large for the mother's dimensions, asynclitism may also be noted.

Asynclitism typically occurs when the baby has trouble negotiating the pelvic inlet and compensates by leading with one side of its head only. With internal exam, the sagittal suture will be high or low in the cervical opening, rather than bisecting it (see illustration "Fetal Asynclitism" on page 149). Asynclitism may signal true cephalopelvic disproportion (CPD); if not, its occurrence often causes relative CPD (see next section). But it may also occur with a baby small for the mother's dimensions, particularly with polyhydramnios and ROM, as the baby may then descend rapidly and settle in a cocked position.

Asynclitism also causes asymmetrical pressure on the cervix.

Another cause for delay may be **cervical edema**. If noted at 6 cm, with the cervix not well applied to the head, rule out the malpresentations just cited. Prone positions can also lead to edema by compressing vaginal tissues adjacent to the baby's head, impairing venous return from the cervix. If edema occurs around 8 cm and the mother has been favoring prone positions, the cervix should thin out rapidly once she is upright. On the other hand, if she has been upright and labor has been particularly painful or intense, edema may be better alleviated by having her take a knees-chest position (with butt elevated).

Sometimes a **cervical lip** is the last obstacle to complete dilation. This is swelling of the anterior portion of the cervix only (the rest being fully retracted), occurring when the head pinches it against the pubic bone. It is most common with persistent posterior babies, due to deflexion. Try repositioning the mother as just described. For a stubborn lip, place ice in the finger of a sterile glove and hold against the cervix. Once the swelling is reduced, or if the lip is soft, you may try to push it back. To do so, position your fingers at the edge of the lip and with the next contraction, push the lip over the baby's head as it descends. Hold it behind the pubic bone, and then have the mother bear down. If the lip is gone, you've succeeded; if not, try again. This may be somewhat painful for the mother: it helps if she is in a semi-squat. It is okay to exert a bit of pressure with this maneuver, but never force the cervix or it may tear.

Occasionally, **tense membranes** or a **tight fore-bag** retard descent and cause an arrest in progress, typically at 7 or 8 cm dilation. You may wish to perform **artificial rupture of the membranes (AROM)**, but first, make sure the head is low enough in the pelvis to prevent cord prolapse (as a rule, it must be at 0 station, but a larger head may fill the pelvis snugly at −1 station). If the head is too high for AROM, you must wait for it to descend. Be forewarned, this may take hours, so be sure the mother is relaxed and active, drinks plenty of water, takes tablespoons of honey, eats if possible, and keeps her bladder empty.

To perform AROM, don a sterile glove, squirt a bit of sterile gel or Betadine (provided the mother is not allergic to iodine) over your fingers, and splint an amnihook between them, keeping the tip protected. As a contraction ends, and with mother propped upright, insert your fingers and push the hook to the bag, pull down on the handle with your other hand to lift the tip, and pull back toward you to snag the membranes. Carefully draw the hook back between your fingertips, and remove your hand slowly. Be sure to take heart tones immediately afterward, and chart.

Do not perform AROM in any other circumstances than cited above. I once made the mistake of doing so with a mother only 4 cm dilated, hoping that descent and pressure on the cervix would stimulate progress. This decision was made after thirty-eight hours of erratic contractions, with another twelve hours of regular, moderately strong ones. A tense bag of waters was forming, and the baby's head (which was small and engaged) was not well applied to the cervix. The mother had a generous pelvis with no anomalies, so I reasoned the forebag was holding the baby up. Surprisingly enough, rupturing the membranes did not bring descent. The real problem was that the mother was still early enough in labor to have active control; she used her excellent abdominal and vaginal vault muscles to hold the baby up so she would feel less pressure on her back. The result of this intervention was **prolonged rupture of the membranes (PROM)**, which, according to the standard of the day, necessitated transport and Pitocin augmentation.

Second stage arrests (addressed at some length in chapter 4) are far less common than those occurring in first stage. Here, too, Friedman's Curve has created false notions of normal progress, in that descent is expected within a certain time frame and in consistent increments. But progress in second stage does not take place in a steady stream any more than it does in first stage. Instead, the baby often stays at +1 or

+2 station for a while as its head molds to the vaginal musculature, and then it may descend quite rapidly. But if you know the mother to have a narrow pubic arch, close-set tuberosities, or a prominent coccyx, see cephalopelvic disproportion in the next section.

If you have determined that there are no physical obstacles impeding progress, consider psychological and environmental dynamics. There are many factors that might cause a mother to resist opening up or letting the baby down. By now, problems revealed at prenatal visits should have given specific clues as to what has gone awry, but here is a general list of possibilities:

- Mother is not feeling enough love, communication, or faith from her partner. (If mother is not partnered, she may have trust/communication issues with her primary helper.)

- Partner or primary helper is unable or unwilling to let go due to inhibitions with self or history with the mother.

- Worries about becoming a parent arise: for the mother, loss of personal attention she enjoyed during pregnancy; for her partner, moving from limbo to new levels of responsibility.

- Mother's awareness of sexual dysfunction, including unknown history of sexual abuse, awakens with the physical-emotional intensity of labor.

- Environment is disruptive: too many people, too many comings and goings, no sense of privacy, or a family friend or relative who is undermining or threatening the mother in some way.

- Baby is feeling hesitant, uncertain of mother's/partner's feelings or its own about being born.

These problems are largely resolved by facilitating intimacy between the mother, her partner or helper, and the baby. Demonstrate helpful techniques of touch and massage during contractions, running oxytocin as you do so. Encourage the mother (and partner, if applicable) to talk to the baby.

As for the environment, the labor room may need to be freshened up (see suggestions in chapter 4). Especially with challenging circumstances, the mother's need for privacy is paramount; explain to supporters that it may be many hours before the birth takes place, and that now is the best time for a break.

In fact, many women want complete privacy in labor but cannot say so (accustomed as we are to accommodating the needs and wishes of others, we may equate the desire to be alone with selfishness or rudeness). Make the suggestion and see how the mother responds.

Sometimes a change of scene is in order. If active labor is just beginning, the mother may benefit from a walk to a nearby park, beach, or wooded area. You or your assistant should accompany her, and someone on the birth team should straighten up the room; remake the bed; bring in fresh tea, water, flowers; and so on while she is out.

Be aware, though, that emotional release is a major catalyst to progress. In the absence of physical impediments, a mother who surrenders all psychological resistance can dilate very rapidly. I have seen a number of women go from 5 cm to complete in less than an hour, spilling out fear and anxiety one minute, easing into sensation the next, and suddenly feeling like pushing. Don't take the mother out for a walk if you sense this kind of release is about to happen!

One of my students told of a birth with a very long second stage; the mother had pushed for more than three hours and was becoming exhausted when the midwives began talking to the baby, telling it to come out. At this, the father broke down and said that it was his fault, his ambivalence, and the baby was born shortly thereafter.

History of sexual abuse (known or unknown) is most likely to manifest in response to pressure on the pelvic floor, especially with rapid descent. The reaction is unmistakable: the mother literally draws herself upward as if trying to get away and is completely panic stricken. Do what you can to soothe her, perhaps get her in water if she is not already, suggest that she place her hand over her vagina (making clear that nothing is entering from outside and that she is in charge) or that she look in a mirror as the head begins to show. Don't be thrown by the intensity of her reaction. Stay strong, stay open, and let her know she is safe.

With any emotionally based arrest, continue to check for signs of clinical exhaustion while encouraging the mother to eat and drink. If she becomes depleted, emotional arrest can quickly deteriorate into physical pathology. Make sure she urinates frequently, as a full bladder can hinder relaxation and descent. Take blood pressure and fetal heart tones regularly, as emotional tension can impact both. Be frank with her (and her partner, if applicable) about any counterproductive behaviors. If physical symptoms of emotional distress begin to manifest, discuss the possibility of transport. This may elicit determination or despair, but a decision must be made promptly. Give the mother a bit of time to consider her options, be encouraging but firm, and the appropriate course of action will soon become evident.

Cephalopelvic Disproportion

The term cephalopelvic disproportion is applied in labor when the fetal head cannot readily pass through the mother's pelvis. When the head is presenting well but is truly too large for the mother's dimensions, we call this **true CPD** (incidence is less than 1 percent). When the head could pass through the pelvis but malpresentation prevents it from doing so, we call this **relative CPD.**

An example of relative CPD is found in the posterior baby (for whom the mother has plenty of room) presenting an excessively large diameter of its head due to deflexion. Referring back to our discussion of the Three Ps in chapter 2, relative disproportion may be eradicated or exacerbated by the degree to which the fetal skull is moldable, the amount of flexibility in maternal tissues and joints, the strength of uterine contractions, and the mother's resolve.

Thus CPD cannot be diagnosed before labor, but if the head bulges over the pubic bone in a rare condition known as **fetal overlap**, it may be suspected. Should the head be easier than usual to palpate in the final weeks of pregnancy, check for overlap by pressing the head toward the sacral promontory and down into the pelvis. If you find "give" front to back with room for descent, rest assured. But if space at the inlet seems limited, try to determine the cause. If the head is posterior and the size of the baby and mother's pelvic dimensions are congruent, deflexion is probably the cause and can be remedied in labor (see page 152, "Posterior Arrest"). But if the head is well flexed and in an anterior or transverse position, consider the possibility of true CPD and plan to monitor labor closely. Yet another option is to induce labor (see "Large for Gestational Age" on page 88).

For the record, failure to engage before labor is not diagnostic as large babies frequently stay at −2 or −3 station until strong contractions bring them down. Extremely strong or weak abdominal tone may also prevent the fetus from aligning with the inlet so that it can descend.

During labor, CPD can occur at inlet (as with a deflexed posterior or asynclitic head), the midpelvis, or the outlet. A pelvis with a flat, heavy sacrum or close-set ischial spines may render passage through the midpelvis difficult, or a reduced pubic arch may result in outlet disproportion. In the last few weeks of pregnancy, encourage the mother to squat for ten to twenty minutes a day to stretch and loosen midpelvic and/or outlet dimensions. Recommend forward-leaning positions when sitting, such as straddling a chair facing its back.

Whenever it appears that CPD might occur, vaginal exercises and massage may also be of benefit. To quote Anne Frye:

> Observations regarding the influence of the pelvic soft tissues on the birth process are highly relevant to the midwifery model of care. The soft tissues are

more easily influenced by maternal distress or relaxation, leading to correspondingly more difficult or easier labors. The flexibility of the pelvic joints is also influenced by the mother's emotional state. That the pelvic soft tissues (rather than the bones) are the primary influence over the movements of the presenting part in the average pelvis underscores the relationship between the maternal emotional state and the physical aspects of labor, and explains the ability of maternal activities and position changes to dramatically alter the course of labor for the better.[3]

Thus relative CPD can be overcome not only by fetal rotation or repositioning, but also with changes in maternal activity or attitude.

How is CPD diagnosed in labor? First, it must seem a reasonable suspicion based on foreknowledge of the baby's size, position, and the mother's pelvic dimensions. **Inlet disproportion** is signaled by arrest at 6 cm dilation, lack of descent past −3 or −2 station, deflexion or asynclitism, and cervix not well applied to the head. Particularly ominous is the cervix hanging like an empty sleeve. Another oddity of inlet CPD is the tendency of the cervix to reclose: I recall several cases where the cervix, hanging loosely during a contraction, spastically tightened up a centimeter or more as the contraction ended. This happens because it has nothing to hold it open, neither the head nor adequate strength in the lower uterine segment. Weak, incoordinate contractions result, and in severe cases, the mother may complain of spastic pains similar to sciatica, running down one leg or up one side of the back.

Midpelvic disproportion presents quite differently. The head may have engaged without trouble, but second stage is prolonged and descent delayed. This is often due to **deep transverse arrest**, in which the head is wedged behind the ischial spines and cannot rotate to the OA (or OP) position.

Outlet disproportion also leads to prolonged second stage but more commonly affects the perineal phase, causing severe early decels or bradycardia, delayed delivery, and tears of the bulbocavernosus muscles or perineum.

What are some remedies for CPD? If at the inlet and caused by malpresentation, you can attempt to manually reposition the head. This is more likely to work with intact membranes, as the baby can more readily move in response to your manipulations. Have the mother get in knees-chest position (with butt elevated) so it is easier to dislodge the baby from the part of the pelvis in which it is stuck. **To correct asynclitism**, press firmly on the protruding parietal bone and center the sagittal suture line. **To secure flexion**, see directions and diagrams in the section "Posterior Arrest," starting on page 152.

If the head is too high to reach, have the mother try **duck walking**. Much as it sounds, she walks in a semisquat position, shifting her weight from one foot to the other. This helps open the inlet by stretching the sacroiliac and pubic joints, at the same time encouraging the baby to reposition itself. For similar effect, have the mother climb stairs two at a time. Ruth Ancheta and Penny Simkin suggest **the lunge**: For this, place a chair on a carpeted floor (so it cannot slide) next to the mother on whichever side her baby is lying. Have her face forward and place the foot nearest the chair onto its seat, perpendicular to her body with toes pointing outward. Continuing to face forward, she lunges sideways with each contraction, moving slowly back to standing as it ends (she can also do this in a kneeling position).[4]

Other maneuvers to try involve the use of the **rebozo**. Stack pillows as for postural tilting (see "Breech Presentation and Transverse Lie" on page 83), stretch the rebozo across the high point of the pillows, and have the mother place her hips over it. Stand over her, straddling her body at thigh level, and pick up both ends. Encourage her to relax completely, and then pull the ends alternately so her hips rock briskly from side to side. You can also use the rebozo with the mother in knees-chest with butt elevated (as suggested in "Breech Presentation and Transverse Lie" on page 83). Or try the "tuschy roll," with mother hands-and-knees and rebozo strung across her hips and upper thighs, ends

Fetal Asynclitism

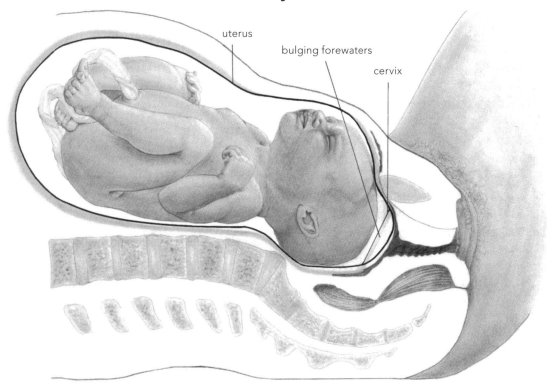

Relative CPD as caused by a posterior position and a deflexed, asynclitic head.

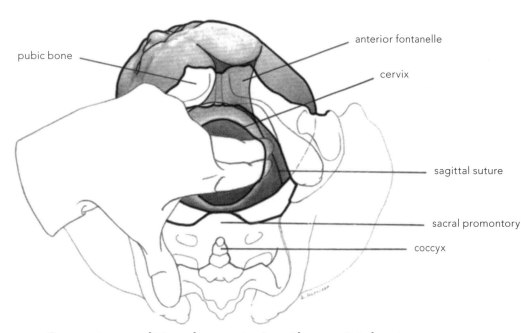

Correct asynclitism by centering the sagittal suture.

twisted like a candy wrapper and then used to rock the hips side to side. Inupiaq Eskimos of northern Alaska use the blanket toss, in which the mother lies in a blanket as strong men at the corners lift and toss her up and down.[5] The Chinese accomplish much the same with **chunging**, an ancient technique that involves two or three people placing their hands on the mother and vigorously shaking her all over (she could be standing and braced for this, in a doorway or leaning against a wall).[6] Yet another possibility is to take the mother for a bumpy car ride, which all too often does not happen until transporting to hospital when it might have been effective in keeping the birth at home if tried earlier.

For midpelvic disproportion and cases of deep transverse arrest, you can use the rebozo to loosen pelvic joints and muscles (mother can be knees-chest or sitting on the toilet) and follow up with the **pelvic press**. For the latter, the mother may wish to squat. Kneeling in back of the mother, place a hand on each iliac crest and press them together as firmly as possible or until you feel some movement. This requires a bit of strength, and is sometimes easier if performed with a partner, who can press with both hands on one hip as you do the same on the other. Pressure on the iliac crests flexes the symphysis pubis and sacroiliac joints, opening the midpelvis so the head can rotate and descend. As you do this, have the mother bear down, even if she is not quite complete. Hold the press for the next few contractions. Have your midwifery partner or assistant check heart tones immediately after each contraction. Results are often quite remarkable.

If this does not work, position the mother in knees-chest, disengage the head slightly from the point where it is impacted (see page 152, "Posterior Arrest"), and rotate the baby to OA (or OP if it will not turn to OA).

The pelvic press is also useful for outlet disproportion, as it opens the pubic arch and increases the bituberous diameter. A deep squat (knees up to the abdomen) serves to accomplish much the same; it can increase the outlet dimension by 20 percent. Use hot compresses to deepen pelvic relaxation and work carefully during delivery to maintain flexion of the head.

Of the three types of CPD, that occurring at the inlet is the most difficult to address. If you cannot reach the head to reposition it and other remedies do not result in descent, you must wait it out. Meanwhile, encourage strong contractions by seeing that oxytocin levels are kept high. Give the mother privacy. If she is partnered, suggest nipple stimulation, kissing, and sex play: if she is single, she can do nipple stimulation herself, and she may want to masturbate. Growing numbers of women report using vibrators in labor for pain relief and pelvic relaxation.

Blue cohosh tincture also stimulates contractions: give a dropperful every few hours, but check heart tones each time to make sure the baby is not overly reactive. In every respect, the mother's Powers are critical: make sure she is well hydrated, changes position often, and feels free to make sounds (open throat, open vagina). If contractions diminish, stop efforts to stimulate labor and support her in getting refueled and rested, with a snack, a glass of wine, and plenty of pillows. When labor starts up again, go into stimulation mode, and after an hour or so, recheck to see if the head has come down.

In terms of time, there are limits. With obstructed labor and prolonged arrest, the lower uterine segment can get so thin that uterine rupture is a possibility—an important consideration with VBAC. But in ordinary circumstances, maternal exhaustion or fetal distress will necessitate transport long before this could occur. The bottom line: mother and baby can endure only so many rounds of hard labor. If CPD is confirmed and all attempts to correct it have failed, take the mother to the hospital. Pitocin augmentation may strengthen contractions enough to effect vaginal birth but can also be traumatic for mother and baby, so transport while both are still in good condition.

After so many hours of difficult labor, pain relief may also be of benefit. Particularly if paired with Pitocin, complete pelvic relaxation via epidural

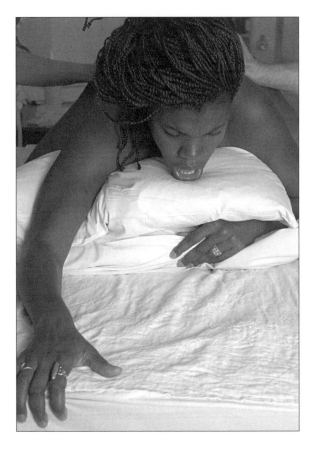

may allow pelvic muscles (and bones) to give just enough to let the head pass through, thus averting a cesarean. Still, these interventions may cause deep disappointment for the mother, both in labor and postpartum. The midwife can help by assuring her that the pain of obstructed labor, with bone wedged against bone, is different from that of ordinary labor and much more intense: she is not "copping out."

If Pitocin and pain relief do not work, at least the mother may be content with knowing that she has tried everything. Seeing a woman through a rough labor that ends in a cesarean is difficult at best, but focus on providing emotional support as you continue to guard her physical well-being. Do all you can to see that her incision is carefully repaired and that the cord is left pulsing as long as possible to ease the baby's abrupt transition. Contact the pediatrician, and prepare to help the mother with immediate postpartum care. Get her up and walking as soon as possible (with staff clearance and support) to speed the healing process and minimize painful gas. Encourage and help her to nurse on demand, and see that she has healthy food and drink brought to her at the hospital. Help pave the way for her homecoming by coordinating the assistance of family and friends. You or your assistant should visit her daily.

Years ago, I served as doula for a woman with an undiagnosed, 9 lb. breech. Her physician recommended a cesarean, and she agreed. Both the father and I were present in the operating room. The mother received an epidural but was unable to tolerate the sensation of numbness in her chest; she felt like she couldn't breathe. So she asked for general anesthesia and was put out. Her husband held the baby immediately, she was taken to recovery, and the baby was taken to the nursery where the father and I took turns rocking and holding it. During the next few days, the mother went through periods of intense depression and paranoia. Even though she had the baby with her, she felt incapacitated, vulnerable to hospital staff, worried about her two-year-old son at home, and extremely disappointed in her experience. One night, she was so upset that she asked me to come stay with her at the hospital. We did a lot of talking in the weeks and months that followed. She repeatedly asked questions about the birth, wanting not just reassurance but exact observations of the baby's behavior, the finest nuances and every little detail I could provide. A year later, I received a picture of myself holding her baby girl in the nursery, along with this letter:

> Dear Elizabeth,
>
> It is a year on the 11th. Thank you so much for all that you gave me. What words can I use to tell you that without you my birth experience would have been really cold, my hospital stay a nightmare, but most of all, I would not have had a true witness to the birth, and how beautifully and perfectly you filled these needs. How I counted on you!
>
> I hope that I am able to give something so wonderful to the great supply of love in the Universe.

Posterior Arrest

Posterior arrest occurs if a baby in LOP or ROP position gets stuck at the pelvic inlet during active, first-stage labor. Posterior positions are common with an anthropoid pelvis, through which the baby may pass without trouble. But with posterior arrest, the occiput snags on the sacral promontory, the head deflexes, and descent is impeded. The resulting lack of pressure on the cervix makes contractions irregular, incoordinate, and weak. Posterior arrest typically occurs at about 6 cm dilation, with station of –3 or –2. Occasionally, cervical edema develops to further compound the problem.

In the past, the only solution I knew was to transport for Pitocin augmentation with the hope that stronger contractions might force descent and rotation. It was frustrating to repeatedly encounter this problem and to know in advance that we would probably end up in hospital. I've had two posterior labors myself, which further motivated me to investigate new ways of addressing this issue.

Assuming there is adequate room in the pelvis and that malpresentation has caused relative CPD, the problem is getting the head low enough to do something about it. What are your options? A **forward-leaning position**, with one foot (on the side where the baby is lying) placed on a low stool or stair, flexes and opens the sacroiliac joint, giving the baby more room to turn. The forward lean (with weight well over and in front of the ischial tuberosities) also makes it easier for the baby to rotate its shoulders without getting caught on the sacral promontory.[7]

Or have the mother try the **butterfly (pancake) position**. For this, she lies on her back, with two people on either side to help her bring her opened legs (bent at the knee) down to the bed and up toward her shoulders. Her bent knees look like butterfly wings, and she will flatten on the bed like a pancake. This is more effective if someone plays "tug-of-war" with the mom, who pulls on a bed sheet or rebozo between her legs so that her chest curls up slightly.

These efforts may cause the head to flex and slide under the pubic bone.[8] The **abdominal lift** does much the same: while standing, the mother laces her fingers under her abdomen as a contraction begins, lifts up about two inches while flattening her lower back (in a pelvic tilt), bends her knees slightly and then pushes in toward her spine about two inches, holding this position until the contraction ends. This is most effective if performed for at least ten contractions.

Or you might use the **rebozo technique**, adding a sharp jerk every few shakes on whichever side the occiput is resting. Try first with the mother in a postural tilt and, if that is unsuccessful, place the mother in knees-chest position (with butt elevated) and use the maneuver described in "Breech Presentation and Transverse Lie" on page 83. According to Doña Queta Contreras, a traditional healer and midwife from Oaxaca, Mexico, this motion sets up a current in the amniotic fluid that helps bring the baby around, along with opening the first chakra (for grounding and connection to the earth).[9]

Meanwhile, the mother will be experiencing significant pain in her back. I've heard it said that back labor is "anterior labor times ten"; be that as it may, pain relief is critical. **Hot or cold compresses** with *very firm* pressure can help, particularly if the pressure is exerted with a downward thrust: place the heel of the hand at the sacral promontory with fingers pointing toward the coccyx and press firmly in and down. Better yet, try the **double hip squeeze**: with the mother in a forward lean, place the heels of the hands on either side of the sacrum in the butt/muscle area (fingers pointing toward the spine) and push hands together. This not only provides pain relief but also opens the pelvic inlet (and thus can also be used for a deflexed or asynclitic head).

In extreme cases, consider the use of **sterile water blocks**, or **papules**. This requires four subcutaneous injections of 0.15 cc sterile water (using a tuberculin syringe) in the sacral area at both dimples near the promontory, and an inch below on either side. Although this causes a very painful burning sensation for about twenty seconds, pain relief then lasts from forty-five minutes to three hours. This alone may prompt spontaneous rotation.

Even if these suggestions do not turn the baby, they may open the pelvis enough to bring it within reach. At this point, you can attempt **manual rotation**. The following technique is based on the work of an Australian obstetrician, R. H. J. Hamlin.[10] (See diagrams at right.)

Begin with an internal exam to establish the baby's position and degree of flexion. You will not be able to find the posterior fontanelle if the head is deflexed but should feel the anterior fontanelle near the pubic bone. Once you have found it, you can undertake maneuvers to flex and rotate the head. But first, you must *slightly disengage the head*, that is, dislodge it from the plane in the pelvis where it is wedged. Do this by spreading your fingers on either side of the sagittal suture, pushing upward on the parietal bones. (I have added this step to Hamlin's technique as I find it makes a big difference in ease of rotation: Anne Frye has termed this the **Hamlin-Davis maneuver**.)

Sometimes dislodging the head is enough to allow flexion and rotation to occur spontaneously. If not, have the mother fully recline (no pillows). Your assistant should kneel, facing you, on the side of the mother where the baby is lying. Keeping the head dislodged, bring both fingers to the *bony edge* of the anterior fontanelle and rotate it to a transverse position. Flex the head by pushing the fontanelle toward the sidewall of the vagina (as if to tuck it back inside the mother) until it is almost out of range of feeling.

Quickly reach for the posterior fontanelle and secure an edge. As you begin to rotate this from transverse to anterior, alert your assistant so she can, at the same time, grasp the baby's shoulder and back, lifting and pushing its body to the anterior position (it is easier for the assistant to do this if the mother turns in the direction you are turning the baby). Once the mother is on her side, quickly check fetal

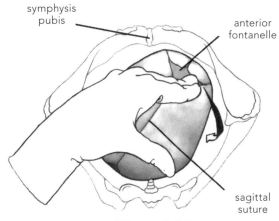

ROP to ROT

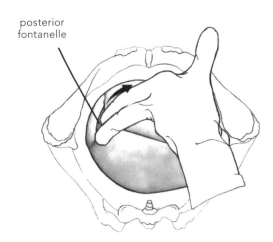

ROT to ROA

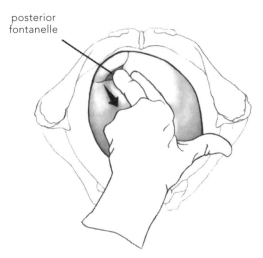

ROA Flexing

heart tones. If all is well, have her sit up, then stand and assume a forward-leaning position to secure the baby in place.

How much force do you need to use? Hamlin used the example of "dialing a telephone" or, in other words, pressure sufficient to maintain flexion during rotation maneuvers. If you feel strong resistance at any point, attempt no further.

If you do not have an assistant to help as above, perform these maneuvers with mother in knees-chest position (with butt elevated). This increases pelvic space and encourages the baby to disengage via the effects of gravity. For this reason, knees-chest may be your best option if the membranes have ruptured. Ordinarily, amniotic fluid provides room for the baby to move in response to your manipulations, but when most of it has escaped, the uterus gets snug around the baby and makes it much more difficult to reposition. If this is the case and you cannot budge the head, the mother might take a shot of whiskey to relax the uterus and/or you could give her a rebozo treatment just prior to rotation.

If you succeed in rotating the baby, check heart tones with every contraction for the next twenty minutes. Then do an internal exam to be sure the baby is still in place. Sometimes the baby reverts to its original position, and it appears that your efforts have been for naught. Do not be discouraged; you may need to make a few more attempts. With each attempt, the baby should flex and descend a bit more, eventually staying in place.

Yet another rotation technique you can try involves (1) dislodging the head slightly; (2) placing two fingers, slightly spread out, on the sagittal suture line; and (3) turning them to rotate the baby. If the baby cannot be rotated to OA despite numerous attempts, consider turning the baby to OP—at least it can descend this way.

Here is an interesting case history. A mother was two weeks postdates; her baby was large and in ROP position. She had a long latent phase of twelve hours, with three more to dilate from 4 to 6 cm. The head was at −2 station and sharply asynclitic, with the right parietal bone presenting. The cervix hung loosely, and I couldn't feel the sagittal suture as it was tucked behind the pubic bone. After a few more hours, cervical edema began to develop, but the head had come down a bit and the suture line was now within reach.

With the mother's agreement, we attempted internal rotation and managed to turn the baby to ROA. It promptly rotated back to ROP but gained a centimeter of descent. An hour later and with good contractions, we tried once more, and this time the baby settled at ROT, −1 station. With yet another try, the baby rotated to ROA, spontaneously flexed its head, and descended to 0 station, cervix 7 cm, at which point we performed AROM to secure engagement. Fetal heart tones were fine throughout, and the baby was soon born in excellent condition. The mother found the procedure to be quite uncomfortable but said that given the choice between procedure and transport, there was no question in her mind.

The bottom line is this: attempt rotation in a timely fashion when mother and baby still have the fortitude to handle it.

Fetal Distress

Abnormal fetal heart patterns during labor have already been covered in chapter 4. In the event of transport for fetal distress, continuous fetal monitoring is likely. This may be external, internal, or a combination of the two.

There are two components of external monitoring, both belted to the mother's belly: an ultrasound unit to assess fetal heart response, and a pressure transducer at the fundus to record uterine activity. Results from the latter are highly inaccurate, as subtle contractions of maternal muscle (with coughing, for example) cannot be differentiated from uterine response, nor can the actual strength of contractions be determined. With internal monitoring, an electrode is attached to the baby's head, and an internal pressure catheter is placed through the cervix and into the uterus to more accurately determine the strength of contractions. Internal monitoring is more likely with fetal distress, particularly if Pitocin is being used to augment labor. In this case, it is critical to see that the uterus is relaxing completely when contractions end. If it is not, reduced circulation can exacerbate fetal distress, and the Pitocin should definitely be turned down or off.

In noncrisis circumstances, **intermittent monitoring** and fundal assessment of the intensity of contractions can be substituted for evaluations by external monitoring. A study published by the American Congress of Obstetricians and Gynecologists (ACOG) showed intermittent monitoring (or assessment of the FHT every thirty minutes in active labor) to be just as efficacious as continuous monitoring. However, this method was used in only 3 percent of cases due to insufficient staffing (for performing and recording these assessments).[11] This is significant in that continuous monitoring may confine the mother to bed, although many hospitals now use telemetry, a remote unit used with both external or internal monitoring systems that allows the mother to be up and moving (there are also watertight units that let the mother be submerged).

Some hospitals utilize **scalp sampling** to further assess the baby's well-being. A small sample of blood is taken from the baby's head, and the pH is tested to determine whether or not the baby is **acidotic**, that is, truly hypoxic. Readings at or above 7.26 are considered normal. Fetal scalp sampling more truly identifies fetal distress than does fetal monitoring—not that the monitor readings are inaccurate, but some babies tolerate stress better than others. Thus, even in the presence of an ominous fetal heart pattern, labor may safely proceed if the scalp sample is within normal range. In short, fetal scalp sampling can make the difference between a cesarean or vaginal birth.

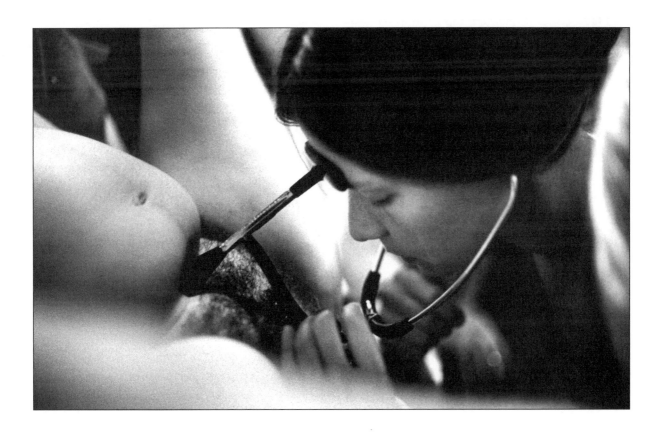

In lieu of fetal scalp sampling, you can use **fetal scalp massage**. Massage should be performed for about ten seconds: a 15-point acceleration of the FHT, lasting fifteen seconds, is said to indicate a pH of at least 7.26.

Cord Problems

Several types of cord problems can reduce blood flow to the baby and cause fetal distress. With **cord entanglement** (cord wrapped around the neck or limbs and body), descent may be inhibited and variable decelerations may result. If these become severe or progress to bradycardia, the baby must be born at once or the mother must be transported, with oxygen at 6 L per minute.

Cord nipping occurs when the cord is pinched between the head and pelvic bones, causing variable decelerations. During first stage, repositioning the mother can shift pressure off the cord and bring the FHT back to normal. But this depends on how low the cord is lying: if the head can move past it entirely, the FHT will return to normal. Otherwise, nipping may progress to cord compression.

Cord compression may be due to either **occult prolapse** (cord low enough in the pelvis to be increasingly compressed by the head as it descends) or **prolapsed cord** (cord at the os, in the vagina or protruding from it). In case of prolapsed cord, *transport at once* (see below). With cord compression due to occult prolapse, variable decelerations may rapidly progress to bradycardia; if so, and the birth is not imminent, give oxygen and transport.

The obstetric disaster of prolapsed cord is associated with polyhydramnios, multiple pregnancy, breech or compound presentation, and transverse lie—conditions where the presenting part is either high in the pelvis or fitting poorly at the inlet. Thus cord prolapse tends to happen in early labor (except with twins, when the second baby is most likely to

be affected). Cord prolapse is occasionally diagnosed in the last few weeks of pregnancy with the discovery of pulsations at the cervix or through the lower uterine segment that are synchronous with the FHT. This finding necessitates immediate hospitalization and a cesarean to save the baby.

If the cord prolapses when membranes rupture (1) call the paramedics; (2) get the mother in knees-chest position (with butt elevated); (3) place your fingers inside her cervix, pushing the head up and away from the cord; (4) place cord *gently* inside the vagina (if not enough room, wrap it in a washcloth soaked in warm water and covered with a plastic bag); (5) give the mother oxygen at 8 L per minute. The first three steps must be done very quickly: hopefully, someone else can call 911 and prepare the washcloth/plastic bag as needed. If there is no one to set up the oxygen, forget it for now. Above all, maintain pressure on the head to keep it from compressing the cord, and *do not remove your fingers until surgery is underway*! If you must transport the mother yourself, lay a chair on the floor and ease her on to it, then lift and tip her head lower than her hips (keep her in this position in the car).

Cord prolapse occurs very rarely, as many of the conditions listed above contraindicate home-birth. But if the head is high in the pelvis near term and the mother calls to report that her waters have released, immediately go and check fetal heart tones to rule this out.

Maternal Hypertension

If blood pressure was elevated in late pregnancy, check every twenty minutes in early labor. You may be pleasantly surprised to find it decrease, as labor can be therapeutic for hypertension (due to high levels of oxytocin and endorphins). But if readings rise steadily and reach 150/100 before the birth seems imminent, transport. Although still within range of

mild gestational hypertension (greater than 140/90 but less than 160/110), you must consider the trend and factor in transport time.

Women with mild gestational hypertension have little risk (only 1 in 500) of developing preeclampsia in labor.[12] But if blood pressure reaches 140/90, screen for symptoms, especially if it has been rapidly rising. At this point, a dipstick for proteinuria is unreliable, as cells present in the amniotic fluid may wash down and give a false-positive reading. Instead, check for clonus/hyperreflexia, and transport at the first sign.

Hypertension also increases risks of placental abruption and fetal distress, so check heart tones every twenty minutes. Push fluids, as dehydration can exacerbate the problem.

Herbal remedies may help to stabilize or lower blood pressure in labor, particularly if they were effective during pregnancy. Tinctures of hops, hawthorn, skullcap, and passionflower are classic for this purpose. Tinctures are better than teas in labor, as they are more potent and better assimilated: placed under the tongue, they are absorbed directly into the bloodstream. Bathing with Epsom salts (magnesium sulfate) can also help lower blood pressure.

In the event of transport, standard procedures for severe hypertension include intravenous magnesium sulfate for the mother and continuous monitoring of the baby. Magnesium sulfate may reduce blood pressure but primarily serves to prevent the changes in brain activity associated with preeclampsia that could lead to convulsions. However, it tends to slow labor and is associated with risks of pulmonary embolism and postpartum hemorrhage. The probable course of events should be discussed with the mother as soon as the problem develops so she will be adequately prepared.

Any woman with severe hypertension prenatally or in labor is at risk for an even greater rise in blood pressure after delivery. Preeclampsia can develop suddenly in the immediate postpartum—be on the lookout for this.

Prolonged Rupture of the Membranes

Prolonged rupture of the membranes (PROM) is challenging to address, in that there is wide disagreement on just how long "prolonged" is in this context. Although it is normal for membranes to rupture at the onset of labor, the concern is that the baby is now at risk for infection because the uterus is no longer closed to organisms present in the vagina. In this respect, PROM is merely a potential complication. The standard of care is to wait no more than twenty-four hours before inducing labor, and some physicians start even earlier to make sure the baby is born before twenty-four hours have elapsed.

The problem with this approach is that it does not incorporate the mother's health, her personal cleanliness, or her environment as relevant factors in her risk status. Women planning homebirth are usually in top condition, and it is a proven fact that risks of infection are much less at home than in the hospital, where patients are routinely exposed to virulent strains of microorganisms for which they may have little or no resistance.[13]

In 1996, a major study on PROM was conducted at the University of Toronto involving 5,041 women from Australia, Britain, Canada, Denmark, Israel, and Sweden. At random, half had their labors induced, and the others were free to wait up to four days for labor to start spontaneously. There was very little difference in outcome for the two groups: about 3 percent of babies developed infection, and about 10 percent were born by cesarean.[14] However, as this study was conducted in hospital with no adjustments made for the health status of the mother or baby, we can assume that the risk of infection is even lower with birth at home.

Yet another study published more than twenty-five years ago by ACOG indicates that infection risks with ruptured membranes increase dramatically twenty-four hours after the first vaginal exam.[15]

This makes sense, for how can we expect to move fingers (or speculum, for that matter) through the vagina without bringing infectious organisms to the cervical opening? Thus it is crucial to *avoid vaginal exams and cultures for as long as possible* when the waters have released. The only exception would be to visually inspect the cervix and vagina for herpes lesions, if the mother has any history.

In my experience, it is not unusual for mothers to go twenty-four hours after the water releases without even starting labor. But to minimize risks of infection, here are some commonsense guidelines for the mother (also given in chapter 4):

- Shower daily (tub baths are fine, too).

- Have no hand-mouth-genital contact.

- Use utmost care when using the toilet, wiping backward and washing hands both before and after.

- Wear no underwear, just clean, loose clothing, and preferably no sanitary pad unless flow is considerable, in which case the pad should be changed often.

- Have plenty to drink to replenish amniotic fluid and keep system flushed.

- Increase dosages of vitamin C, up to 2 g per twenty-four hours, or 250 mg every three or four hours.

- Eat good-quality, nonconstipating foods to keep energy levels high.

- Take temperature readings every three or four hours, reporting any elevation at once.

You may want to order lab work to check for white blood and elevated banded cell counts (generated in response to acute infection). However, it is possible for the mother to be only minimally infected, while the baby is decidedly septic. If this is the case, fetal tachycardia will result. Once membranes have been ruptured for twenty-four hours, check fetal heart tones regularly.

Your response to early release of the waters should include close phone contact with the mother during the immediate postrupture period, to check on her morale and to make sure she is following guidelines for avoiding infection. Avoid exams and internal manipulations unless there is genuine need—definitely not before advanced active labor. If you must check, use Betadine or other antiseptic solution with sterile glove, and do not insert your fingers into the os.

If the woman is known to be GBS positive, these guidelines change considerably. The Centers for Disease Control and Prevention (CDC) recommend that GBS-positive mothers receive antibiotics within eighteen hours of ROM. This is up to the mother as a matter of informed choice: if she wants antibiotics, administer them by IV; if she declines, a pediatrician should see the baby as soon as possible, and you must watch for signs of infection.

Whenever risks for neonatal infection are increased, make certain the mother understands normal newborn behavior. An experienced pediatrician colleague says the first sign of newborn infection is failure to nurse. Any baby who acts listless or irritable should be checked at once by a pediatrician.

Unusual Presentations

Vasa previa. This is an exceedingly rare complication in which placental or cord vessels present at the cervical os. This can happen with a velamentous cord insertion or if vessels extend beyond the edge of the placenta, running through the membranes and across the cervix to an accessory, **succenturiate lobe** of placental tissue. If membranes rupture at this location, the mother will hemorrhage and the baby could die. Diagnose this complication with the discovery of a pulse near the cervix in late pregnancy, particularly if unusual changes in the FHT are noted after the exam. If not discovered in pregnancy, vasa previa is usually identified in early labor. Otherwise, if membranes rupture and bleeding is noted, give the mother oxygen and rush to the hospital.

Face presentation. This is relatively rare, occurring once in every 250 deliveries. In fact, careful prenatal palpation should have alerted you to this long before the birth. With a face presentation, the deflexed head is quite noticeable unless the baby is posterior (in which case the occiput is out of range). If you discover this before the head is down in the pelvis, make an attempt to secure flexion (see illustration, page 59), bearing in mind that face presentation may be caused by cord around the neck deflexing the head as the baby descends. Proceed slowly, with continual assessment of the FHT.

Another cause of face presentation is true CPD. Do your best to make sure this is not the case, lest you waste precious time and energy at home.

The mechanics of face presentation require that the baby be born OP. Although labor may begin with the baby anterior, descent cannot occur in this position because the brow will impinge on the symphysis pubis. When the face begins to show, hold back the baby's brow by applying counterpressure to the perineum until the chin escapes—it must not get caught behind the pubic bone. Obviously, the occiput will put extra strain on the perineum. Tearing is common with face presentations; you may not be able to prevent it. Suction is usually necessary because the baby is facing up and may thus get a nose full of fluids as the head births. Have resuscitation equipment ready.

The newborn will probably have considerable bruising and swelling, indications for arnica and vitamin K. Also watch for breathing difficulties due to tracheal edema.

Brow and military presentation. These deflexed positions of the head can be remedied prenatally during the last few weeks of care. If they are discovered in labor by internal exam, you may be able to flex the head with internal maneuvers. See "Posterior Arrest" on page 152 for instructions.

Compound presentation. Most of the time, this means that a hand is presenting alongside the head, a condition known as **nuchal arm.** Compound presentation is usually discovered as the head is birthing, but it depends on how far down the hand extends. The biggest problem with compound presentation is the likelihood of perineal lacerations, as the head and arm together create an unusually large circumference. You may be able to avoid this by gently pinching the baby's finger before the head crowns, which may cause it to retract its hand. If this doesn't work, prepare to extract the arm so the shoulders can be born. The easiest way to do this is to grasp the hand and manually restitute the head while bringing the arm across the chest and outward (see illustration on page 160).

Membranes presenting at delivery. This is more a quirk of delivery than a complication. If the membranes bulge from the vagina at birth, they usually rupture with extension of the head. But if the rupture occurs higher in the uterus, **delivery in the caul** may result, with intact membranes enveloping the face and obstructing breathing unless removed. Cross-cultural beliefs say that birth in the caul brings good luck; however, the sensation of pushing water bag plus baby is quite intense! If the mother asks you to break the bag, warn her immediately before doing so, as the release of pressure can come as quite a shock.

If the bag is left intact and the baby is born in the caul, immediately hook a finger into the membrane below the chin and peel it back over the face so the baby can breathe. My daughter was born in the caul, and my midwife used a sterile receiving blanket to catch and lift the membrane edge, to which it adhered. Whatever you do, be sure and quick.

Shoulder Dystocia

Shoulder dystocia is a serious complication that can jeopardize the baby's life. It occurs when the anterior shoulder is impacted behind the pubic bone, usually because the shoulder girdle is too broad to negotiate the anteroposterior dimension of the pelvis. With

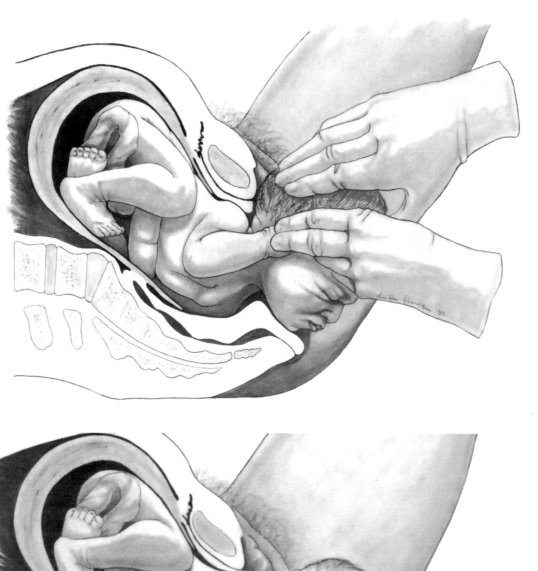

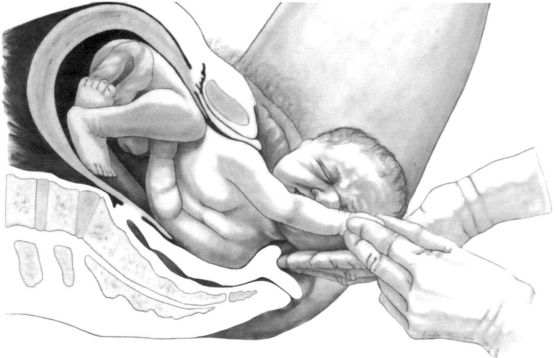

Extracting the Nuchal Arm

the baby stuck in the birth canal, chest compression impairs venous return from the head and can lead to intercranial bleeding, brain damage, and death unless the problem is remedied swiftly and competently.

It is easy to panic with this complication, but less likely if it has been anticipated beforehand. The mother with a baby large for her pelvic dimensions is a prime candidate for shoulder dystocia. So is a mother with diabetes, as **macrosomia** (baby's body large relative to head size) is common with this condition. Nevertheless, if the head can pass through, so can the shoulders, although you may need to do a bit of maneuvering to make this happen.

Here is the usual course of events. An unusually large head passes over the perineum, then pulls back or retracts against it: this is the **turtle sign**. Due to tension on the neck, there is **no restitution**. Both these occurrences are due to shoulders too high in the pelvis to allow the head normal freedom of movement. At this point, the **baby's color rapidly deepens to dark purple**. Despite the mother's pushing efforts, nothing changes and a diagnosis is made.

Immediately have the mother roll over to her hands-and-knees (the **Gaskin maneuver**). This will often shift the baby and bring the shoulders spontaneously. If not, this position will promote pelvic relaxation and enhance your ability to maneuver. Next, use the **Rubin-Davis maneuver**, reaching inside the perineum for the posterior shoulder, placing two fingers *in front of it* (at the juncture of the chest and armpit), and *pushing the baby backward* to the oblique diameter of the pelvis (about 30 degrees). This dislodges the anterior shoulder and the baby is free to birth spontaneously.

Note that I have added my name to Rubin's on this maneuver, for although we both use rotation to the oblique, he does so with fingers behind the shoulder, pushing the baby forward. I find the above technique more effective in that the shoulder girdle stays rigid, affording better traction for turning the baby.

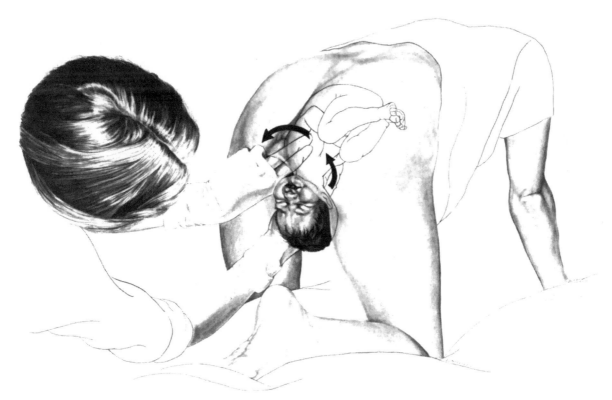

Managing Shoulder Dystocia

An alternative to hands-and-knees is the **McRoberts position**, in which the mother is fully supine with her knees hyperflexed to her shoulders. This lifts the pelvis off the bed or floor, increasing flexibility of the joints and available room to maneuver. Next, rotate the posterior shoulder by lifting the baby's head toward the pubic bone, placing two fingers behind the posterior shoulder, and moving it to the oblique position. (With the mother in this position, collapsing the shoulders by pushing from behind is best because gravity has them pressed deeply into the pelvic floor.) Usually this will bring the baby out, but if not, extract the arm (**Jacque-mier's** or **Barnum's maneuver**) to further reduce the girth of the shoulders. Do this by splinting the upper arm with two fingers, sweeping it across the chest, then grasping the hand and bringing the arm out.

In either position, **suprapubic pressure** (heel of your hand immediately above the pubic bone) can be applied in conjunction with your rotation efforts to help dislodge the anterior shoulder. Press inward and at an angle to complement the direction you are turning the shoulders with your other hand.

The worst case of shoulder dystocia I ever encountered was forewarned by a midwife who visited me a few days prior to the experience. She told me of a recent experience where none of the maneuvers mentioned above had worked. "Well, what did you do?" I asked, and she said, "We pulled and prayed until finally, the baby came out." This sounded like a panic scene I would just as soon avoid, but sure enough, a few days later. . . .

The mother was of small stature. She had been artificially inseminated and knew nothing about the father. At her last prenatal, fundal height was 40 cm. After a long labor, the head birthed smoothly about three-quarters of the way without a tear, but I had to push the perineum back over the chin, and there was no restitution. As the face rapidly turned purple, we had her move to hands-and-knees.

My senior apprentice was assisting; this was to be her first catch. She attempted the Rubin-Davis maneuver, but reported that she could not reach the posterior shoulder. She tried again with suprapubic pressure, but no change. So I stepped in, and indeed, the posterior shoulder was impacted high in the sacrum curve, in a rare condition known as **bilateral shoulder dystocia**. I instinctively called for both strong suprapubic and fundal pressure, figuring that strong suprapubic pressure would keep the anterior shoulder from being further impacted, and fundal pressure would bring the baby down enough so that I could reach the posterior shoulder (I've termed this the **Davis maneuver**). I then rotated the baby to the oblique and it was born. Although it needed resuscitation, it was fine shortly thereafter (Apgars 2 and 8). But the mother tore all the way through her rectum; I had done an episiotomy out of panic and it extended badly.

My junior apprentice said later that she had seen the "Angel of Death," and it certainly felt to me for a time like we might lose the baby. But I let go of my fear, and with this, adrenaline shot through me and I knew what to do. And yes, I guess I prayed, or at least offered up my total concentration.

Along these lines, students want to know how much time they have to get the baby out with shoulder dystocia, and I always answer, "None." There is no time to waste on ineffectual procedures: you must act immediately with the most potent response possible.

This next case was a comanaged hospital birth with one of my favorite backup obstetricians. This mother had experienced a difficult posterior arrest and transport with her first birth and chose hospital birth this time in case she wanted pain relief. She started out in the alternative birth room and progressed to about 6 cm, then opted for an epidural and was transferred to labor and delivery. She dilated rapidly to complete but slowed dramatically in second stage.

The physician was concerned, but he decided to leave the room because he noticed that she did better when he was away. Although she was hooked to a fetal monitor, I suggested she squat on the floor by the bed, and the baby descended and crowned immediately. I called for assistance as the head was born, and it soon became apparent that the shoulders were stuck. Both the physician and I were quite disoriented: he was used to handling this with the mother reclining, and I was used to having her roll over to hands-and-knees, which the tangle of monitor tubes and wires prevented. He told me to "pull down, down, down" on the head, until fearing I would damage the neck, I said, "No, you do it, you know what you're doing." Apparently he did not, because he began twisting the head this way and that, and I realized he was panicking. Suddenly, my mind cleared: I pushed his hands aside, applied suprapubic pressure, and directed him to go for the posterior shoulder, with which the baby promptly delivered.

Later, as he was completing the chart he pointedly asked me, "What would you call that delivery position?" The mother had actually been sitting on the lap of my partner who was kneeling behind her, so I suggested the term "supported squat."

"Hmm," he responded, "Sounds good . . . and that was suprapubic pressure with rotation to the oblique, was it not?" A nice gesture of acknowledgment, to top off a most challenging comanagement experience.

According to some texts, it may happen that you have no problem reaching the posterior shoulder but cannot rotate the baby. Based on the mechanics of shoulder dystocia, this makes no sense to me, for if the head has just passed through the vagina, the tissues should be pliable enough to allow the body to turn easily. Perhaps this occurs when forceps or suction has been used, and the tissues have had little time to stretch and relax. In any case, **breaking the clavicle** (collarbone) will collapse the shoulder girdle and facilitate delivery. Although this is a horrifying prospect, it is preferable to brain damage or death.

To break the clavicle, position two fingers against its anterior surface, position your thumb posteriorly, and push it forward between your fingers (one doctor who used this procedure relayed that the

clavicle "snapped like a matchstick"). Breaking the bone outward minimizes the risk of puncturing the lungs. A pediatrician should see the baby immediately, but do not worry: clavicles heal very readily.

Check any baby who has had shoulder dystocia carefully for bruising, injuries to the clavicles, or **Erb's palsy** due to nerve trauma. The latter is usually caused by pulling on or twisting the head: maneuvers unlikely to be effective, for if the shoulder is stuck behind the pubic bone, what possible good can these do? Erb's palsy may be detected with an asymmetrical Moro reflex (see "Newborn Exam," page 137). Severe dystocia is an automatic indication for vitamin K. Consult a pediatrician at once if anything is abnormal.

This is often a "crash-and-burn" complication for the midwife: it can take a while to recover from it. By the second-hour postpartum, you will be totally exhausted from running so much adrenaline. It is almost impossible to drive safely under these circumstances, so eat and rest (or sleep) before getting on the road.

Surprise Breech

Even if you have decided you cannot assist breech births, it is wise to memorize and practice an emergency routine. How does surprise breech occur if the midwife has palpated assiduously? If the baby is extremely posterior, the sides of the head may feel remarkably like the iliac crests of the hips. Firm maternal abdominal muscle, excess fat, or extra amniotic fluid may also confuse your evaluation. When in doubt, do an internal exam: the feeling of hard round head is quite distinct from that of the soft, irregular butt. If you are still unclear, order an ultrasound.

On rare occasions, the vertex baby turns breech at the last minute, especially if high in the pelvis at term. Suddenly you have a surprise breech on your hands and may not have time to transport. Be ready for this.

Assisting Breech Birth

The core dictum for assisting breech birth is simple: hands off the breech! In virtually every breech I have witnessed or assisted, the baby has birthed so rapidly that there was no time or need for manipulation. In the majority of cases, just follow these guidelines.

1. *Warm up the room!* This is critically important in breech birth as the baby's body will be exposed to air for an extended period unless the birth occurs in water.

2. *Let the mother follow her instincts in choosing a birthing position.*

3. *If the mother is pushing forcibly, suggest that she breathe her baby out.* Not that she must hold back, but rather, she should let her body do the work and support it with her breath. If she pushes in a panic, the baby's body may be out before the cervix is dilated enough for the head to pass through. This is less a concern if she is birthing in water, but if not, the baby will attempt to breathe when the body and cord are exposed to air, and the head must be free to deliver at this point.

4. *Do not support the baby's body: let it hang free to promote flexion of the head.* Have the mother lift the baby up to her as the head delivers.

Here are several guidelines for unusual circumstances.

1. *If the baby emerges with its butt to the mother's pubic bone and does not advance, nudge the legs to the antero-posterior position.* Do this by placing a finger at the iliac crest, then rotating gently. This should prompt further descent of the body.

2. *If the baby has birthed to the umbilicus and the cord is pulled tight, create a bit of slack.* If the cord is under the pubic bone, move it to the side. Do this very gently, though, as handling the cord can cause spasm and constriction of vessels.

3. *If the shoulders are not birthing, feel at the back of the baby's head for a possible impacted arm.* If you discover this, turn the baby's body toward the elbow of that arm to free it.

4. *If the baby is not OA after the birth of the shoulders, rotate it to this position.* Grasp the baby at the hipbones only, as undue pressure on internal organs could cause serious damage.

Note the advantages of water birth for breech: it alleviates the concern about keeping the cord and body warm to delay breathing until the head is born. Water also provides a medium of support that makes it easier for the baby to negotiate its way out with no assistance from you.

An excellent reference on breech birth is Maggie Banks's *Breech Birth: Woman-Wise*, available directly from the publisher, Birthspirit, online at www .birthspirit.co.nz.

Amniotic Fluid Embolism

Embolism is the entry of foreign matter into the bloodstream. When this material enters the lungs, it causes obstruction or constriction.

The exact cause of **amniotic fluid embolism (AFE)** is unknown. It can occur with abortion, amniocentesis, and amnioinfusion. During labor, hyperstimulation of the uterus is a factor. Pitocin is implicated, but Cytotec even more so: it hyperstimulates the uterus so greatly in some women that microscopic hemorrhage sites open and AEF occurs. Women with uterine scarring are more at risk, particularly those with previous cesarean section and less-than-thorough repair. It is also associated with preeclampsia, placental abruption, and placenta previa.

There is also some evidence to suggest that AFE causes hyperstimulation by setting off a catecholamine reaction. Whatever the mechanism, maternal mortality is as high as 60 percent. Thankfully, this complication is rare, with incidence of 1 in 13,000 births in the United States.[16]

Symptoms generally occur when the mother is in hard labor and include gasping for air, a drop in blood pressure, depressed cardiac function, hypoxia, seizures, and DIC. Call 911, administer CPR with oxygen, and have your assistant start an IV. Or, if the mother has given birth, apply bimanual compression, as she is likely to bleed out.

If born within fifteen minutes, 67 percent of babies survive intact.[17]

Hemorrhage

Hemorrhage is a complication we would all rather avoid. Thus it is crucial to take an exhaustive medical history and do thorough prenatal screening, including appropriate lab tests, so women likely to hemorrhage may be identified and treated, or risked-out in advance if necessary. All women should have a complete blood count at the initial visit, with a repeat at the onset of the last trimester. An adequate HCT/HGB reading ensures maximum resilience if bleeding does occur with the birth.

A history of postpartum hemorrhage does not necessarily contraindicate homebirth. Mismanagement of third stage (after the birth but prior to delivery of the placenta) is so common that you must rule this out to realistically assess the mother's risk. If she recalls, "I was fine right after the birth, but then the doctor pulled on the cord; it really hurt, and I started to bleed a lot," you can assume the hemorrhage was iatrogenic. Additional information about measures required to stabilize her, such as medications, IV, or transfusion, will give you a more complete picture of the extent of the hemorrhage and her recuperative abilities. Nevertheless, history of postpartum hemorrhage (or excessive bleeding following injury, surgery, or dental work) should be investigated via screening for clotting factors. These

tests are numerous and complex to interpret, so get medical consultation on this.

Yet another factor in postpartum hemorrhage is close-set child spacing, that is, the mother has given birth to several children in quick succession without adequate time to fully recover. Childbearing and breastfeeding can take their toll on a woman's body: if abdominal muscle tone is not restored, the uterus may not be able to contract effectively with a subsequent birth. Assess the mother's general appearance in terms of fitness and vitality. On this basis, recommend abdominal exercises or aerobic activities (like brisk walking or swimming) to help her get in shape. You may also wish to suggest herbal or homeopathic remedies. Cayenne pepper (three to six capsules daily) boosts circulation and elimination. Alfalfa tablets taken regularly during the last weeks may also help, as alfalfa is rich in vitamin K, which facilitates the clotting process.

Intrapartum bleeding. There are two principal causes of bleeding during labor: placenta previa and placental abruption. Rarely, bleeding is caused by uterine rupture or by rupture of a vessel with vasa previa (addressed in "Unusual Presentations," earlier in this chapter).

Placenta previa. This has already been discussed in chapter 3. For review, this refers to placental implantation low in the uterus, either over the cervix or at its edge, so that separation and bleeding occur with effacement and dilation. It is commonly diagnosed in the last trimester of pregnancy by painless spotting or bleeding, and appropriate management is determined at that time.

Placental abruption. Also discussed in chapter 3, this is a premature separation of the placenta before birth occurs. This poses grave danger to both mother and baby: the more the mother bleeds, the more the baby's oxygen supply is reduced. The only way to control the hemorrhage is by immediate cesarean, unless the abruption is marginal or the mother is about to give birth. Here are the symptoms:

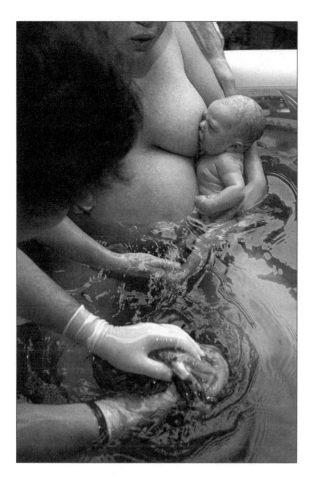

and keep a close check on the FHT. The pain may be due to incoordinate uterine action, but transport immediately if it becomes persistent or acute.

Uterine rupture. In spontaneous labor, this is extremely rare, particularly if the uterus is unscarred. It occurs when the normal process of retraction goes on and on until the lower uterine segment becomes so thin that it tears. It is associated with the following:

- Improper use of uterine stimulant drugs
- Obstructed labor due to true CPD, transverse lie, fetal anomalies, or vaginal tumors
- Grand multiparity with prolonged labor or improper uterine stimulation
- Uterine abnormalities
- Pendulous abdomen with resulting malpresentation
- Overdistension of the uterus from polyhydramnios or multiple pregnancy

Uterine rupture can also be caused by invasive procedures like external version, fundal pressure, or manual removal of the placenta, particularly if the mother had uterine surgery (including cesarean) within the last few years. If rupture is impending, the mother will be anxious and complaining of pain, with pulse elevated and blood pressure low. If the baby has not been born, fetal distress will be noted. When rupture occurs, the mother may cry out or report that something has given way inside her and will rapidly go into shock due to internal bleeding (face and lips white; thready, erratic pulse; cold sweat). Vaginal bleeding may or may not be evident. Treat the mother for shock and give oxygen at 10 L per minute. Transport immediately!

Third stage hemorrhage. This refers to an excess of two cups or 500 cc blood loss after the birth of the baby but before delivery of the placenta. Estimating blood loss is not easy for beginners; try pouring a measured amount of liquid on an underpad (some midwifery instructors use a mix of liquid starch and red food color) to get an idea of what one

- Severe, persistent abdominal pain (different from the ebb-and-flow sensation of contractions)
- Abdominal tenderness (abdomen rock hard to the touch)
- Fetal distress (with FHT pattern indicating hypoxia)
- Blood appearing at the outlet (will not occur in the event of concealed abruption, as blood loss is trapped behind the placenta)

Any woman with sudden and persistent abdominal pain, whether accompanied by bleeding or not, must be transported at once and should be given oxygen and treated for shock.

If a woman complains of sharp but sporadic pain, apply heat to the affected area of the uterus or two cups looks like. Do not forget that clots must be added into the measurement.

There are three principal causes of third-stage hemorrhage: (1) partial separation of the placenta, (2) cervical lacerations, and (3) vaginal lacerations. Partial separation of the placenta is the most life threatening of these, as blood loss is usually greater than with lacerations and more difficult to control. With the placenta distending the uterus, blood will continue to flow from vessels exposed at areas where it has already separated. The only solution is delivery of the placenta, which permits uterine muscle fibers to contract fully and close off the bleeding vessels.

Although time is of the essence, you must first *determine the cause of bleeding.* Quickly rule out **cervical or vaginal lacerations.** Cervical lacerations are unlikely, as they are associated with the use of Pitocin, Cytotec, forceps, and vacuum extraction, but they may occur if mother is less than healthy (borderline anemic, tissues friable) and the birth was precipitous. Vaginal lacerations deep enough to involve small arterioles (which bleed in gushes similar to those with partial separation) may also occur in these cases, or with a deflexed head, compound or face presentation, or persistent occiput posterior. Check for lacerations swiftly but thoroughly, dabbing with sterile gauze at any torn areas. If it appears that an arteriole has ruptured, clamp an artery forceps where the blood flow is most concentrated and use tie-off suturing to control bleeding (see "Suturing Technique," page 174). If blood also appears to be flowing from the uterus, treat this first as it is potentially life threatening.

Partial separation of the placenta has several causes. The most common is incoordinate uterine action caused by "fundus-fiddling" attendants. If left alone, the uterus will clamp down uniformly and fully release the placenta in the vast majority of cases. But if it is poked and prodded, only certain areas contract, releasing only these portions of the placenta.

Other factors include prolonged or precipitous labor from which the uterus is too fatigued to separate the placenta in a single effort. Rarely, portions of the placenta are morbidly adherent and resist separating, even if contractions are strong and coordinate. This is due to a condition known as **placenta accreta** (or in more severe cases, **increta** or **percreta**), which may involve little or all placental tissue (see "Retained Placenta," page 171).

Bleeding without lengthening of the cord, and no apparent urge on the mother's part to expel the placenta, signal partial separation. To make a diagnosis, don a sterile glove and follow the cord to the cervix. If the placenta is lying over the os, it is indeed separated and can be expelled by the mother's efforts, or you may use controlled cord traction to remove it. But if your fingers trail up through the os and into the uterus, you have diagnosed partial separation and should (1) give the mother tincture of angelica, (2) begin vigorous nipple stimulation (if the baby is not already nursing), and (3) administer 10 to 20 units of Pitocin by IM injection (or by IV if you are able). These measures serve to contract the uterus and will hopefully expel the placenta in the next few minutes. (Do not worry that Pitocin will close the cervix. It contracts the longitudinal fibers of the uterus only, not the circular ones at the cervical os.)

How you proceed from this point depends on the amount of blood loss. *If blood comes in small, occasional gushes, only a small portion of the placenta has separated.* Should you attempt to remove it manually, you might encounter large sections morbidly adherent and impossible to detach, and significant blood loss will occur as you distend the uterus with your hand. Eight minutes after the initial dose, give another injection of Pitocin (you can alternately inject 10 cc saline solution with 10 units Pitocin directly into the cord if it has been cut). After several minutes, follow the cord to the cervix to see if the placenta is present. If not, assess blood loss to this point. Anything over two cups is considered a hemorrhage; some women go into shock at the loss of four cups. Figure transport time and make a conservative decision.

If you decide on transport, you must ride in the ambulance to continue to assess blood loss and monitor the mother's condition, as paramedics are not trained to handle this complication (they will treat her for shock, warmed with blankets, feet elevated, and oxygen given by mask). Continue to repeat Pitocin injections at eight-minute intervals to control bleeding and keep her stabilized. If she begins bleeding heavily during transport, you must manually remove the placenta then and there.

If blood loss is torrential from the start, **manual removal** is your only option. There is no time to transport: the mother could die if you delay. Fortunately, heavy blood loss means that a considerable portion of the placenta is separated, thus manual removal should not be difficult. Make sure the placenta is not already separated and lodged behind the cervix, in which case it can be easily grasped and removed. If it is still attached, proceed to remove it. Don a fresh, elbow-length, sterile glove, pour antiseptic over it and insert through the os, using your other hand at the fundus to prevent the uterus from being forced upward. Slip your hand between the uterine wall and the separated portion of the placenta (which will be hanging free), then pry the rest off, using the edge of your hand like a spatula. Once you have detached it, skim the uterine wall for any fragments, grasp the placenta, and bring it out. Your assistant should give Methergine and/or Pitocin, and vigorous uterine massage should be started at once.

Assess the mother's blood loss and vital signs. If her blood pressure is low, if she looks pale or feels cold and clammy, or if her pulse is erratic, give oxygen and transport, treating for shock. If she is stable, push fluids, keep her warm and quiet, and continue to assess vital signs. The placenta should be examined carefully to be sure it is complete. If there is any question, take the mother to the hospital immediately for a consultation (she may need a D&C).

If in the midst of manual removal you discover that sections of the placenta are morbidly adherent, remove as much as you can by peeling cotyledons away from the membranes on the part of the placenta that is hanging free. Reducing the volume of what is retained will help reduce bleeding. If the mother continues to bleed heavily, give Methergine as a last resort. This may close the cervix, but it will also cause very strong contractions that can save the mother's life by minimizing blood loss during transport, particularly if she has lost more than three cups of blood and transport time is longer than twenty minutes.

In contrast to the above recommendations, **active management of third stage** has become the standard of care throughout the world. In this, the mother is given an injection of Pitocin with the birth of the head, followed by cord traction (regardless of whether or not the placenta is separated), and all too often, manual removal. This procedure should never be routine; it can be painful for the mother and may lead to postpartum infection. Manual removal should only be performed as a *lifesaving measure.* The one component of active third stage management that may make sense is Pitocin injection, particularly for anemic mothers. It is essential for those who have been induced or augmented, as they will not experience the surge of Pitocin naturally occurring with delivery.

I once had intuitive foresight of a partial separation. After the mother called to tell me labor had started, I lay down to clear my mind and focus on last-minute tasks when an inner voice said clearly, "There's going to be a partial separation." I protested that there were no risk factors for it. "And besides," I argued, "I've handled this before. . . ."

In a tone deadly serious and chilling, the voice responded, "You've never handled ANYTHING like this before. . . ."

Now I was frightened! I called my assistant and told her what had happened and then put it out of my mind to get ready for the birth. During labor, we kept a close eye on the mother's hydration and urination, and had Pitocin (20 units) drawn up in advance.

It paid to be prepared. The baby delivered beautifully, and then torrential bleeding began. I followed the cord, felt it meet the placenta just inside the cervix, and thought, "Oh good, it's right here," but as I attempted to grasp it, I realized the cord was inserted at the placenta's edge and the upper margins were still attached. Before I knew it, I was manually separating a very sticky placenta. I had my assistant give the prepared injection as blood literally poured down my arm, pooling under my elbow. I felt like I was on "automatic pilot," but the process was soon completed. The uterus firmed up immediately, and the mother was stable with blood loss of four cups.

In retrospect, I was very glad for this warning, though it raised concerns about recognizing and trusting my intuition, which led me to further study this subject. Now I consider my intuition to be a great asset to my work and give thanks for this powerful initiation.

Fourth stage hemorrhage. This refers to blood loss in excess of two cups or 500 cc after the placenta has delivered but within twenty-four hours of the birth. Roughly 80 to 90 percent of cases are due to a condition known as **uterine atony** (lack of tone). Still, you must rule out other causes of bleeding before proceeding with a remedy, unless blood loss is torrential (covered later in this section).

Begin by **ruling out cervical or vaginal lacerations**. Also **see if the mother needs to urinate**, as a full bladder can cause postpartum hemorrhage by preventing the uterus from descending into the pelvis and contracting fully. Ask the mother if she feels like going to the bathroom, or palpate the bladder to see if it is enlarged. A few drops of peppermint oil in the toilet bowl or tap water running at the sink may help her let go.

Also **rule out sequestered clots**, which form when the uterus does not clamp down firmly after the placenta delivers. In this scenario, small clots distend the uterus just enough that more bleeding and clotting occur, on and on in a vicious cycle until the mass can reach the size of a fist. The best way to deal with sequestered clots is to prevent them. Massage the uterus firmly after the placenta delivers or, better yet, have the mother birth the placenta in an upright position so internal organs compress the uterus automatically. Suspect sequestered clots if the uterus feels slightly enlarged or if a slow trickle bleed begins after the placenta delivers and then gradually increases. Check for clots by doing a sterile exploration at the cervix, and remove them by scooping them out with your fingers. Follow up with the uterine massage.

In managing fourth stage hemorrhage, it is important to realize that oxytocic drugs, herbs, or homeopathic remedies cannot help a uterus filled with clots or one prevented from contracting by a distended bladder. Oxytocics work for uterine atony, caused by long or precipitous labors that render the uterus too exhausted to clamp down efficiently. Overdistension of the uterus from polyhydramnios, a large baby, or multiple fetuses can also cause uterine atony. Respond with fundal massage and oxytocic agents, or **a bit of raw placenta** (also rich in oxytocin) placed at the mother's gumline. These measures should be effective unless a pathological condition inhibits coagulation (which should have been screened out beforehand).

If you are faced with a seemingly uncontrollable fourth stage bleed—that is, uterine massage and medications do not work—immediately call for help while giving the mother oxygen and **bimanual compression**. Besides the internal method illustrated on the next page, you can perform this maneuver externally by grasping and lifting the uterus firmly with both hands, then pressing them together as firmly as possible. Treat the mother for shock and give fluids (by mouth or intravenously).

When dealing with a woman who is hemorrhaging, keep her attention focused on the here and now. This means commanding her to stay present, to look you or her partner in the eyes, or to touch and speak to her baby. In truth, you must call on her to rally her vital force, particularly if she is drifting or fading out. This is one reason why prenatal communication

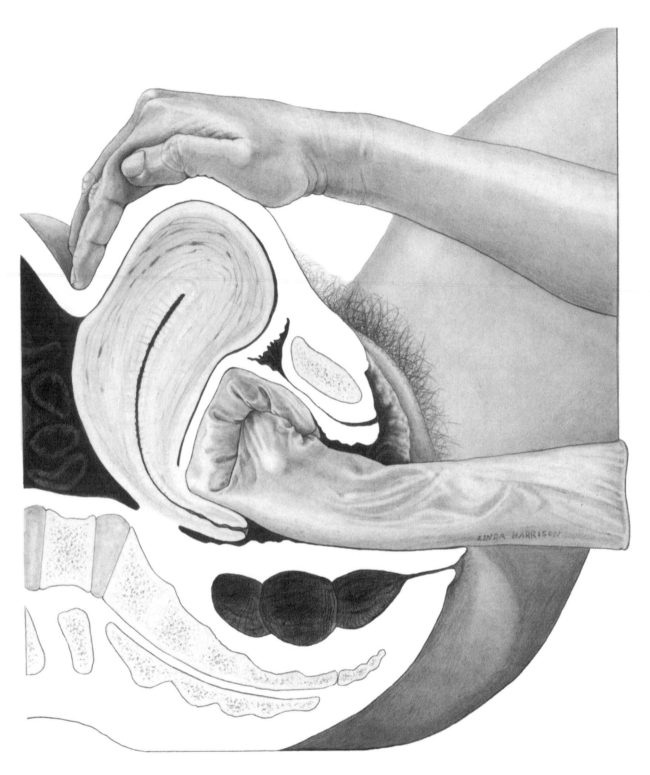

Bimanual Compression

must be authentic: you need to have channels open and ready to be activated in case of this kind of emergency.

To illustrate: Here is the experience of my former midwifery partner with her own second birth. She lived in the country up a rough road, and when her husband drove down to get the midwives, she birthed precipitously. After birthing her placenta, she began bleeding heavily and somehow managed to inject herself with Pitocin. She later confided, "You know, Liz, I really got how women can just slip away when they bleed like that. I was already so high from the birth, and it would have been really easy just to check out completely. It was the coziest, warmest, most delicious feeling—it just felt so good." I never forgot this, as only then did I fully appreciate how firmly and passionately the midwife must tell the hemorrhaging mother to stay present.

This links to an experience I had with a young Venezuelan mother who had just given birth precipitously. During their pregnancy, she and her adoring partner told me repeatedly, "If there is anything wrong, just tell us and we will fix it." I thought them a bit naive but delighted in their devotion to one another. Soon after birthing her placenta, the mother began to bleed quite heavily. I checked her bladder and massaged her uterus but could find no obvious cause, at which point I encouraged her to nurse, gave her some tinctures, and prepared the Pitocin. Her partner turned to look at me and asked, "What is wrong?"

"She's bleeding too much," I said, "I'll have to give her an injection."

"Wait a minute," he said. And as though it were scripted, they joined hands, looked into each other's eyes, and began to chant, "*No más sangre, no más sangre*" (*sangre* is Spanish for *blood*). The bleeding stopped as abruptly and completely as if someone had turned off a faucet. And that was that!

Sometimes you have a case of **slow trickle bleeding**: a lazy, sporadic flow, which, barring other factors, may reflect the mother's emotional state.

Brazilian homebirth physician Ricardo Herbert Jones advises, "Postpartum trickles are like tears from the uterus—you can help the mother stop bleeding by asking her how she is feeling."[18] Give this a try, but if the mother is emotionally withdrawn, take a strong stance and tell her to stop bleeding. Have her touch and talk to her baby. Give her something sweet to drink, with plenty of praise and encouragement. Tinctures of blue cohosh and shepherd's purse may help: give a large dose, a dropperful of each under the tongue.

Watch the slow trickle bleed very carefully. It may start and stop repeatedly, so blood loss must be reassessed continuously. If in excess of 750 cc (three cups), you must transport, even though the situation may not appear critical. You may need to give Pitocin or Methergine as much as forty-five minutes after the birth if blood loss has accumulated to 500 cc and the mother shows no signs of stabilizing. Experts on the subject repeatedly advise, "It's rarely the torrential hemorrhage, but the slow trickle bleed that kills." Stay alert, and do not leave the mother until blood loss has been fully controlled for at least an hour: longer if it exceeded 600 cc.

Retained Placenta

The placenta usually comes away from the uterine wall with the first strong contractions following the birth. This may take twenty minutes or more, as the uterus must recover its strength and reduce in size sufficiently to shear the placenta away. Absence of the characteristic **separation gush** is a definite sign to wait and see.

Watch for emotional signs of separation: the mother may suddenly become distracted from her baby or throw you a questioning look. If physical signs concur, tell her that it is time to birth the placenta and help her into an upright position. If you stick to this routine, you'll find the placenta usually delivers within the first half hour postpartum.

Certain circumstances may interfere. One is prolonged labor, which can leave the uterus so exhausted that it can't quite finish its job. If the mother is tired and the baby not yet nursing, offer tinctures of cohosh and angelica. After an hour or so, you may wish to administer Pitocin IM. If none of these works, there may be a problem of abnormal implantation.

The condition of **placenta accreta**, in which the placenta implants abnormally into the endometrium, argues against cord traction in any circumstance where placental separation is not clearly established. An unforgettable picture in *Williams Obstetrics* shows a fatal case of an **inverted uterus**, pulled completely out of the vagina with placenta still attached. Placenta accreta was once quite rare—in 1980, the rate was 1 in 2,500—but by 2006, this climbed to 1 in 210, due to the increase in cesarean section.[19] Depending on the amount of tissue affected, a D&C may be sufficient to remove a placenta accreta, or **hysterotomy** (opening the uterus for surgical removal of the placenta) may be required.

Rarely, the placenta invades the **myometrium**, or muscle layer of the uterus. Known as **placenta increta**, this condition is associated with incomplete repair of the cesarean incision. A more extreme form is **placenta percreta**, in which the placenta invades not only the uterine muscle but adjacent tissues or organs. Thus a midwife assisting a VBAC may wisely request that the mother have an ultrasound to make sure the placenta is not imbedded at the scar site. Placenta increta and percreta may necessitate **hysterectomy** (removal of the uterus) if there is no other way to facilitate separation; in fact, percreta is associated with a 50 percent maternal mortality rate.[20]

Sometimes **maternal inertia** stalls placental delivery. I recall a birth that went quite quickly; we arrived when the mother was 9 cm dilated. She had established deep intimacy with her partner, and despite our closeness to her prenatally, my partner and I felt like intruders. She birthed with little assistance, and then we waited (and waited) for the placenta. Two hours later, after nursing her baby and taking tinctures repeatedly, she went into the

Giving an Injection

1. Take a moment to steady yourself.
2. Flick the ampule to get all the medication into the base and break the tip off and away from you, being careful not to touch the edges.
3. Remove the syringe from the package.
4. Remove the needle cover, place the needle into the ampule—checking to see that the tip of the needle is all the way into the ampule to avoid drawing up any air—and pull back the plunger to draw up the solution.
5. Pointing the syringe upward, quickly tap the sides to bring any air bubbles up, then press the plunger to remove air and bring the medication to needle level.
6. Locate the outer, upper quadrant of one hip.

7. With your left hand, cleanse the injection site with an alcohol pad, and then hold the area firmly, with the skin spread flat.
8. Plunge the needle in about three-quarters of the way, in one quick movement.
9. Draw back on the plunger to see if a vein has been entered. If blood comes up, push the needle in a bit more and check again.
10. If clear, inject slowly, pushing the plunger all the way down to the base.
11. Draw the needle out quickly in one smooth movement and put pressure on the site with a cotton ball until the bleeding stops. You may cover the area with a spot bandage.
12. Dispose of needles and syringes in the sharps box provided by your lab.

bathroom and delivered the placenta by herself. She came out and handed it to us, saying good naturedly, "Here's what you wanted!"

Some women resist letting go of the placenta because it represents the last vestiges of pregnancy, or the last barrier to motherhood. Focusing the mother on the beauty of her baby will often bring the placenta. A bit of encouragement—"Let's just get the placenta out, and you'll feel so relieved"—may be all she needs to let go.

How long is it safe to wait? As long as there is no bleeding, the uterus remains firm, and fundal height is stable, you can wait several hours. Beyond that, an extended watch may cause anxiety and fatigue for both the mother and her attendants. Also, the cervix eventually begins to close, which may present an obstacle to placental delivery. Infection is another potential danger, as the cord extending from the vagina may permit germs to migrate to the uterus. At two to three hours, discuss going to the hospital, and after another twenty minutes or so, transport.

Assessment and Repair of Lacerations and Episiotomy

One of the most interesting facets of my student years was observing the different ways midwives and doctors sutured. Also interesting were decisions regarding when and when not to repair. After observing respective healing time and discomfort with various techniques, I developed my own suturing protocol (as presented by my mentor, John Walsh, in the "Suturing Technique" sidebar on page 174).

Episiotomy is rarely justified except in cases of fetal distress necessitating immediate delivery. An episiotomy may be easier to suture than a laceration, but you must cut through muscle, whereas lacerations are often superficial. Episiotomy weakens the musculature unless perfectly repaired and causes much greater discomfort and slower recovery.

With the vast majority of births, the perineum is intact. Otherwise, there may be minor abrasions, none of which require stitches. These are most likely to occur on the labia as torn skin with smooth and intact flesh underneath. Suturing these is unwise, because stitches will not hold unless imbedded in the flesh.

Sometimes a minor internal split of the bulbo-cavernosus muscle occurs, even though the perineum remains intact. If bleeding can be controlled with a bit of pressure (using sterile gauze), you need not suture. Internal tear edges will meet and join together as long as the split is no more than halfway through the muscle. First-degree perineal tears also heal by themselves if the mother takes good care of them.

But be sure to make a thorough and honest assessment of each and every laceration. Unfortunately, there is a strange status quest among midwives regarding the ability to do tear-free births; do not let this prevent you from suturing when it is clearly necessary. Sometimes the mother will be more comfortable if sutured, especially if tear edges do not **approximate**, that is, fit together easily. (For more on aftercare of the perineum, see chapter 6.)

Infant Resuscitation

This topic should be discussed with the mother (and her partner, if applicable) before the birth. Begin by citing the conditions in the baby that would require it. Explain that some occurrences like placental abruption, or cord accidents due to prolapse, true knot, or velamentous insertion, may result in fetal demise despite your best efforts. Describe resuscitation procedures in enough detail so that if they become necessary, the mother (and her partner) will know what is taking place and can support your efforts.

Beyond infant, child, and adult CPR, the CPM credential requires certification in neonatal resuscitation. The American Heart Association and the American Academy of Pediatrics offer courses on

Suturing Technique
John Walsh, MD, midwife

Unlike most obstetricians who prefer to make an episiotomy (with endless rationalizations), midwives take great pride in helping the mother maintain an intact perineum. This is the hallmark of a good midwife and is genuine proof of her patience. Nevertheless, tears occur commonly and sometimes surprisingly. A nine-pounder slides out without a nick, while a five-pounder creates a second-degree laceration unexpectedly. Often the head births exquisitely, only to have the shoulders do damage because of some urgency. And what does it gain a woman to have a wonderful birth at home only to have to pack up, drive to the hospital, and be sutured by strangers who may receive her with rudeness or even hostility?

Every midwife should learn to suture and do it without recoiling. It is one of those skills with an aura of mystery about it. This is probably because suturing is considered to be within the scope of surgery, with firsthand experience not easy to come by. Although it is a skill acquired by seeing and doing under the guidance of a teacher, it requires understanding and rehearsal before actual practice.

It is essential to set up properly for the procedure, or you will not be able to do a good job. The mother should be made comfortable on the bed's edge. She should have a clean, dry underpad

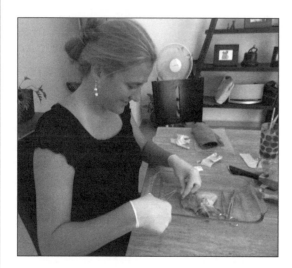

beneath her. You must have excellent lighting; carry your own lamp and extension cord or forehead-mounted system to eliminate this worry. Also, you must get in a comfortable position as you begin—your back will definitely begin to ache, and sweat will pour down your nose. This is really hard work.

The first step in repair is careful examination. Wear sterile gloves for this. It may be necessary to place several gauze pads in the vagina to aid exposure and sop up the oozing that can obscure your landmarks. Roll up the gauze and insert like a tampon. Just don't forget to remove it when you are done—it will be practically invisible because it will be blood soaked. Take your time to be certain you see the full extent of any tears or bleeding sites. Don't assume that everything is okay—you must look.

If the mother is uncomfortable during the exam, give local anesthetic now, starting with lidocaine spray or gel, then subcutaneous injections of lidocaine (1 or 2 percent). Wait a few minutes for it to take effect. Meanwhile, see that the mother is well supported with pillows, holding her new baby and not paying much attention to what you are doing.

Let the mother know that lidocaine does not completely anesthetize tissue and she may feel moderate pressure or pulling sensations, although these should not be painful. This worries some women, as they are afraid your next movement will hurt a lot. Avoid doing anything suddenly, and the mother will begin to relax and stop anticipating pain.

The basic suture kit needs to contain these instruments and supplies:

- *Two needle holders.* To avoid touching the needle after a stitch is made, a second needle holder is used to grab and transfer the needle to the needle holder being used for the repair. Five-inch Baumgartners are probably the best. The tips are small and serrated to hold the needle tightly without slipping. Hemostats cannot be used because the balance and the grip as the needle is driven through tissue make a subtle but important difference in doing a good job.

- *A Russian forceps.* Many midwives prefer this tool to a second needle holder (used as described above).
- *A tissue forceps.* These look somewhat like tweezers but are called forceps. Semkin-Taylor or Addsons are good choices, as they are very delicate. Tiny, interlocking "rats teeth" at their tips enable you to hold and lift tissue nicely without pinching or destroying membranes. Thumb forceps or dressing forceps are not suitable for handling skin, and the usual tissue forceps found in medical supply houses are too large and clumsy to do precise and careful work.
- *Two or three mosquito hemostats.* As their name implies, these are hemostats with small tips used for clamping small "bleeders." They should never be used for anything else.
- *Scissors.* A pair with sharp/sharp tips is used for cutting suture material precisely. This should not be the scissors used during delivery or for cutting the cord.
- *4 by 4 sterile gauze pads or sponges*
- *Betadine solution*
- *Suture material.* Generally, 3-0 chromic gut on a Ct-1 or Ct-2 half-circle needle (tapered, not cutting) is most useful. The designation "3-0" refers to the diameter and tensile strength of the suture. A 5-0 is smaller, weaker; a 1-0 is thicker and stronger. A 4-0, $^3/_8$ circle is best for more superficial tears; it pops through skin easily but can bend if used for deep muscle sewing. The needle is swaged onto the suture material so there is no "eye" or bump of thread to pull through tissue. By the way, catgut really comes from the submucous, connective tissue of sheep intestine. It dissolves in five to seven days, unless impregnated with chromic oxide, which prevents it from decomposing so readily. A new suture material, Vicryl, is increasingly preferred to catgut as it is less likely to irritate tissue (this may be the material of choice for vegans).

Your instruments should be kept wrapped until local anesthetic has been given. Suturing must be done by sterile technique. This may seem complicated and difficult to organize at first, but practice makes perfect. It is essential to have an assistant, and you both must know exactly what to do. In the following explanation, the one doing the suturing will be "A" and her assistant will be "B."

1. A opens her pair of sterile gloves and puts them on, then places the sterile inner wrapper down to serve as the sterile field.
2. B (ungloved) opens the outer suture wrapper and drops the sterile suture packet on the sterile field, then does the same with the sterile gauze pads and the syringe (this should be 10 cc, 23 gauge, 0.75-inch needle).
3. A takes the sterile instruments (needle holders, Russian forceps, scissors, mosquito hemostats, and tissue forceps) and places them on the sterile field.
4. B applies lidocaine gel or spray to the wound (without touching it), then wipes the lidocaine top with an alcohol pad.
5. A picks up the syringe and draws up an amount of air equivalent to the amount of lidocaine she wishes to inject—5 to 10 cc. B holds up the bottle; A injects the air through the rubber stopper and then draws up the lidocaine. A and B must be careful not to touch each other's hands or tools; this requires a delicate choreography between them.
6. A now begins injecting lidocaine around the edges of the wound and prepares to suture.
7. B puts on sterile gloves and assists by holding the labia open while A does the suturing. She can also reach for gauze and dab while A is stitching.

A word now about injections: Always rule out an allergy to lidocaine by reviewing the mother's medical history. And read the package literature that comes with lidocaine, especially the part about side effects. If the mother says she feels peculiar after you have injected, stop everything and assess the situation carefully. Every now and then, a woman may have a reaction that is simply one of distaste for shots and needles. True drug

continued >>

reactions are rare but emotional reactions are common. Make sure that is all it is. If she is feeling faint, suddenly says she feels hot and shaky, or has a metallic taste in her mouth, watch for signs of shock. Take blood pressure and pulse, monitor skin color, check the uterus for firmness, and so on.

Injecting is easiest if you start at the **apex** (top) of the tear inside the vagina and work downward. Inject directly into the sides of the laceration, parallel to the skin. Try not to plunge the needle all the way to the hilt, as that is its weakest point. Inject no more than 1 cc at a time, pulling the plunger back each time to make sure you are not in a vein. It takes a surprising amount of force to squirt medication into tissue. Be patient; if you inject too quickly, it will sting. The tissue may become somewhat distorted by the anesthetic, so when you are finished injecting, reassess your landmarks.

Now clamp your needle so it is perpendicular to the needle holder and curves away from you. If you are right-handed, the point should be to the left. Once the lidocaine has taken effect, start a row of continuous sutures at the apex inside the vagina. Your tissue forceps grasps the left side, the point of the needle is placed about 0.25 in. from the right edge, and a bite of tissue is taken, moving right to left. The needle pops through the other side and is clamped in the middle by your second needle holder or Russian forceps. Unclamp the original needle holder, and then pull the suture through until you have a short end of about 3 in. Reclamp the needle with the first needle holder, set all down on your sterile field, and triple-knot your first stitch, trimming the short end to 0.25 in.

Now make a series of stitches as above, about 0.375 in. below one another. Pull slightly on the strand as each stitch is placed, so the edges to be closed next come easily into view. It also helps to reapproximate edges (hold them together) every stitch or two, to make sure they are matching up correctly. The last stitch should be placed just inside the hymenal ring. Do not knot: just cut the suture to leave an end of about 4 in. (you will later tie this to the strand used to repair the perineum).

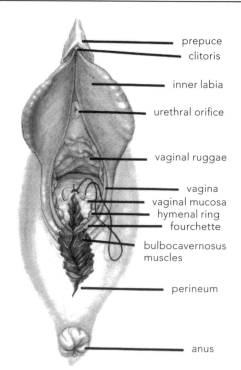

prepuce
clitoris
inner labia
urethral orifice
vaginal ruggae
vagina
vaginal mucosa
hymenal ring
fourchette
bulbocavernosus muscles
perineum
anus

Anatomical Landmarks

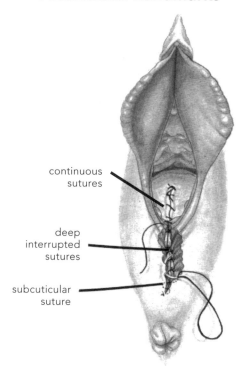

continuous sutures
deep interrupted sutures
subcuticular suture

Repair Techniques

Next, join the deep muscle tissue with a series of two or three interrupted sutures. These will bring the edges of the skin closer together, evenly distributing tension and eliminating dead space. Start at the top and work your way down. The first of these, where the tear is the deepest, should be done in two parts, one bite on each side (like halves of a circle—the first from the outside in, the second from the inside out). These stitches should be parallel to the vaginal floor; be sure to keep your needle holder vertical to avoid entering rectal tissue. The first stitches are triple-knotted, with both ends cut. Your final stitch should be triple-knotted too, but do not cut both ends—leave the suture string attached.

Now close the superficial layer just under the perineal skin with subcuticular stitches. Your first stitch goes on the right, parallel to the skin, from the level of the last internal stitch down to the bottom of the tear. Run a second stitch upward on the left side (again, like halves of a circle). To continue to go upward, you must reverse the needle position in your needle holder, that is, the point of the needle should be on the opposite side of how it has been thus far. Make your stitch on the right, then switch the needle again to move up the left, and so on. Place your final stitch so the point comes up just inside the hymenal ring, opposite the loose end. Pull each loose end separately until snug, then triple-tie together, and trim.

Here are some basic principles to keep in mind for any type of suture job:

- *Close lacerations (no matter where they are) in layers—muscle to fascia to skin.* The basic idea is to eliminate tension in any one spot.

- *Eliminate dead spaces between layers.* Otherwise, oozing can occur and a small (or large) hematoma can form. These terribly painful swellings can cause the repair to fail. Dead, empty spaces are weak and prone to infection.

- *Don't suture too tightly or you will impair circulation.* Anticipate slight tissue swelling after you complete the repair, and compensate by not sewing too tightly. Do not use too many stitches either, as each interferes with circulation to some extent. Vaginal tissue is highly vascular and good at healing itself.

- *Check your landmarks very carefully and repeatedly.* If you have waited several hours to do a repair, edema may confuse the picture. Double-check what goes with what. Go slowly. The bulbocavernosus muscle at the mouth of the vagina is an important landmark; it should be united very meticulously. Also, if the tear is deep, make certain that the levator ani muscle encircling the anus has not been torn either partially or completely. Repair of a third-degree laceration is strictly a job for the experienced.

- *Sutures should be placed so that the depth is greater than the width.* This fundamental principle of suturing produces a closure where the edges meet correctly; it is important to figure out why this is so.

- *Be careful never to clamp the suture with the needle holder, as it may break at this site.* Suturing is easier if you wet the suture with Betadine before beginning and as needed as you work. This keeps the string from sticking to itself (and to your gloves).

- *An assistant can be very helpful by cutting sutures as they are placed.* This saves you the movements of laying down the needle holder and forceps to pick up the scissors. Hold both strands tautly as your assistant prepares to cut. She takes the scissors and then, with the index finger pointing down the blades, opens the scissors tops just slightly, places them slowly on the strands 0.25 in. from the knot, and quickly snips. If the tails are cut too short, they may slip, whereas long ends cause irritation by poking adjacent tissue.

If there is swelling after the repair, give the mother arnica and have her apply alternating warm and cool compresses to stimulate circulation. Ice packs should only be used if swelling is extreme. Make sure to tell the mother to rinse the area each time she uses the toilet, using warm water with a squirt of Betadine. Have her keep the repair dry by exposing it to sunlight, a light bulb, or with a hairdryer. She should not use vitamin E or other oils on the wound, as this keeps wound edges from adhering to each other. If you have done a good job, the majority of the healing will take place in a few days.

neonatal advanced life support (NALS): for information, call (800) 242-8721 or contact the nearest branch of the American Heart Association. It is important that you inform the mother of your training in this regard.

Much has been said already about monitoring during labor so that fetal distress is not allowed to persist and deepen into depression. The most common cause of last-minute distress is severe head compression, which seldom necessitates resuscitation if the baby is born promptly. However, the baby's tolerance for this is based on many factors, including its health status and that of the mother and whether labor has been prolonged. The baby of a clinically exhausted mother may react suddenly and severely to head compression in the final stages of labor. As stated earlier, moderate bradycardia or early decels to 60 BPM or less are indications for immediate delivery.

When a baby is born in a compromised condition, the top priorities for stabilizing it are **warmth** and a **clear airway**. Regarding the latter, it is crucial to appreciate the folly of trying to resuscitate a baby that is chilled. Naked and wet, it will lose body heat rapidly unless placed on the mother's belly and covered, head to toe, with two or three flannel blankets (preferably oven-warmed). Suction as indicated, but be careful not to stimulate the gag reflex by placing the bulb syringe too far back in the throat.

Unless at risk due to stressful labor, postmaturity, prematurity, or intrauterine growth restriction, a baby with a hypoxic phase of fewer than ten minutes will usually come around quickly. Minor, last-minute depression causes no significant change in blood pH (acidosis) that might hinder spontaneous recovery. Remember that the baby will continue to receive oxygen from the mother as long as the cord is left pulsing: this allows time for complex internal changes that establish respiration. This transition takes longer for some babies; it is not abnormal for twenty seconds to elapse before significant respiratory efforts are made.

Neonatal depression falls into two categories. **Primary apnea** (apnea means without breath) describes the baby who has not been hypoxic for long, but has already made gasping/respiratory efforts while in utero in an attempt to compensate. Stimulation and blow-by oxygen (holding tube by the nose) should bring this baby around (see below, Apgar 6 at moment of birth). But the baby who has suffered a greater degree of hypoxia and has made a second round of gasping/respiratory attempts is in **secondary apnea**. It will not attempt to breathe on its own again, *so waste no time with stimulation*. This baby needs **positive pressure ventilation**, via mouth-to-mouth or bag-mask resuscitation, and possibly **chest compressions** (see below, Apgar 2 or less at moment of birth).

Assessing at the moment of birth allows you to prepare for resuscitation. For although Apgar scoring is officially performed at one minute, we don't wait that long to help a baby in distress and so assess immediately. The highest Apgar possible at this time is 9—with 1 point off for color, as incomplete circulatory changes mean that even the healthiest baby will have blue hands and feet. All this baby needs is warmth.

A baby with a 6 Apgar at the moment of birth—2 points for heart rate but 1 for everything else, color bluish, a bit floppy, with minimal respiratory efforts—most likely experienced a long, difficult labor or a very rapid one: it is either exhausted or missed the stimulation and drainage that more time in the birth canal would have provided. This baby needs warmth, possibly suction, and stimulation via firm and loving massage at the base of the spine and up the back. It should be against the mother's skin for continued warmth and contact. And ask the mother to talk to her baby! Neonatal intensive care nurses report that babies' oxygen levels surge upon hearing the sound of the mother's voice. These techniques should bring a response within fifteen to twenty seconds; if not, try a **seesaw motion** of rocking the baby from head to toe. This affects

For Parents: In Case of Transport

- *For the mother:* don't panic! It is easy to feel despair and loss of control on arriving at the hospital. But you have a better chance for a good outcome if you stay open and relaxed.

- *For the partner:* If your partner is exhausted or nearly so, don't expect her to make complex decisions about hospital routine or physician recommendations. Here is where all your study and investigation during pregnancy really pays off. The better you know your stuff, the easier it is to respond to suggested procedures. And you can always ask your midwife for ideas or support.

- *For both of you:* Ask for what you want or enlist your midwife's assistance in doing so. You have only one birth of this baby; don't hold back! The hospital can be an intimidating place, but just because the routine runs a certain way doesn't mean it can't be altered. For example, you can definitely refuse the following:

    Wearing a hospital gown

    People running in and out of your room continually

    Attendants talking during contractions

    Bright lights in the labor or delivery room

    Routine IV

    Routine episiotomy

    Having the baby taken away from you immediately (barring emergency complications)

- In the event that the baby requires care in the nursery and the mother cannot go with the baby due to need for repair or other surveillance, her partner (or doula if she is not partnered) should go to the nursery and maintain verbal and physical contact with the baby (warming units have holes to put hands through) until the mother is able to join them.

- If you are unsure about any recommended test for your newborn, ask your midwife or pediatrician. Don't be railroaded into a package treatment; let them convince you that each test is truly necessary for the baby's welfare.

- If you must stay in the hospital, activate your postpartum support system immediately. Don't think you can wait until you get home— you need it now! Have fresh fruit, vegetables, bread, cheese, water, and so on brought in daily, as hospital fare is inadequate in quality and quantity for a breastfeeding mother.

- Don't hesitate to ask for privacy. Routine checks on mother and baby occur on a regular schedule, but unless they are truly necessary because of some specific concern, refuse this constant monitoring or you will never get any rest! You may also find that as shifts change and new nurses appear, each will have some suggestion about wrapping, feeding, or caring for the baby. Offer your thanks, but explain that you prefer to figure things out yourself. If they press you, reassure them that you are fine and they need not worry. Otherwise, you can go crazy with input and may lose confidence in your natural mothering abilities.

- If you have been in the hospital for a few days due to some complication, be prepared to be absolutely exhausted when you get home. You don't get much sleep in the hospital anyway, but combine this with the stress of transport and the adjustments to your newborn, and imagine how tired you will be! Arrange it so no one is there when you first get home, except siblings and their caretaker.

- Take it easy on the processing; it may take some time before the whys and the wherefores of transport become evident. If you start to feel emotionally overwhelmed, call on your midwife.

diaphragmatic pressure to stimulate respiration. Remember to keep the baby warm: change dampened blankets promptly.

Hospital response to the slightly depressed baby is quite different. As duties are sharply divided by scope of practice, the obstetrician must immediately pass the newborn to the neonatal team. This requires premature cord clamping, which further compromises the baby. The neonatologist then places the baby in a warming unit, applies mechanical suction to its nose and throat, and, more often than not, bag-masks it even though it is already breathing. Time and again, I have watched babies deteriorate rapidly with this treatment. It is noteworthy that in all this, stimulation is usually overlooked—no one touches the baby. Sometimes I do it myself, while encouraging the mother to talk to the baby from across the room.

The baby born in secondary apnea, with Apgar 2 or less, is easily identified by its shockingly white and completely limp appearance, with no respiratory efforts whatsoever (as heart rate is the last to go, it may receive from 2 to 0 points in this category). Wrap this baby immediately in warm blankets, and as soon as suction is complete, administer pocket or bag-mask resuscitation with oxygen. Often the baby will open its eyes and look straight into yours before it begins to breathe, which opens your heart and greatly boosts your concentration. If the heart rate is less than 60 BPM (Apgar 1) or there is no heartbeat (Apgar 0), begin cardiac massage. A friend or the partner should call the ambulance at once.

Sometimes babies make gurgling noises with resuscitation. Depending on degree, you may need to repeat the suction (use a DeLee for best results). Rarely, globs of thick mucus are lodged in the throat and must be quickly removed with a fingertip. But don't fuss too much with this: securing ventilation is your top priority.

If the five-minute Apgar is less than 7, keep working to get the baby stimulated and engaged,

and redo Apgar readings every five minutes until you have two in a row of 8 or higher.

Circumstances of newborn stabilization are not always black and white. I have seen a few babies birth in fine condition and then rapidly deteriorate due to a lukewarm reception from the parents. Sometimes the mother is so exhausted that she cannot muster welcome for the baby. Or perhaps the baby is of undesired or unexpected gender. Use your heart in moments like these: "What a gorgeous girl (or boy) you have!" Or to the sibling standing by, say enthusiastically, "You have a sister (or brother)!" Love kindles life—it's just that simple—and the midwife must be ready to bring this to bear if need be.

I had an experience along these lines that I have never forgotten. The baby was born after an hour-long second stage and trouble-free labor. Heart tones were good throughout; the scalp tone was pink. No

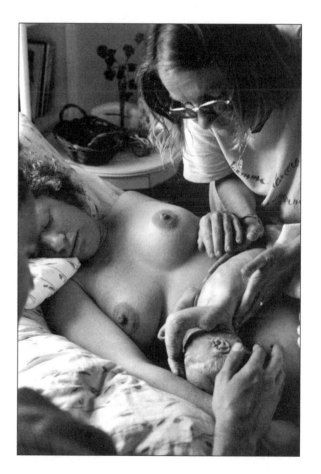

meconium in the waters, but there was a very tight cord around the neck, which I felt obliged to cut. The shoulders then birthed without delay, so there was no reason to expect what happened next.

Although the Apgar was 6 at birth, the baby lost what little muscle tone and color it had and respiratory efforts became irregular. Stimulation seemed to help, and the baby pinked up a bit with DeLee suction (it actually sucked the tubing). I thought the baby had made it then, but instead it proceeded to go pale and flaccid. I tried a few breaths with pocket mask, to which the baby responded mildly (although it had never really stopped breathing after the initial stimulation). The one-minute Apgar was 4. I tried more stimulation, but the moment I stopped, the baby began to fade away again.

Several minutes had gone by, so I decided I would take the baby and give it all the energy I could muster (I also had my apprentice call 911). As I took the baby in my hands and began the diaphragmatic seesaw, someone in the room observed that the baby had not yet opened its eyes. At that it winked its lids, and I began to swing its body slowly from side to side, hoping to prompt it to take a peek. Not much of anything, and I was beginning to panic. Then I recalled that its strongest response had been sucking on the DeLee, so I put my little finger in its mouth. A wave of desperation and tenderness swept through me as I began to speak, "Come on in, baby, it's not so bad here, come on, *please* come in." At that, it started sucking, opened its eyes, and looked right at me, and then turned nice and pink. Meanwhile, the paramedics arrived, but soon realized that nothing but observation was needed and left shortly thereafter.

How to explain the baby's in-and-out behavior? Likely causes, such as prematurity, infection, or maternal drug use, did not apply. However, there was a great deal of emotional tension between the parents regarding their relationship and the baby. The father had been unfaithful repeatedly during pregnancy and had made no adjustment whatsoever to his new responsibilities. Just moments after the birth, he literally moved to the far side of the room, and the mother froze up completely. I think the baby simply felt unwanted. The father would not connect with it at all; the mother would not speak to it when I prompted her. No wonder it was tentative! This was why, when I gave it my finger to suck, I instinctively said, "It's not so bad here . . . come on in."

This experience overwhelmed me as I came to realize that the baby's life was entirely in my hands—that I alone would make the difference in its decision to live. I had never been in this position before and still recall the confusion of searching for the baby's soul, hoping to give enough love and energy that it would want to stay. I definitely learned the importance of clearing up serious personal issues between parents in advance. As it turned out, the parents separated shortly after the birth, and the woman moved out of the area. But she kept in touch and proved to be a loving and devoted mother.

In any marginal situation like this, be sure to maintain an extra-long postpartum watch. Check the baby carefully and repeatedly (especially the heart and reflexes). Do not leave until the mother is warmly attentive and the baby is glowing. Contact the pediatrician and arrange to have the baby seen as soon as possible.

Fetal Anomalies

Fetal anomalies can be genetic in origin or may be caused by certain viruses, chemicals in the environment or workplace, radiation, street drugs, or pharmaceuticals. The following are useful references:

- A current edition of the *Physician's Desk Reference* will help you identify teratogenic effects of over-the-counter and prescription medications.

- The Organization of Teratology Information Services (OTIS) is an excellent resource on teratogens of every kind: reach them at (866) 626-6847 or at www.OTISpregnancy.org.

- The March of Dimes Birth Defects Foundation, at (888) 663-4637, which provides information on parent support organizations.

The most common fetal anomaly is heart defect. Minor defects like cleft palate or clubfoot are undetectable until birth, while more serious ones like spina bifida (exposed spinal meninges) may be discovered by blood tests and ultrasound in early pregnancy (see chapter 2). Although generally detected by AFP screening, palpation in late pregnancy may disclose hydrocephaly (enlarged cranium) or anencephaly (little or no cranial vault, with extremely large, long limbs).

Whenever a baby is born with anomalies, parents need to see, touch, and bond. Most mothers readily embrace their babies regardless of defects, often noting the beauty of other features. Just be sure to stay in close proximity to the mother (and her partner) until you are certain they have noticed the anomalies. Avoid pointing these out unless they are clearly in denial; in which case, do so simply and gently,

without discourses on causes, treatment, outcome, and so on. This information will surely be requested later: let the parents set the pace.

Occasionally, a mother rejects a severely deformed infant upon its arrival. If so, comment on the many perfect features of the baby. This provides a foundation for bonding without forcing her to confront the anomalies immediately.

Some midwives feel an odd sense of shame when assisting the birth of a baby with anomalies. This is probably a carryover from medieval days, when midwives were accused of practicing dark arts and causing fetal deformity. But it is also possible to feel all the joy and wonder as when assisting a normal baby—maybe more so. A midwife friend of mine related, "I had always been afraid of assisting a baby with deformities, but when it finally happened, I felt thrilled by his beautiful spirit and was very welcoming. He had many anomalies, but his body was secondary. I was shocked at how open I was to him, almost as if his imperfections made

---

Principles of Infant Resuscitation

If the baby is born limp and floppy, with a white body, do the following:

1. *Have your assistant or a family member call 911.*
2. *Provide warmth.* Wrap the baby with blankets and cover the head.
3. *Clear the airway.* Suction mouth with bulb syringe or DeLee if necessary.
4. *Move the baby to a flat surface and position so the chin is up but not overextended.* Otherwise, the airway will be occluded.
5. *Begin ventilation.* Place a mask unit over the baby's nose and mouth and give two slow breaths, allowing for exhale in between. Watch the baby's chest—it should rise and fall as you

work. If not, make sure you have a good seal over the nose and throat.

6. *If necessary, do full CPR.* Have your assistant take the baby's pulse, and if below 60, begin cycles of 15 chest compressions to two breaths, with approximately 120 compressions per minute (or as close to that as possible). Give compressions by placing both thumbs on the lower half of the sternum (just below the nipple line), pressing in about a third the depth of the chest. Switch to your bag-mask unit (hooked to oxygen) as soon as possible.
7. *After thirty seconds, briefly stop and recheck pulse.* Discontinue chest compressions once the heart rate reaches 60 BPM.

---

him more perfect in some way. This touched my heart profoundly."

You may also feel sadness, but your most crucial task is to open your heart and stay in the moment. You have plenty of time later to find your own support, but your initial reaction sets the tone for the mother and her supporters to begin making an adjustment.

Most anomalies require no immediate treatment, except for heart defects (indicated by cyanosis and respiratory distress) or spina bifida. In both cases, the pediatrician should be contacted and the baby transported to the hospital at once. With heart problems, keep the baby warm and give blow-by oxygen; with spina bifida, cover sinuses or exposed meninges with sterile gauze soaked in warm saline solution. Although not urgent, a baby with other anomalies should be seen as soon as possible as there may be other internal defects not readily detected by cursory examination.

Stay in close contact with the mother—not just for weeks, but for months. Do whatever you can to connect her with resources for information and support. This is certainly one area where the Internet has been a boon, as those who once suffered in isolation can now go online and find chat groups of others in the same situation. As mentioned earlier, there are also numerous national and international support organizations dealing with specific anomalies (see appendix B).

If anomalies are so severe as to be incompatible with life, take your cues from the mother and her partner. They may or may not want to transport, and you are obligated by professional ethics to respect their wishes. On the other hand, you must also give life support and call the paramedics if the baby appears viable. (See the next section on "Stillbirth and Neonatal Death" for more information.)

Stillbirth and Neonatal Death

Often death is caused by severe deformity, and it is clear that there are only moments of time for greeting, acknowledgment, and letting go. It is a blessing that birth generally leaves us refreshed and exhilarated, so if death occurs soon after, it is in a positive, open framework.

It is different when a baby is stillborn, especially with no apparent defect. Depending on when the baby died, the mother will either be in shock or already grieving as she gives birth.

Many women considering becoming a midwife hesitate at the thought of losing a baby. Is it the tangle of emotions, fear of accusation, or confrontation with death itself that is so frightening? Remember that birth and death are both high-energy, transitional states, and the guidelines for moving through them are virtually identical. Losing a baby is incomprehensibly tragic but easier if you stay emotionally present and connected. Help the mother touch and claim her baby: encourage her to save a lock of hair, take foot- and handprints, or take photographs. If she has a name for the baby, encourage her to use it. Bear witness to this rite of passage. Don't give consolation; there will be time for that later on.

The coroner must be notified of any stillborn infant weighing 500 g or more. Autopsy is at the discretion of the coroner. But if it can be established that the baby has been dead for some time, autopsy is optional. The coroner releases the body to a funeral home of the mother's choosing. With hospital stillbirth, the physician signs the death certificate: out of hospital, this is the coroner's task.

It is very difficult for the mother in the first few days postpartum. Hormone fluctuations compound her grief, which intensifies as her milk begins to flow. Suppress lactation with sage tea and by binding the breasts. Spend time with the mother and her supporters daily for the first few weeks. During these visits, friends and family may stop by and will look to you for reassurance and support (and they will have lots of questions). Just being there as a witness and friend, ready to listen, is your most important task right now. The mother may want suggestions on how to talk to siblings about death. See to her recovery by guarding her privacy, if need be. Take care of yourself, and get plenty of rest.

After assisting her first stillbirth, a midwife colleague related that she was both surprised and honored that at the memorial, each guest made a point of speaking not only to the parents and the reverend but to her as well. Be prepared to play an important role in this event. Learn to recognize the stages of grief—denial, anger, bargaining, depression, and acceptance—and be ready to share your observations with the mother as appropriate.

At some point, encourage her to make a scrapbook or write a chronicle of the birth and death. Expect to be in touch with her for many months and make it a point to call regularly and see her whenever she chooses. Contrary to popular belief, grieving is often a lengthy process comprised of rounds—some more vivid and painful than others—that may continue for a lifetime.

Notes

1. E. A. Friedman and B. H. Kroll, "Computer Analysis of Labor Progression," *Journal of Obstetrics and Gynecology* (British Commonwealth) 76 (1969): 1075–79. E. A. Friedman and B. H. Kroll, "Computer Analysis of Labor Progression II, Distribution of Data and Limits of Normal," *Journal of Reproductive Medicine* 6 (1971): 20–25.

2. Leah Albers, "The Duration of Labor in Healthy Women," *Journal of Perinatology* 19, no. 2 (1999): 114–19.

3. Anne Frye, *Holistic Midwifery*, vol. 2 (Portland, OR: Labyrs Press, 2004), 50.

4. Ruth Ancheta and Penny Simkin, *The Labor Progress Handbook* (Oxford, UK: Blackwell Science Ltd, 2000): 154–56.

5. Frye, *Holistic Midwifery*, vol. 2.

6. Frye, *Holistic Midwifery*, vol. 2.

7. Jean Sutton, "Occipito-Posterior Position and Some Ideas of How to Change It!" in *Midwifery: Best Practice*, ed. Sara Wickham (London: Elsevier Science Limited, 2003), 97.

8. Elizabeth Bachner, private correspondence, 2007.

9. Doña Queta Contreras and Doña Irene Sotelo, Midwifery Today conference notes, Oaxaca, Mexico, October 2003.

10. R. H. J. Hamlin, *Stepping Stones to Labor Ward Diagnosis* (Adelaide, Australia: Rigby Ltd., 1959).

11. American College of Obstetricians and Gynecologists. ACOG Practice Bulletin. Clinical Management Guidelines for Obstetrician-Gynecologists, Number 106: "Intrapartum Fetal Heart Rate Monitoring: Nomenclature, Interpretation, and General Management Principles), July 2009.

12. B. M. Sibai, "Diagnosis and Management of Gestational Hypertension and Preeclampsia," *American Journal of Obstetrics and Gynecology* 102 (2003): 181.

13. Henci Goer, *The Thinking Woman's Guide to a Better Birth* (New York: Berkley Publishing, 1999), 210.

14. M. E. Hannah et al., "Induction of Labor Compared with Expectant Management for Prelabor Rupture of the Membranes at Term," *New England Journal of Medicine* 334 (April 1996): 1005–10.

15. M. F. Schutte, P. E. Treffers, G. J. Kloosterman, and S. Soepatmi, "Management of Premature Rupture of Membranes: The Risk of Vaginal Examination to the Infant," *American Journal of Obstetrics and Gynecology* 146, no. 4 (June 1983): 395–400.

16. H. A. Abenhaim, L. Azoulay, M. S. Kramer, and L. Leduc, "Incidence and Risk Factors of Amniotic Fluid Embolisms: A Population-Based Study on 3 Million Births in the United States," *American Journal of Obstetrics and Gynecology* 199, no. 1 (July 2008): 49 e.1–8.

17. Frye, *Holistic Midwifery*, vol. 2.

18. Ricardo Herbert Jones, Midwifery Today conference notes, Oaxaca, Mexico, October 2003.

19. Cunningham et al., *Williams Obstetrics*, 23rd ed., 777.

20. Frye, *Holistic Midwifery*, vol. 2.

Liam Andrew
Shannon Anton, CPM

We watched the moon rise slowly from inside the jeep. The moon rose slowly, and slowly I watched every detail of her round, white fullness so pronounced. The speed of my life, every movement and interaction, has been altered to reflect the slow pace of grief. Next to the moon I can see a few people leaving the church. I wonder why they don't notice the moon right there, only then I realize she is behind them—concealed yet right there on the horizon, suspended silently in front of me, looking me right in the eye. I am familiar with this feeling in my heart. It is what I feel for an old, old friend that I have loved well but have not thought of for too long. Nostalgic and strange, because someone else now has died and that sadness is again permeating my days, slowing them until I can see the beauty in everything. Sometimes I must be slowed so very much before I can see it clearly; then there it is and the moment can pass to the next.

A few days ago, I walked in the park and crossed the land bridge between the ponds. On the sand were the usual folks, plus ducks and turtles, which always skitter into the water as I approach with my dogs by my side. A single turtle stayed on the sand, making no move toward the water. I was quite close before I realized she was still there, looking at me, unwavering. Her eyes found my gaze and held it. I stopped. It was a long moment of slow stillness. The scent of the pond, the sand, the lush green on the banks became like a fog around me and mixed with the heat of hiking. I took a step forward to steady myself in her gaze. Once there I continued on, walking fast away from her because, I told myself, the dogs would bother her. Uh huh. And now I think of her stare and know that today I could meet her gaze completely.

What I remember most from Susan's pregnancy is her smiling face above her growing belly. We laughed easily during our visits. Her baby moved in response to our feeling his knees, his back, kicking us while we listened to his heartbeat. We guessed sometimes he was a boy, sometimes a girl. The Blessingway brought my assistant Jane and I into the circle of loving closeness that surrounds Susan and Mark.

Susan called me at 6 a.m. On the phone she was nervous and giggly, contractions woke her around 4 a.m. after not much sleep. We talked, and I planned to come when she called me back, or if I hadn't heard from her by 10 a.m., I would come by and check in. I arrived at their house around 11 a.m., and Susan was in early labor. She was kneeling on the floor with her elbows on the bed, beginning to be uncomfortable during her contractions. I worked to help her stay relaxed during them, to breathe deeply and loosely. She moved into the ease of that without struggle, and as she did, the contractions became longer. I took her blood pressure and we agreed to listen to the baby's heartbeat after the next contraction.

Susan leaned back on the bed and I pressed the fetascope to her belly. I heard nothing, and seeing from the shape of her belly that the baby was still posterior, continued to listen in other places, guessing how the sound of the heartbeat might travel around folded arms and legs. I sat back to stretch and saw with some surprise that the bottom half of her belly was covered in the small ring-shaped indentations left by my fetascope. I had still heard nothing.

I grabbed my Doppler from my bag and explained that I wanted to use it to try and hear the baby; Susan agreed. I listened. I heard nothing. I asked Susan if she'd been feeling the baby move and she said she thought so, though as the contractions became stronger it might have been the start of each contraction that she had thought was movement. I jiggled her belly, rubbing the baby's knees, hoping for a kick to let me know all was well. Nothing. I put my Doppler on the charger, thinking maybe it wasn't working properly, and sent Susan downstairs for a glass of juice to try to wake the baby up.

continued >>

A few minutes later, we tried to find the heart-beat again, this time downstairs on the couch where we had always done prenatals together. I told myself that she hadn't been flat enough upstairs to hear easily. With the fetascope I again heard nothing, covering her lower belly once more with round indentations.

I went upstairs to get my Doppler again, and while I was in the bedroom I felt that same unsteadiness I'd felt with the turtle. I told myself I'd been on my knees too long and now I'd run up the stairs, no wonder. But once downstairs again with the Doppler, still I could hear nothing of the baby's heartbeat. Out of frustration both with the technology in my hands, and the feeling that at this point, I might not know the heartbeat if it bit me, I held the Doppler to my own heart and heard it clearly: boom . . . boom . . . boom.

Satisfied the Doppler was working, I held it again to Susan's belly. The words "silent uterus" rose up from somewhere deep in my mind. I thought how strangely accurate they were: I could hear no sound at all. Susan had felt nothing of movement yet, and was beginning to believe she might not have felt the baby move since the night before; she and Mark had spent time together, feeling the baby kick.

We went back upstairs so I could do an internal exam. I thought if I could stimulate the baby's head, he might give us a kick. We worked between contractions, Susan lying back while I reached with my fingers to find her cervix opened three centimeters and a bulging bag of water in front of her baby's head. The baby's head itself was slightly overlapping at the sagittal suture, and I thought the edge of the suture line had a jagged, shard-like quality to it. The baby's head was still high in her pelvis, high enough it seemed odd that there would be molding now, already. When I pressed against the head, I could feel a wrinkly, loose scalp over the crown. Thinking back now, things seem obvious, but then it seemed that nothing made sense.

I tried one more time to hear the baby's heartbeat and when I could not, I said to Susan and Mark, "This has never happened to me before, it's just never taken me this long to hear heart tones. We haven't felt the baby move and I don't know what else to try. I think we need to go to the hospital and try to get the baby on the monitor."

Susan and Mark agreed. I added, "We'll probably get there and find the heartbeat right away and I'll feel like an idiot, but I don't care. I'll go call now while you get things together."

I went downstairs and phoned labor and delivery. The voice on the other end was familiar, and when I identified myself, she said, "Shannon, it's Jan Randall. How are you?"

In a moment's passing my mind flashed through my experiences with Jan; she'd apprenticed with me for a short time. I recalled the sense of her at my shoulder as a young, single mom pushed her baby out after a few short hours of labor, the mom's laboring sounds and then the baby's cries echoing off the high ceiling of her Victorian apartment, grayish morning light filtering through tall windows. I also remembered her very pregnant body just a few months ago: she'd given birth at home herself, to a healthy baby boy.

Realizing time was doing that amorphous thing it does around birth (and death), I came back to the present, to Jan, and in the same breath I laid out everything that had happened so far. When I came to not having any other ideas except coming in, she agreed. She said it was a slow day there and she could take care of us herself; she wanted to keep things low-key for Susan and Mark.

I called my apprentice and gave her a brief version of what was happening. She would meet us at the hospital.

We drove on the freeway. I followed Mark, and as we drove, I thought to myself how good it was that we were staying in the exit lane, since we were going so slowly. I glanced at my speedometer and was surprised to find it at 60 mph. I looked around—even knowing this I would have guessed our speed at around 30 mph. I backed off Mark's bumper to a reasonable distance, vaguely aware that something was definitely up. I was in an altered state now and felt a sense of something important to come.

On arrival, we made our way to labor and delivery. The ward was quiet. No one was willing to meet my eye directly, and while one nurse handed us a clipboard with admission forms on it, she turned abruptly on her heel and retreated behind the desk. I felt as if everyone there had heard of our concern and no one was quite sure how to respond to us in this limbo time of not knowing. So to be respectful, no one engaged with us. I stayed by Susan and Mark while they wrote down the few lines of information needed.

Jane arrived. Then Jan came over to us and greeted us warmly, showing us all into a room. She made explanation of the technology at hand, reminding Susan that it takes a while sometimes to find the heartbeat with the monitor. Jan swept slowly across Susan's lower belly. She paused at intervals, waiting, looking at the monitor, listening for the familiar and reassuring blip of heartbeat. Nothing. She told Susan and Mark that she liked to have a second person try before being convinced that we couldn't get anything on the monitor. Jan looked at me and asked if I'd like to give it a try. I took the sensor in hand and repeated the search. My sense of the baby was obscure, not like usual when I have an idea where to try and hear heart tones. I knew I was in the right area but it still felt off, like I only thought I knew where to listen.

After searching across her belly again, I asked Jan, "What's next?" She recommended a sonogram; Susan and Mark agreed. Jan went to get a doctor, and we waited. The room was quiet. I didn't know what to say to fill the space, so I said nothing. We waited together quietly. Inside myself I was feeling a dread certainty; I hoped I was wrong and I hoped I wasn't too transparent.

The door squeaked open and Jan returned with a doctor following. The doctor came directly to look Susan in the eye and introduce herself. "I'm Dr. Frazier. I've brought a sonogram machine with me so we can have a better look at your baby. Is that all right with you?" Her voice had the kind steadiness that I knew from other transports when we'd worked together. I felt relieved to see her on duty, a friendly and familiar face. I felt like we were being buffered by a soundness of community that surprised and comforted me.

As Dr. Frazier moved the sono probe across Susan's belly, I held my breath. She was quiet, looking hard all around. Then she swept over the baby's ribcage and I could see clearly the brightly lit ribs

in silhouette around the heart. There was only stillness. No movement, no heartbeat.

In a tone of voice that was kind but left no room for possibility, Dr. Frazier said, "I'm looking right now at your baby's lungs and heart, and I don't see any movement. The baby's heart is not beating. Your baby has died."

Susan and Mark were stunned, my eyes were already tearing, and I felt no breath in my own body.

After a brief pause, Dr. Frazier asked Susan, "Have you been laboring a long time?"

Susan's reply was like a reflex, "No! It's just really started."

"When did you last feel the baby move?"

"Well, I thought I was feeling movement with every contraction, but as the contractions got a little stronger, I think I was feeling the beginning of them, maybe not movement. But the baby was moving a lot last night, we both felt it." Susan looked at Mark, and they held hands a little tighter.

"This is intense news I'm giving you, and I have to tell you, I've been up all night. So before I say for certain, I'd like another doctor to have a look, just to be sure. Is that all right with you?" I knew that Dr. Frazier was willing, hoping to be wrong. But I also knew what I saw on the sono screen, what I sensed as time went on. I could appreciate her wanting to be wrong, knowing but not wanting to believe, but still, knowing.

For the next hour we hung in a limbo that felt like days. Susan couldn't really let labor go on, she couldn't quite begin grieving, she couldn't feel all was well. The sono machine sat blindly against the wall, waiting with us. At one point Susan said, "Second opinions are good. We'll wait."

At long last, three doctors entered the room together. Dr. Frazier introduced Dr. Jones and Dr. Irwin. It was Dr. Irwin who repeated the sonogram and at 3 p.m. confirmed the baby was dead. There was a long moment of shocked silence, and then we all began to cry. The doctors excused themselves, saying softly that we could have all the time we needed and to come get them when we were ready to talk about a plan.

continued >>

The door swung shut and Susan and Mark, holding each other, began to wail. I felt the wall against my back. Cool, solid, I slid down to sit at its base, the floor rising up to meet me. I could not look at Jane for a long time. My face was wet but I wasn't sure if I was crying. Jane caught my eye and crawled over to put her arms around me. We both sobbed.

I remember thinking how empty I could still feel with someone's arms around me like that. It wasn't Jane's embrace that was empty: it was the emptiness of loss that I remembered couldn't feel any better no matter who held me. That is the forlorn truth about grief. It's just in you until it's not anymore. It seemed tragic to have it fill me again, to know the hard path of its eventual leaving, that path stretching out long and lonely before us all, especially before Susan and Mark.

We mourned hard for the first hour after the news of their baby's death. At the end of that time, Susan's labor was beginning to pick up; she was getting practical. She looked at me squarely and, not asking for confirmation, said, "I still have to birth this baby, right?"

I was standing close to her and Mark. I forced my voice out of my body, "Yes."

Susan looked first at Mark and then at me again and nodded, "Okay."

"Should I go and get Dr. Frazier now?"

"Yes."

I moved through the door and down the hall. The lights were too bright; the skin on my cheeks and around my eyes was strangely tender; coming to the nurses' station I felt my eyes squint. Dr. Frazier was reading my chart on Susan. I sat down next to her and waited for her attention to turn to me. Another of those long moments passed.

"Hi, how're you doing?" she asked. I could only inhale and nod my head a little. She spoke directly, this time to me, "You gave her good care. There isn't anything you should have done that you didn't."

At this I had tears on my face, "Well, something like this happens, I have to wonder. . . ."

Dr. Frazier took my hand and said, "She received excellent care from you. I'll tell her the same thing. If she'd been our patient she wouldn't even be here

yet. She's forty-one weeks, but that isn't enough for our postdates protocol to set in. You did a good job." She paused and added, "And we're not gonna do anything about this." I realized she was referring to having me investigated or arrested, and I couldn't believe how far that was from my mind. The thought of having to protect myself right now was too much. I just could do what I was doing. I felt so still inside, like movement or speech required incredible intention.

I sniffed and thanked her: "It's really nice of you to say that."

She nodded. "One of the docs here had a daughter getting top OB care at Stanford; at thirty-nine weeks her baby died. They don't know why. We may not find out either." She turned back to the chart and asked, "Is she ready to talk?"

"Yes, I came to get you."

We walked into Susan's room and all attention turned toward the doctor. She spoke in soft tones and laid a hand on Susan's arm. The contractions were getting stronger. Dr. Frazier and Susan briefly discussed the options: staying here to have her baby or having her baby back at home. Then I heard Dr. Frazier tell Susan that there wasn't anything she should have done that she didn't do, that she had gotten excellent care with her midwives. Then she left us to the decision making.

The door closed and Susan asked me if I would still help her have her baby at home. I said, "Of course. We'll be wherever you are. If you stay here, we'll stay. Whatever you want to do is really okay." She asked if she could have her friends come to the hospital. Her contractions continued to get stronger. It seemed too difficult to return home at that point. I went to call Peg and Jackie.

For the next twenty-four hours, the labor of birthing and grieving coexisted. Alternately each would fill the room—laughter and tears. Friends and family came to call, more like after a death than in preparation for a birth. None of it felt wrong.

Susan worked with her contractions, breathing, moaning, sighing, until the last bit of cervix was dissolved around her baby's head. She felt pressure enough to make her want to push, and as she bore down she felt the need to be more upright. She pushed well that first time, very vertical, using the squatting bar and coming a bit onto her feet at the end of the bed. After that contraction, I felt inside to check on the baby's descent and position.

Another contraction came quickly, and as I was removing my fingers from Susan's vagina, I could feel the bones of the baby's head shifting suddenly and sharply beneath the scalp. The molding was extreme and the scalp loose over it. The edges of bone felt sharp and shard-like, as I remembered from before.

I thought of a squirrel I'd skinned after a road kill and how the skull was fractured into a hundred tiny sharp pieces. The sound those pieces made when I shifted the squirrel in my hands, it traveled not through the air to my ears but instead vibrated through my fingers and up my arms. Like broken glass but denser, like stoneware, but hydrated and suffused with the stuff of living. It was a sensation of sound in my body. The baby's head bones made a similar clicking and grinding.

For one frightening moment, I could imagine the baby's head coming apart, the bones tearing through the scalp and compressing together flatly. I motioned to Jane to help me position Susan in a more reclining posture, allowing more space toward her sacrum for the baby's head to descend, removing direct pressure from the pubic bone.

She pushed again in this new reclining position, and I felt the need to check once more to assure myself that the worst was not happening. The baby's head then felt normal, still sharp around the edges but molding in a reasonable way.

Susan pushed a bit more. Suddenly, we could see the baby's head through her labia! I brought Mark down on the floor with me; on our knees we watched as more of the head gradually appeared. This baby had a good amount of dark hair, wavy and wet.

I felt inside again to see how the head was molding, how it was moving the bands of muscle out of the way toward crowning. I was afraid again of what might happen to the baby's head if I wasn't careful. I began pressing evenly on the muscle bands at Susan's vaginal opening. All I could think was, "I don't want the baby's head to come apart." I thought then, "Wow, I wonder if all bottoms feel this tight before the baby's really pressing more

toward crowning? I never ever do this. Why am I doing this?" I stood up and stood back, thinking, "Geez, girl, get a grip!" I looked around and saw Anne, our nurse, standing nearby. I whispered in her ear, "Have you been to a stillbirth before?" She nodded yes.

"How careful of the head do I have to be?"

"Oh, not very."

I looked at her with my heart and so completely trusted her that I just moved back to the floor, beside Mark, and knew I'd be all right, the baby would be born without damage, and Susan could see and hold her baby without ugliness or horror. I felt a huge worry leave my body. I was warm and relaxed all at once. The world around me slowed again.

I looked at Mark and said, "We'll do this together so neither one of us will be alone." He nodded and smiled a little.

Susan continued to push. Each time, the baby moved a little bit. I was glad to see the gradual movement; her bottom was stretching perfectly with the gentle pressure of the baby's head. Even though the head had begun to come around the pubic bone with her pushes, between contractions it would slip back up again. Susan could feel this and felt at first like she was losing ground. I assured her that with the next contraction, the baby would move right back down again. A bit of a running start. Susan laughed at my joke and I realized what joy and expectation filled the room.

When the baby stayed in view between pushes, I kept pressure on the occiput of the baby's head to help keep it flexed, and to protect Susan's urethra and inner labia. There was a lot of give in her perineum; she was stretching around the baby's head beautifully. She reached down around my hands and felt the bulge of baby's head and smiled like when you just can't believe something so wonderful is happening.

Susan slowly crowned her baby's head. Little by little, the baby was born to his forehead. Mark's forehead, the baby had Mark's forehead! A long pause for the next contraction, and then the baby's nose and finally mouth and chin were born. Dark

continued >>

fluid drained from the baby's nose and mouth. I said to Mark, "The airway is getting squeezed clear now, this is really normal." Mark, not taking his eyes off the baby, nodded.

I felt along the baby's neck and found the cord, loosely there. I pulled an easy loop but it wasn't enough to go over the head. I reached for the first cord clamp and said, "The cord's around the neck and we need to cut it. Mark, do you want to cut it?"

"No, no, go ahead," he said. A little more time went by as I reached for the second clamp and then the scissors and said, "Okay, Mark, you wanna cut it?"

"Oh . . . sure, why not."

I held the cord by the clamps and he slid the scissors under, along the baby's neck. My fingers protected Susan and the baby. Mark cut the cord and helped me unwrap it from the baby's neck.

The next contraction and push didn't change anything. I carefully reached inside along the baby's back to find the shoulders completely unflexed. The usual sweep that brings unflexed shoulders together only moved loose bones in their joints; the baby had no real form. Utter lack of muscle tone allowed movement away from my hands rather than my hands shaping the baby's movement. With two hands I gently rotated the shoulders, and ever so slowly the baby restituted to face the right.

I heard Dr. Irwin ask me if I wanted suprapubic pressure, and heard my reply, no, the shoulder was right here. Concentration consumed me. I had to support every bit of the baby's birthed body or it would fall loosely to the bed. Susan continued to push and slowly, slowly the baby's body was born completely.

Mark helped me hand the baby up to Susan's belly. We all stood around the edges of the bed, around Susan and the baby. I don't know what we expected; no one was prepared for such a beautiful baby. We all just stared with awe for a moment before tears began to fall. We cried hard in those first minutes. Mark lifted the baby's leg to see, boy or girl? He was a boy. Susan and Mark said his name right away: Liam Andrew. He was named. He was their son.

I looked down as I cried, and tears splashed on my left breast. I'd been in the same dress for two days; the weight of the cotton had the neckline plunging, my bosom quite exposed. The sensation of Liam's birth was so much on the surface of my body; the sensation of the tears on my breast filled and startled me. It somehow echoed on my skin, the sadness in my heart. I was transfixed with the moment: I could see birth and death, the cycle of life before me. I was filled with a deep and abiding trust in life. It was a moment when everything came together vividly to make sense, to make a whole; it was also a moment of blinding grief. Susan was glowing, triumphant in her birth, ravaged and grieving in her son's death. So much all at once. It was a sacred and perfect time. I hope never to experience it again; I pray never to forget its influence.

We stayed together for five hours after Liam's birth. We held him, prayed for him, bathed and dressed him. We took photographs. We even laughed.

After having seen Susan and Mark the next day, I stopped on my way home to get food for my dog. When I returned to my car, it wouldn't start. It was a hot day and everything remained in slow, vivid motion. Moment by moment passed as I stared at the brightness in the air around me. The last thing I wanted to do was deal with a towing company. I just wanted not to talk to anyone. I left my car and began the two-mile walk home. I headed for Golden Gate Park, for home on the other side.

Walking felt heavy but good. Everything was blindingly bright. I think I walked with my eyes closed, the heat searing through my eyelids in a swirling red density. I'm sure I was not alone.

I strayed from the present just as I crossed the polo field. By the time I skirted the ponds and was overcome with the moist smell of the mud, the tall grasses and their whispering shuffle, I was back in Iowa, following another dirt path, and headed for the short track. I recalled that bright day well. Skeater wore no helmet; he rounded a corner on his cycle and met Roger head on. Literally. Skeater collided with Roger's bike and then his helmet and landed finally in the soft grass of the field. It was my first true loss. Grief held my hand as I crested the sandy bank of the pond. Today the turtles won't meet my eye; they skitter into the water and are gone. That rich muddy smell, all heady and ripe: I recognize the scent of decay, of loss and turning under. I am relieved to name it. I am comforted by the familiarity of it. I give a nod of greeting to my old dead friends and see Liam among them. All those nice boys together.

As I broke through the line of grass and found my feet on asphalt, I was at once confused. I spun around, reeling, really, and the foreground popped back into focus. It is 1995. I am a midwife. I have a place on my left breast that is ablaze. That is where the grief leaks out, where it exactly meets the light of day. Darkness to light, inside to out. It is a small opening, like for a pinhole camera, and the view is incredibly sharp.

A few days later, in the chair with Natasha leaning over me, needle buzzing in hand, I read the sign on the wall that says "Yes, it hurts," and I think, "But not that bad." She asks me something, and I don't know how to reply; it was a simple question I can't recall now, but what I did say was, "I'm a midwife and I had a stillbirth in my practice. Liam Andrew Brooks O'Donnel." She paused and looked at me closely. She didn't look away, but she went back to my breast, back to her work. It's a beautiful tattoo. Tending it was both painful and validating. Something physical hurt, but I could put salve on it and it felt better. At least on the surface.

CHAPTER 6

Postpartum Care

Postpartum care is the last frontier for midwives and those concerned with maternal well-being. Far too many mothers are virtually abandoned after a day or two of the most rudimentary care. We therefore refer to the first three months following birth as the "fourth trimester," with the understanding that pregnancy and birth are transformative experiences culminating in this crucial phase of reintegration.

Preparation for the fourth trimester should begin prenatally. Nothing is more important than connecting pregnant women with one another, or better still, with those who have recently given birth. Group prenatal care (see page 235, "Setup and Administration") or childbirth preparation classes may help to facilitate this, but however it happens, it is not optional. Once the baby is born, you will move on with your practice, and the mother will need other mothers for counsel and support. This is especially crucial if she has few friends and none of them have children. Mothering in the first few months is made up of many mundane concerns, and contacts with others in the same phase, even if not the most profound of intimacies, will serve a great purpose.

For all its sweetness, this is one of the most challenging times in a woman's life. It has wisely been said that the challenges of pregnancy and birth are but preparation for the enormous adjustments postpartum. I often tell women that the first six weeks of caring for a newborn is the hardest work they will ever do. That we treat new mothers as if nothing has changed, expecting them to be back on their feet or at work in a matter of days, is the height of denial. In nearly every society but ours, continuous care is provided at this time; the mother's only obligation is to stay in bed and focus on the baby.

Mothering the mother leads to her full recovery. Good care lets her move through the challenges of this period gracefully, and her child reaps the benefits of her increasing security in her new role. Care of new mothers assures survival of the species, but more than that, it positively affects the quality of life for all of us.

Postpartum customs of certain Native American and Indonesian cultures literally make sure that the new mother is not left out in the cold. Adequate heat is the centerpiece of care, as new mothers are perceived to be greatly opened by birth and thus susceptible to chill and loss of energy. If needed, a fire is built near or even under the mother's bed so she can remain unclothed and fully at ease. In Mexico and Guatemala, she is treated to a **temescal** (steam bath with herbs) just days after giving birth. In contrast to the numbing isolation endured by most mothers in the United States, these women are surrounded by female friends and relatives who feed, counsel, and joke with them. In the Philippines, a new mother is believed to be in such a state of grace that if she dies in the first forty days postpartum, her soul will automatically be in heaven.

When a woman is not well cared for, there are complex and often long-term effects on her body, personality, and sexuality. If she is forced out of bed or back to work too soon, overproduction of adrenaline will derail her recovery. Without sufficient rest, postpartum recovery is prolonged and often incomplete.

Although the roots of postpartum depression are largely biological, there are emotional factors, too. This period is characterized by a degree of personal loss, which is often unexpected and may be quite painful. Single friends may find it hard to relate to the baby, and the primary relationship, rather than reverting to what it used to be, is likely to be strained by worry and fatigue. Old routines and ways of handling the most basic tasks must change, and privacy becomes a thing of the past. Depending on the mother's work situation, the family may also lose income. Mix in a measure of chronic fatigue, and the ground for depression is laid.

Postpartum adjustment is so much easier if the mother learned while giving birth that control is just an illusion. But if her birth experience was less than optimal, she may remain confused on this point and find it hard to surrender to the demands of mothering. Thus it is critical that you help her debrief her birth experience. She may want to discuss the birth as early as day one and may need to do so repeatedly over the next few months. This is particularly true if the birth was difficult or disappointing: she needs to grieve, and you must support her in this. (Preparing the mother for debriefing is covered in "Home Visits," page 60.)

Even if her birth was trouble free, she will be vulnerable and impressionable for some time. Well-meaning but misguided advice sinks deep: criticism is not easily forgotten. Do all you can to protect her from negative influences while seeing to her needs for physical and emotional warmth.

Day-One Visit

Begin this visit by appraising the environment for order and cleanliness. If laundry or dishes have piled up or if the refrigerator is bare, get things organized. See what the mother has been eating and drinking (there should be a jug of water at her bedside). The room should be comfortably warm, and baby things readily available. If she has not showered yet, help her do so. Ask how she has been feeling in general: any dizzy spells, exhaustion, or emotional upsets? Her report will largely be influenced by what kind of help she is receiving from her partner or friends.

Stress her need for a full ten days of absolute rest, following her body's signals for sleep and nourishment just as she did while pregnant. Explain how high levels of oxytocin released with breastfeeding prompt uterine involution (the return of the uterus to its pre-pregnant size) and retoning of the vaginal muscles, but if she is overactive or stressed, the release of adrenaline will inhibit this process. In other words, the more she rests and lets her body recover, the sooner she will look and feel her best. This message bears repeating as it is critical to her recuperation.

On the other hand, she should walk several times daily, even if just up and down the hallway. Good circulation in her legs helps prevent **thrombophlebitis** (see "Thrombophlebitis and Pulmonary Embolism" on page 211).

Herbs and Homeopathy Postpartum
Shannon Anton, CPM

Keep the room warm immediately following the birth and do not give the mother cold drinks. If a newly postpartum woman has to warm her body after a chill, or if she has to warm up the contents of her stomach, she is wasting vital energy. Her entire course of postpartum recovery can be greatly affected by these factors. Her energy at this time is precious. Respect and conserve it.

Postpartum Bath

If a woman has been consistently stable in the immediate postpartum hours, I offer her a healing postpartum bath. Here is a recipe, contributed by midwife Janice Kalman and originated by the Chico midwives:

Boil one large bulb of *garlic* in a big pot of water for twenty minutes. Turn off the flame and add dried herbs: one handful *comfrey* leaves, one handful *witch hazel* solution, half a handful *uva ursi* leaves, several slices of dried or fresh *ginger root*, half a handful of *yarrow flowers*, and a large pinch of *rosemary*. Steep covered for at least twenty minutes. In the meantime, scrub the tub thoroughly and rinse carefully. Paint the entire surface with Betadine and let stand twenty minutes. Rinse tub completely. Run warm (not hot) water to fill, include a large handful of sea salt, and strain the herbal concoction into the tub. The mother and baby may both get in the bath, provided someone stays with them constantly.

Afterpains

These can be very painful and distracting for the new mother. Strongly brewed *ginger* tea brings relief from afterpains. Pour one cup boiling water over three to five slices of fresh *ginger* and steep five to ten minutes. *Motherwort* tincture also eases afterpains—begin dosage at half a dropperful and increase as needed.

Herb Pharm makes an excellent herbal compound tincture called *Hellonias Viburnum* that greatly relieves afterpains. Take one dropperful as needed.

Prolapsed Uterus or Cervix

Sometimes a woman's cervix comes down to her introitus after giving birth. If so, reglove and gently push the cervix back up to its usual position. Instruct the woman to stay in bed as much as possible and to begin exercising the pelvic muscles. In addition, homeopathic *sepia 200C* offers vital support.

Homeopathic *sepia 200C* is also indicated when a woman reports feeling her insides dropping or sagging when she walks or stands. Have her take this several times a day and continue to rest in bed.

When there is uterine, bladder, or hemorrhoid prolapse, or when a woman seems especially exhausted and compromised in the weeks postpartum, it indicates compromised liver **chi** (or strength). Recurrent yeast infections also indicate weakened liver chi. Refer the mother to a skilled practitioner of **traditional Chinese medicine (TCM)**. It is worth noting that uterine prolapse at any age can usually be corrected with TCM.

Healing after Cesarean Section

Homeopathic *staphysagria* promotes healing after a cesarean or any surgical procedure. *Staphysagria 30C* taken several times a day will support full recovery. When painful symptoms ease, discontinue use.

Nipple Soreness

Expressing a few drops of milk and rubbing it into the areola will help sore nipples heal. Also allow nipples to air-dry after nursing or expose them to sunlight. If nipples are cracking and bleeding, try homeopathic *graphites 30C*, taken several times a day.

Milk Fever and Mastitis

Because most engorgement and milk fevers emerge during the night, I ask my clients to have four homeopathic remedies on hand: *arnica*, *bryonia*, *phytolacca*, and *belladonna*, all in the over-the-counter potencies of 6x or 30C.

When the breasts are full, tender, and hot to the touch, getting the baby to nurse or expressing a bit of milk so she or he can latch on is crucial. In addition, try homeopathic *bryonia 30C* and *phytolacca 30C*, alternating every twenty minutes until engorgement symptoms resolve, usually in a few hours. *Echinacea tincture*—half a drop per pound of body weight—can be taken several times a day, when the breasts are engorged, to prevent the onset of mastitis.

Compresses

Compresses can stimulate the flow of milk, preventing it from backing up and becoming infected. Warm water may be used, but steamed, fresh *comfrey leaves* or strong tea compresses are more therapeutic. Keep compresses on for twenty minutes. Whole, raw *cabbage leaves* (which steam on the breast) may also be used and should be left until they soften. During this time, the mother may cry and express concerns, disappointments, or fears. Be present and ready to listen. Also have something warm available for her to drink.

Fever with Engorgement

Engorgement or lumpy soreness in the breast accompanied by a rising fever can be resolved with homeopathic *belladonna 30C*, taken every twenty to thirty minutes. Fever should reduce to normal in the subsequent few hours, and the homeopathic remedy can be discontinued.

Meanwhile, the mother must also nurse or express milk from congested areas. Coating the breasts with *aloe vera* helps reduce the risk of secondary infection. Doses of *echinacea tincture* also support the body in healing mastitis. Make sure she is well hydrated, well nourished, and getting complete rest.

Building the Milk Supply

Galactagogues help women maintain an abundant supply of breast milk. They may be helpful to any mother having a difficult time recovering from birth. A classic galactagogue is *dark beer*; have the mother drink one a day. *Hops* in tincture form can also stimulate milk production.

Another old remedy is *fennel/barley water*. Boil half a cup pearled barley in three cups water for twenty-five minutes. Save the *barley water*, and reheat it (do not boil) to make *fennel tea*, with one teaspoon *fennel* to one cup *barley water*. Do not steep the tea longer than thirty minutes.

Drying Up the Milk Supply

As midwives, we sometimes help women who have miscarriages or stillbirths, or for some reason choose not to nurse their babies. Still, they will have milk. To help ease engorgement, follow the instructions above. In addition, have the mother bind her breasts with a long, stretchy wrap. Cold compresses also act to dry up the milk (though cold in any form undermines postpartum healing). Drinking *sage* tea is a dependable method for reducing milk production, and two drops daily of *pokeroot tincture* minimizes engorgement.

Extended Postpartum Bleeding

Some women continue to have bright-red spotting after six weeks postpartum. To remedy this, try *shepherd's purse tincture*, half a dropperful twice a day for up to a week. *Moxa* therapy applied midline between pubic bone and umbilicus (known as the conception vessel) and over the sacroiliac joints supports uterine involution. Referral for TCM is appropriate.

Umbilical Cord Care

A few drops of *echinacea tincture* on the newly cut cord stump is a reliable way to treat the umbilical cord. You may also use *goldenseal tincture* or breast milk. Treat the cord several times a day until the stump falls off.

continued >>

Jaundice

Traditional Chinese medicine offers a very effective remedy for newborn jaundice, which parents can obtain from a Chinese apothecary or herbalist. Simmer this root and swab the liquid inside the baby's mouth. One or two applications will usually clear jaundice.

Colic

A few teaspoons of crushed *fennel* or *caraway seed tea* can greatly relieve the discomfort of colic. Try light pressure and warm compresses on baby's belly, or bringing its feet slowly up to its ears several times. Clockwise massage in a sweeping motion above the belly button may also be effective.

Homeopathic remedies are fairly specific. Most common is homeopathic *chamomilla*, followed closely by *nux vomica* and *mag phos*. Highland makes a colic formula, available at most natural foods stores (their teething remedy is also excellent).

Misalignment of the skull or spine may also be implicated in colic. Have the baby see a chiropractor with pediatric expertise (newborn adjustments are more like massage than manipulations).

Some babies find great relief in this simple exercise: With the baby on its back, grasp the thighs and lift the feet toward its head, like during a diaper change. Continue to roll upward and raise the baby until it is hanging upside down. Really! Now wait and watch it move; it will rotate its back this way and that. When it seems finished, gently let it down: first touch its head down; then roll down shoulders, back, and butt; and then let its legs uncurl. Babies particularly benefit from this exercise when it is offered daily.

Always wash your hands thoroughly upon arrival and before examining the mother. Use aseptic technique when handling the baby and universal precautions when in contact with any secretions. Things to check include the following:

1. *The nipple, for soreness or cracking.* If soreness is developing, evaluate the way the baby is taking the breast. Explain the asymmetric latch (more areola drawn in at the lower jaw than at the upper), and recheck the frenulum. See that the mother is lifting the baby to the breast and that it is not hanging from the nipple. Although you may have discussed this with her already, she may have received conflicting advice from friends or relatives. Reassure her that she need not limit how long the baby sucks but must always make sure that it is taking the nipple correctly. If the nipples are cracked, suggest a bit of topical vitamin E between nursing sessions, and stress how important it is that she continue to nurse often: she can begin with the least affected breast, then switch to the more tender side once she has had letdown.

2. *The uterus, for normal involution.* It should be just below the mother's umbilicus and should feel firm, not tender. Massage it briefly to expel any clots, and have her sit up for a few minutes before checking her flow.

3. *The lochia, for color, amount, and odor.* **Lochia** is postpartum shedding of excess endometrium. On day one, expect **lochia rubra**, or red-brown flow in amounts like a heavy menstrual period. The odor should be fleshy, like menstrual blood.

4. *The perineum, especially if there has been swelling, tearing, or suturing.* Swelling should be gone; if not, suggest that she continue alternating warm and cool compresses, but also make certain she is rinsing her perineum twice a day with warm water and a bit of Betadine. If swelling has increased and she complains of pain, check for a hematoma (see "Hematoma" on page 210).

This is also a good time to assess for **cystocele** or **rectocele**. With these, the vaginal walls pooch forward at the introitus, usually from prolonged or very intense pushing. If the pooch appears at the perineum, it is a rectocele, due to weakening or straining of pelvic floor muscles. If the pooch appears near the urethra, it is a cystocele, due to straining of vaginal vault muscles. In either case, have the mother resume the **elevator exercise** (see page 60), and reassess at seven days.

If she had stitches, check to be sure they have held. Repaired edges should be clean, dry, and pulling together (if not, have her apply fresh aloe vera or bottled gel). Signs of infection include inflammation, pain, and discharge; if these are noted, consult a physician.

If the mother complains of tenderness but the area looks healthy, suggest **sitz baths** three or four times daily. These can be taken in a sitz bath unit (which sits over the toilet seat) or as a shallow bath in a regular tub. Plain hot water is fine, although adding ginger solution to the bath will increase circulation and relieve itching. Use an entire root (sliced thin) for a large pot of water, simmer twenty minutes, strain, and divide into several portions for a day's supply.

Also see if she has had any discomfort with urination. Remind her to pour warm water over her vaginal area as she urinates and check her temperature, to rule out urinary tract infection (see below). See if she has had a bowel movement, and if not, recommend fiber-rich foods. If she had stitches, fear that they might tear with bearing down may be causing her to hold back; if so, suggest counterpressure with a folded tissue.

5. *The mother's temperature record.* If elevated, she may be dehydrated or may have a systemic, urinary tract, uterine, or perineal infection. Rule these out one by one. If there is perineal pain, check for a hematoma.

6. *The mother's pulse.* If elevated, see considerations in item 5.

7. *The mother's blood pressure.* This is particularly important if it rose during or immediately after labor. If elevated, check for signs of preeclampsia and consult with backup as indicated.

8. *The baby's cord stump.* It should look clean around the base, not red or swollen. Be sure that whoever is diapering the baby is folding the top edge back so urine won't irritate this area and is swabbing the cord regularly with alcohol or hydrogen peroxide. Remove the cord clamp only if the stump is completely dry.

9. *The baby's skin color, inspecting for jaundice.* Depress the flesh on the baby's chest and extremities, checking for yellow undertone. Jaundice is unusual on day one and should be immediately referred to a pediatrician. Depending on degree, the baby may need a **bilirubin count** (see "Jaundice," page 205).

10. *The baby's skin consistency, for dehydration.* If the baby's wrists and ankles look cracked and wrinkly, it needs to nurse more often. Dehydration can develop rapidly in very hot weather and is more apt to be a problem with postmature or IUGR babies who have very little subcutaneous fat. Also note the temperature of the skin: if overly warm, see that the baby is not overdressed, and take its temperature.

11. *The baby's elimination pattern.* It should have passed meconium by now and should be urinating frequently (if the mother is using disposables and is uncertain of the latter, have her line them with tissues to more accurately gauge the amount.) If the baby has not had a bowel movement by forty-eight hours, consult a pediatrician.

12. *The baby's nursing pattern and behavior.* Sleepiness (especially after a long labor) is normal for the first day. Lethargy (characterized by drowsiness, disinterest in nursing, and lack of muscle

tone) is of concern. The lethargic baby should be seen by a pediatrician immediately, particularly if the mother's temperature is elevated or if neonatal jaundice is noted.

Also ask parents about the baby's cry. If they report a high-pitched, catlike wail, and the baby is at risk for **hypoglycemia** (see section later in this chapter), do a heel stick for glucose levels and refer if needed. If in conjunction with jaundice, it is urgent that a pediatrician see the baby immediately.

13. *Anything unusual in the newborn exam.* Reevaluate if parents have not yet seen a pediatrician.

The main purpose of the day-one visit is to see that the mother is off to a good start: relaxed, happy, comfy with her baby, and well cared for. If she looks frazzled or unhappy, you must try to find out why, as most women are in bliss at this point. On the other hand, her partner may be exhausted, finally registering the strain of lengthy labor support and loss of sleep. If so, suggest they send out for dinner (if not covered already), spend time in bed with the baby, and take the phone off the hook until they feel a bit more stable. Also suggest they place this message on their answering machine/cell phone and on the front door: "We had the baby, it's a _____, we're fine but tired, enjoying our babymoon. Please call in a few days so we can plan to have you over."

See if the mother wishes to talk about the birth, and make yourself fully available for this discussion, wherever it may lead.

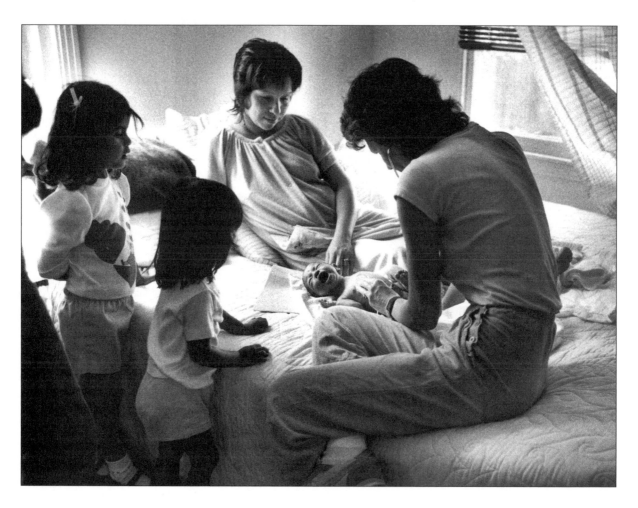

If minor concerns are noted on day one, make sure the mother understands the indications that should prompt her to contact you at once. Plan to visit again on day two; even if she says she feels fine by phone, you must make your own assessment. Indications to see her before then include pain in the perineal area (with repair), elevated temperature, excessive blood loss, newborn lethargy or irritability (depending on degree, the baby may need to see a pediatrician immediately), difficulties breastfeeding, or extreme mood swings. If everything is normal on day one, a phone call on day two is sufficient.

Day-Three Visit

By day three, the challenge of integrating newborn care with daily life has become evident, and emotional meltdown is common. At the same time, hormone surges that initiate lactation may increase the mother's instability, causing tears to flow just as her milk comes in. The baby must make its own adjustment to breast milk and so may experience fussiness or crying spells. All of this plus deepening fatigue can greatly exacerbate emotional distress in both parents. Day three is truly the point of reckoning: the birth is over, the baby is here, and nothing is the same. Particularly if the mother's partner has been handling all household responsibilities, he or she may be at the point of collapse. This may leave the mother feeling stranded; if so, see that her postpartum support system is fully activated.

This is an excellent time to give the mother a ritual bath. See the herbal recipe and instructions suggested by Janice Kalman and the Chico midwives in the "Herbs and Homeopathy Postpartum" sidebar on page 194. As an alternative, clean the tub, run plain warm water, float rose petals on the surface (if available), light candles, and put on music (mother's choice: perhaps something she listened to during the birth) to create a beautiful ceremonial moment of honoring the mother in her new role. With this, discussion of the birth may begin (or resume).

To best facilitate the mother's processing of her birth, you might pose the question, "Are you happy with your birth, or is there anything you wish had been different?" Of course, you must be entirely relaxed and receptive if you expect her to be fully honest with you. If she doesn't have much to say, be patient: there will be plenty of time later on to talk things through. For now, just encourage her to express whatever she is feeling—this is prime time for emotional release.

You may also want to offer this special rebozo treatment, as suggested by traditional Guatemalan and Mexican midwives. Have the mother lie on her back on a flat surface (like a carpeted floor) in a warm room. Place the center of the rebozo under her head, making sure it is folded neatly (not bunched up). Kneel on the floor facing her head, with an assistant on the other side. Cross the rebozo over her forehead and, with each of you taking one end, pull firmly and hold for at least a minute.

Then move the rebozo down to her shoulders, lower ribs, waist (gently), hips, thighs (just above the knees), calves, and ankles. Each time, cross the rebozo, pull taught, and hold. When she is ready to get up, instruct her to turn to her side and push herself up with her hands, to help keep her ribs closed.[1]

Oh, how mothers love this! It feels like a full body massage but also serves to "bring the bones back together," as the traditional midwives say. Both physically and emotionally, the mother feels held and hugged by the rebozo; the treatment is soothing and helps counter the propensity to chill. Advice varies as to how often this should be performed— some midwives say not until the mother has had some emotional release, and so prefer to wait at least until the mother's milk is coming in and she has discussed her birth a bit.

Be sure to do these checks on the day-three visit:

1. *The breasts.* Engorgement will be evident by visual examination, but stay alert to any reddened areas. If engorgement is a problem, make sure the mother is nursing on demand and with

proper positioning. Have her soak her breasts (or whole body) in warm water, as this will stimulate the release of any backed-up milk. Then show her how to express milk.

Many women find this easier if they oil the entire breast. Have her use long strokes toward the nipple, working down from the collarbone with one hand and up from the base of the breast with the other. If she feels lumps, have her work from behind them. This may hurt at first and she may need to go slowly, but make sure she applies enough pressure to bring the milk out: up to ten sweeps may be necessary before milk appears at the nipple. Demonstrate the proper way to get the flow started by grasping the edges of the areola, pressing inward, squeezing together, and then pulling toward the nipple.

Another tried and true remedy for engorgement is the application of cold cabbage or steamed comfrey leaves, left in place for twenty minutes. Have her repeat this periodically throughout the day. For lingering engorgement, she can try hot ginger compresses under her arms or in the upper, outer quadrants of her breasts.

If her nipples are cracked, check the baby's latch. Recommend vitamin E on the nipples between nursing sessions. Cold cabbage leaves tucked against the nipples may also provide relief.

2. *The uterus, the lochia, the perineum, and so on.* Recheck the perineum only if the mother has complaints or concerns. Ask if she feels any vaginal pressure or dragging sensation when out of bed, and if so, remind her to do the **elevator exercise** (see page 60). Also ask her if her blood flow has been consistent—any clots, heavy bleeding, or dark-red blood? By day three, the flow should be a bit lighter than before, beginning to change from lochia rubra to a pinker **lochia serosa**. Palpate the uterus for enlargement, and note any tenderness that might indicate infection (check the odor on her pad if you are concerned).

3. *The mother's temperature.* Elevation to 101 degrees is normal at the time the milk comes in. Nevertheless, rule out urinary tract, systemic, or uterine infection by checking for symptoms (see "Day-One Visit").

4. *The cord stump.* You can definitely remove the cord clamp by now, or if it has been a lotus birth, the cord should have come away cleanly by this time.

5. *The baby, for jaundice.* A bit of a yellow tinge is normal in the face and down to the nipple line, but unusual in the extremities. Ordinarily, excess bilirubin is diluted and flushed from the system by breast milk. If the baby is very yellow, have the mother place him or her in a sunny window, as sunlight helps the liver conjugate and eliminate bilirubin. Make sure the baby is nursing long and frequently, and check again the following day (also see "Jaundice" on page 205).

6. *The baby, for dehydration.* This is particularly important if jaundice is present.

7. *Baby's behavior, nursing pattern, crying pattern, and so on.* See items 5 and 6 above and 8 below.

8. *Mom's relationship to nursing.* This is crucial. Make certain that she is not trying to get the baby on a schedule or limit time at the breast. Replace any notion of structuring the baby's need for food with a sensual, loving approach based on trusting the baby's instincts. The sensation of letdown varies from mild tingling to a sexual sort of release, and some women experience orgasm while nursing. Try to promote a positive feeling around letting go with the baby.

9. *Sleeping arrangements.* Check to see what has evolved. If the baby is in bed with the mother, how does her partner (if applicable) feel about this? If the baby is in a basket or crib, how does the mother feel about getting up to nurse? Is she getting enough sleep? Is someone in the home willing to get up and bring the baby to her?

10. *Sibling/partner behavior.* If there are siblings, see whether they are relying on the mother for care, and if they seem to resent the baby. Suggest ways to involve them in baby care so they are all are on the same team, or for younger sibs, suggest special snacks or toys at nursing times. If the mother is partnered, see if he or she is counting on the mother for household management or food preparation when her need for rest should be the priority. Share your observations and reiterate her need for support: if not from her partner, then from others.

You may receive a phone call from the mother after this visit, especially with regard to the last four points above. Amazingly enough, conflicts about discipline may already have arisen between the mother and her partner (or relatives). Men, in particular, often worry that the baby will be spoiled by too much attention, too much contact, too much love. Some respond by setting limits on how much time the baby spends with the mother or insist that it be left to "cry it out" when it fusses, which exacerbates the problem.

Whether due to cultural conditioning, fear, or simple jealousy, this misguided approach to parenting should be set aside as soon as possible. Explain that the mother has literally enveloped the baby for nine months, its every need immediately met. It has no experience of waiting to be fed or held and when upset, cannot know that its mother (or father) is in the next room. Babies need all the security they can get—there is no such thing as too much love for a newborn!

Help the mother and her partner see that by surrendering to the sensitivity and vulnerability engendered by love, they will be stronger and wiser in the end, and their baby will grow to be a loving, secure child. Encourage them to relax and get to know the baby through touch, play, and gentle massage (also an antidote for colic). Advise them to set a time each day to share their feelings and concerns, to be concluded with cuddling. Do all you can to generate a container of protection for the burgeoning family. Let them know that you care and that they are doing fine.

Also help the mother honor her need for alone time. Have her pinpoint what that might look like: a shower by lunchtime or time outside in the afternoon? Strategize with her supporters on how she can get this time each day.

As with the day-one checkup, anything unusual is best followed up by a house call rather than by phone. Otherwise, if everything is normal, a phone chat each day is sufficient until your next visit.

Day-Seven Visit

By day seven, the mother's partner (if applicable) may be back at work, and friends and relatives may be busy again with their own concerns, leaving the mother feeling depressed and forgotten. Her

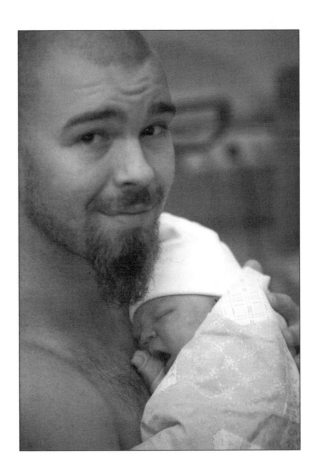

emotions remain volatile, and her energy is nowhere near pre-pregnant levels. If she has been entertaining well-wishers or doing more around the house than she should, she will be even more deeply exhausted. A definite sign of overactivity or stress is **increased lochia flow** or change from serosa back to rubra. *This mother needs help*: enlist several close friends or relatives to clean the house, do laundry, get the shopping and errands done.

Once again, she may wish to discuss her birth. This may be instrumental to her recuperation and ability to relax and enjoy her baby. Graciously accept any feelings of resentment, frustration, or sadness she may express, and try to respond without being defensive. Pay tribute to her strengths and downplay her shortcomings, if any.

Listen closely to the scope of her personal difficulties. Most mothers have no idea of how relentless mothering will be until it is upon them. Under these circumstances, it is hardly surprising that many experience postpartum blues. But you must differentiate this from depression: the blues diminish as time goes by, but depression, as characterized by increasing withdrawal and inability to cope, gets progressively worse and worse. Know that there are times when professional intervention is indicated (see "Postpartum Depression," page 213).

By day seven, physical recovery should be evident:

- If the mother had perineal repair, the skin should be closed by now.
- Lochia flow should have notably decreased.
- If she has been exercising her pelvic muscles, cystocele or rectocele should be diminishing.
- Breastfeeding should be established.

Assess the mother's emotional condition as well, and provide referrals if indicated. Do your best to help her with any difficulties during this visit, as you will not see her for several weeks unless she calls for help.

Even though it may seem early, you should broach the topic of sex. Advise the mother to have nothing in her vagina until her lochia flow has stopped; if she had stitches, she should see you before going ahead. Encourage her to listen to her body (as always) in making decisions on when she is ready.

Over the next few weeks, see her at once if she calls to report extreme fatigue, exhaustion, continued bleeding, or sensations of pressure or dragging in her vagina when she is up and about. These are symptoms of poor healing that must be addressed promptly if she is to recover.

Three- to Six-Week Checkup

The timing of this visit depends on the mother's rate of recovery. If her flow ceased at least a week prior to contacting you, you can assume her uterus is well involuted, her cervix is firmed up, and she is ready for her final checkup.

A critical reason for this checkup is to give the okay for sexual activities involving penetration, along with suggestions on how to make these as pleasurable as possible. Suggest plenty of lubrication, as breastfeeding causes dryness and fragility of the tissues, no matter how intense desire may be. If appropriate, raise the issue of birth control. Although rare, ovulation can occur as early as six weeks postpartum: I have known several mothers who conceived at this point without resuming menstruation and in spite of breastfeeding exclusively.

If the mother had stitches, the timing of this checkup is also determined by the condition of her perineum. Before she comes in (and if she is willing), ask her to wash her hands and gently insert two fingers to see if the area is still sensitive to pressure. If so, she is probably not ready for sex (or contraceptive fittings). Second-degree tears can take a while to heal completely, and if her lochia flow has stopped and she is feeling fine, no need to worry. See her no later than six weeks, though, for if adequate healing has not taken place by this time, you must determine the reason.

Emotional conditions may also precipitate scheduling this visit sooner than later. For example, if a woman calls at three weeks to report feeling depressed or emotionally incapacitated, see her at once, even though her physical recovery may be weeks away.

Depending on the size of your community, this may be the last time you see the mother for a while and your last chance to assess her recovery. Note her energy level and general demeanor: is she happy, in love with her baby, and at peace with herself? If she seems weak or ailing in any respect, speak to her about your concern. Energetically, she should be drawn back together by now: self-contained, whole, and well. If you have any doubt of this, continue to keep in touch.

Things to check at the final exam include the following:

1. *The uterus.* It should be out of range of palpation except by bimanual exam. If it is enlarged, she is probably still bleeding, indicating poor recovery. Prescribe rest, long relaxed nursing sessions to allow oxytocin to do its work, optimal nutrition with plenty of calories, supplements as indicated, and involuting tea or tincture of black haw and shepherd's purse.

2. *The cervix.* It should feel firm, closed, and situated high in the vaginal vault as with the initial pelvic assessment. However, some women do not regain their pre-pregnant cervical position and tone until cutting back significantly on breastfeeding (when introducing solid foods to the baby).

3. *Internal muscle tone.* This should almost be back to normal by now if the mother has been doing vaginal exercises. If not, explain the importance of strengthening the pelvic muscles to keep the uterus and other internal organs in their proper positions. Check for tone in two areas: high in the vault and just inside the vaginal opening. Often a woman has good tone in one area but little in the other. Review vaginal exercise techniques (see page 60).

4. *Lacerations or episiotomy.* Healing should be complete, although there may still be tenderness with labial skin splits as newly formed skin takes time to toughen up. This may cause some discomfort with sex, but adequate lubrication and creative positioning can help.

   If the perineum feels rigid with scar tissue, encourage the mother to do perineal massage to soften the area, using evening primrose oil. This procedure can be emotionally and physically reassuring for any woman nervous about having sex again.

5. *The abdominal muscle tone.* Have the woman lie down, place your fingertips along the juncture of abdominal muscles running from the umbilicus to pubic bone, and then have her lift her head and shoulders. Check for gaping; women typically have about 0.5 in. separation at this point. If the separation is greater, suggest abdominal exercises, starting with single leg lifts and progressing slowly to half sit-ups (with knees bent). You might also refer the mother to postpartum exercise or yoga classes or suggest she meet informally with several other new mothers for exercise interspersed with baby massage and conversation.

6. *The breasts, for tenderness or lumps.* It is said that the hormones of pregnancy can accelerate abnormal cell growth if any is preexisting. Even if the mother has seen a physician since the birth, she may not have had a thorough breast exam. This is also a good time to review self-exam with her.

7. *The cervix, by Pap smear.* For the reasons stated above, do a repeat Pap even if the mother was screened in early pregnancy.

8. *The hemoglobin or hematocrit.* This is especially crucial if the mother appears weak or exhausted or has a history of hemorrhage either with the birth or during the postpartum period.

9. *The diet.* A new mother often forgoes her physical needs in deference to the baby's. She hardly has time to eat, let alone cook. Her partner may offer to take on meal preparation but may not be aware of the nutritional demands of breastfeeding. If the mother complains of chronic fatigue, nervous irritability, or upper respiratory infection, suggest more protein, more calories, good sources of vitamins B and C, and trace mineral supplements. If her hematocrit is less than 37 or hemoglobin below 12 (nonpregnant standards), treat her for anemia with nutritional recommendations, herbal tinctures or teas, and supplements.

10. *Adjustment to parenting.* This is a broad category of evaluation, but a few well-chosen questions will reveal any disturbing trends. Ask the mother how she is sleeping, as this is critically important to her long-term well-being. According to a study by Kaiser Permanente and Harvard Medical School, mothers six months postpartum who slept five hours or less per day had a threefold higher risk for substantial weight retention (11 lb. or more) at their baby's first birthday than those who slept seven hours or more per day.[2] Ask how she and her partner (if applicable) are getting along and how she is coping with the challenges and frustrations of mothering.

The Baby:
Complications and Concerns

Cesarean-Born Babies

Babies born by cesarean may have difficulty latching on and establishing breastfeeding, depending on whether general anesthesia was used and how long the baby was separated from its mother. As midwife, it is critically important that you pay attention to the breastfeeding relationship, and assist the mother in attaching to her baby if bonding was disrupted.

Evidence shows that babies born by cesarean are 58 percent more likely to develop obesity as young adults. This appears to be correlated to lack of exposure to the mother's vaginal flora, which with vaginal birth, colonize the baby's intestinal tract in a beneficial way.[3] This lack of exposure also puts the baby at risk for colic, asthma and eczema.[4] To offset this negative effect, probiotics for babies are now available.

Hypoglycemia

Hypoglycemia refers to abnormally low blood sugar levels. A measurement of 50 to 60 mg glucose per 1 ml blood is normal for a newborn, but anything below 30 is of serious concern. Infants at risk are those (1) large for gestational age, (2) small for gestational age, (3) premature, (4) postmature, or (5) whose mothers were diabetic. Otherwise healthy babies who were hypoxic during labor or depressed at birth are also at risk. Symptoms include lethargy, irregular respirations, inability to regulate body temperature (hypothermia), refusal to nurse, irritability (high-pitched cry), and tremors. (**Hypocalcemia** has similar symptoms but is much more rare.)

If the baby is at risk, do a **dextrostix** to check glucose levels. This is done by heel stick, with a drop of the baby's blood collected on a special reactive strip and tested for glucose levels. If at or just above 45 mg, have the mother nurse the baby as often as possible, and give it water with a little molasses (1 teaspoon per cup) every few hours, preferably after a nursing (using an eyedropper or the tip of a small spoon).

Central nervous system damage can result if blood glucose levels are insufficient, so recheck daily until levels are normal. Some babies require more aggressive treatment than fluids by mouth, such as IV therapy with hospital surveillance. Consult with a pediatrician if blood glucose levels dip below 45.

Meconium Aspiration

Any infant with moderate to heavy meconium at birth is at risk for serious respiratory problems. Listen carefully immediately after the birth for any sign of lung obstruction. If the baby is breathing rapidly, be alert to other signs of respiratory distress syndrome: nasal flaring, grunting with exhale, retractions of the chest and abdomen, and cyanosis. If any of these are present, give blow-by oxygen (holding an oxygen tube to the baby's nose) and immediately contact a pediatrician to arrange for transport.

If the baby seems congested but not otherwise compromised, help it breathe more easily by providing steam. Close up the bathroom, turn the shower on hot (full force), and sit with the baby in the room until you hear its breathing ease (if there is no shower, use a sink or steaming kettle). You may also wish to apply percussion to help clear the lungs. Place the baby on your lap with its head down, back exposed. Tap sharply with two or three fingertips in each quadrant of the lungs, particularly in any area that sounds obstructed.

If the baby resumes a normal breathing rhythm and is stable for several hours, and the mother and her partner understand warning signs of further trouble, check back again the next day. But if the baby remains congested despite the use of steam and percussion, contact a pediatrician immediately.

Transient Tachypnea

This is a temporary condition of the newborn involving abnormally rapid respirations. Normal rates are 40 to 60 breaths per minute; with tachypnea, rates may increase to 120 breaths per minute. Transient tachypnea is caused by delayed absorption of fetal lung fluid. By itself, it is not a significant problem.

However, tachypnea is associated with several serious conditions: respiratory distress syndrome, meconium aspiration, and sepsis. If there are predisposing factors for these conditions, contact the pediatrician (who may want to meet you at the hospital for x-rays). Otherwise, the problem will resolve spontaneously with a bit of time, but you must stay with the baby until its breathing is back to normal.

Neonatal Infection

If the mother had fever or foul-smelling fluid during labor at a point too late to transport, or if fever and uterine tenderness develop postpartum, the baby should immediately see a pediatrician to be screened for sepsis. This is particularly important if the mother's GBS status is positive. Cultures will be performed on the baby, and because some of these take up to seventy-two hours to return, prophylactic antibiotic treatment is recommended. Considering that one of the first symptoms of GBS infection is apnea (cessation of breathing), hospitalization may also be advisable.

The septic baby may show a variety of symptoms: lethargy, irritability, jitteriness, fever, and dehydration. Tachypnea is a sign of sepsis, as is cyanosis. If the baby appears to be infected, cultures of the spinal fluid may be recommended in order to rule out meningitis.

In the event of prolonged hospitalization, your support and reassurance can help the mother establish and maintain her milk supply while continuing the bonding process. Above all, help her stay as close to the baby as possible: it is more than overwhelming to face the fact that the baby may be very ill and to watch painful tests be administered repeatedly. She will need the expertise of a good pediatrician as well as your continued presence and encouragement.

Jaundice

Neonatal jaundice is no longer the concern it was a decade ago. We now recognize the vast majority of cases to be **physiologic jaundice**, unassociated with the dangerous rise in bilirubin characteristic of pathological types.

What causes physiologic jaundice? While in utero, the baby's need for oxygen is met by a high percentage of red cells in its bloodstream, higher than in most adults. Once the baby is breathing, it no longer needs all these red cells, so the excess are broken down for elimination. A by-product of this process is **bilirubin**, which imparts a yellow tinge to the baby's skin. Physiologic jaundice usually manifests on day two or three postpartum and is remedied when the mother's milk comes in and flushes the baby's system clean.

One significant factor in increased physiologic jaundice is altitude—babies at ten thousand feet are four times more likely to have excess bilirubin than infants at sea level. It is also more common in premature infants, infants with bowel obstructions, or those with infection.

Another kind of jaundice that seldom requires treatment results from **ABO incompatibility**. This phenomenon is similar to RH sensitization: if blood from an O-type mother transfers to her A- or B-type baby during the birth, the baby will have more trouble eliminating excess red cells and so will have excess bilirubin. **Breast milk jaundice** is yet another nonthreatening condition caused by a hormone in the mother's milk that can interfere with the baby's ability to process bilirubin. Unlike most other varieties of jaundice, it manifests after the milk comes in.

In contrast to the above, **pathological jaundice** may be caused by liver disease, an obstructed bile duct, infection, or RH hemolytic disease. This is easily differentiated from physiologic jaundice in that it manifests at birth or within the first twenty-four hours. However, jaundice from ABO incompatibility may also appear early. To be safe, refer any jaundice at birth or on day one to a pediatrician. If the jaundice is pathological, high levels of bilirubin may be nearly impossible for the baby to eliminate and may seep into the basal ganglia of the brain, which leads to **kernicterus**, or permanent brain damage. Signs of kernicterus include lethargy and a high-pitched cry.

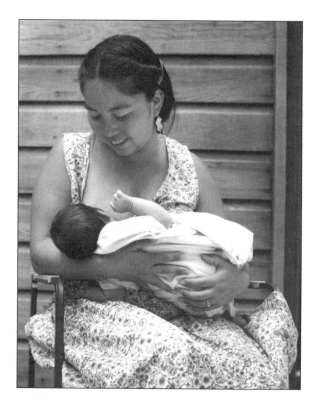

Depending on the degree and type of jaundice, the baby may be hospitalized for treatment—placed under **bili-lights**, with periodic blood draws to assess bilirubin levels. If bili-lights are used, it is crucial that the baby's treatment be properly supervised, as dehydration, burning, and possible genetic damage can occur with excessive exposure. Jaundiced babies are also at risk for infection.

Physiologic, ABO, and breast milk jaundice are essentially normal and self-correcting but may cause the baby to become lethargic and disinterested in nursing. If so, and the characteristic yellow tinge noted on the baby's face and neck runs no lower than the nipple line, encourage the mother to nurse often and expose the baby to sunlight (with body naked and eyes protected) for thirty minutes, twice daily. In my experience, babies kept in dark rooms for the first few days of life have higher bilirubin levels than those liberally exposed to sunlight. Contrary to medical opinion, physiologic jaundice is unrelated to late cord clamping.

Babies born to mothers whose labors have been induced or augmented with Pitocin must be watched carefully. Pitocin competes with bilirubin for binding sites, rendering elimination difficult. The same is true of vitamin K and certain drugs like diazepam, sulphonamides, steroids, and salicylates. If the baby's extremities appear jaundiced, consult a pediatrician.

Circumcision

Circumcision is a controversial procedure. It is no longer routine; in fact, the American Academy of Pediatrics now states that circumcision cannot be justified on medical grounds. Nevertheless, the practice is ancient: it is portrayed in Egyptian murals and has long been a central rite in Jewish traditions. Circumcision has been practiced mostly by cultures in hot, dry climates, with water for bathing at a premium. But today, and particularly in the West, it is a custom perpetuated chiefly by fathers wishing their sons to look as they do. If the mother and/or her partner are considering circumcision, they should carefully weigh the pros and cons before making a decision.

Circumcision is a surgical procedure. It is often done without local anesthetic, so the baby must be strapped spread-eagled in restraints. The skin adherent to the tip of the penis is severed and cut back to completely expose the glans, and then clamps are placed to control bleeding. Sometimes a Plasti-bell device is used instead, which clamps and cuts off blood flow to the foreskin, causing gradual tissue necrosis. In either case, the pain is severe. Babies generally cry so hard with this procedure that they can scarcely breathe. Possible physical side effects include infection (several deaths have been documented), and penile sloughing necessitating reconstructive surgery.

Knowledge of the procedure is enough to persuade most parents of its dangerous and emotionally traumatic nature. Some opponents of the procedure, many of whom are nurses and physicians, deem it a form of sexual mutilation or even child abuse. But

what about the alternative: the uncircumcised penis? What about the supposed dangers of infection, and what are the basics of care?

The foreskin covers and adheres to the glans for the first year or two, at which point the boy will pull it back as he becomes aware of his genitals. Parents should not pull back the foreskin for any reason, as this can trigger a vicious cycle of bleeding and infection. Once the foreskin is moveable, they can remind the boy to pull it back in the tub or shower to clean beneath it—this is as simple as cleaning under the fingernails or cleaning secretions from the folds of the female labia.

There is continuing debate regarding the effect of circumcision on sexuality. On an uncircumcised male, the foreskin captures the first drops of moisture secreted with arousal; then, as erection increases, the foreskin pulls back and the glans is automatically lubricated. Evidence shows that circumcised men require more stimulation to become and remain sexually aroused.[5] This makes sense, as the foreskin preserves the sensitivity of the glans, which may be dulled on the circumcised penis due to constant friction with clothing.

Returning to some fathers' concerns about their sons appearing different from them or from other boys, it comes down to this: if we agree that circumcision is a violent and potentially harmful procedure, we must break the cycle of its use. In all fairness, we should really leave the choice to the boy himself: it is his body, and he can decide in the future if he wants the procedure done. My personal feeling is this: if nature had intended man to be without foreskin, baby boys would be born this way.

Nervous Irritability/Colic

Dealing with a colicky baby requires the same patience and endurance as giving birth. However, if labor has been unusually difficult or postpartum assistance minimal, the mother may feel overwhelmed if the baby is frequently fussy. Above all else, help her maintain her objectivity so she will not project feelings of guilt or resentment onto every anxious cry the baby utters. Suggest that when her patience is at an end, she use labor-coping tools such as deep relaxation or deep breathing. Reassure her that it takes a while to get to know the baby's signals, but she will soon be able to differentiate fatigue-based cries of overstimulation from those for food, diaper changing, or simple contact.

Have her pay attention to the timing of crying spells and see if there is any correlation to her own tense times during the day. In many cases, crying and fretting reach a peak around 6 p.m., when the mother may be busy making dinner and trying to share the day's events with her partner, who has just come home from work. The baby feels the confusion and stress of it all and reacts by crying excitedly. If such

is the case, perhaps evening transitions can be made more gradually, with conversation between partners saved for later in the evening. Alleviate dinner hassles by relying on soups, stews, or casseroles that can be made while the baby naps and reheated later.

Sometimes, in spite of every effort, nothing seems to work. Most of the time, the baby will soon outgrow its initial crankiness, but on the other hand, babies' temperaments run the gamut from intensely high strung to quietly content. Along these lines, I believe that a baby's nature is fully evident at birth: I can think of many occasions when I have run into a family whose birth I assisted years earlier and sure enough, the personality of the baby I remember is there in the child before me. In other words, babies are unique and have their own journey to make in life, with their own style of coping. If you are

---

For Parents: What to Do When the Baby Cries

- If the birth was complicated by malpresentation or shoulder dystocia, or if manual manipulations of the head were performed or molding was extreme, consider cranial-sacral therapy. This gentle realignment of the baby's head, neck, and spine can work wonders.

- Try nursing in peace and quiet, without jiggling the baby around (best if baby is sprawled across mother's body as she leans back).

- Have the baby's sleeping place somewhere quiet but still close to the center of activity.

- If the baby wakes when set down, try nursing lying down and then quietly getting up once the baby is asleep.

- Let the baby spend lots of time in a baby carrier positioned near your heartbeat.

- Establish a ritual break period for yourself, when your partner or other supporter completely takes over for an hour or so (immediately following a nursing is best). Use that time to rest, take a shower, call a friend, or otherwise rejuvenate.

- If the baby seems to have gas (pulls its legs up sharply, its stomach rumbling), try giving warm catnip tea by bottle or eyedropper (also see the massage technique in "Herbs and Homeopathy Postpartum" sidebar, page 194).

- If all else fails and the baby is crying hysterically, try running the shower or turning on the dryer or vacuum cleaner. High-frequency sounds may be calming if the baby is very upset.

---

reasonably certain the mother is doing the best she can, advise her to relax and accept what is. Otherwise, chronic anxiety or frustration can sap her emotional reserves and hinder her recuperation.

Minor Problems

- *Diaper rash.* After carefully cleaning the baby's bottom, natural oil should be applied with each diaper change. Aloe vera gel (for wet, open sores) and calendula cream (for chafing or inflammation) are also effective. Some mothers report that **Bag Balm** (intended for use on livestock to reduce teat inflammation) is a miracle diaper salve. Sometimes diaper rash is the result of improper diaper laundering: a buildup of ammonia can cause repeated episodes of rash unless the residue is removed by bleaching. To prevent this, soak diapers in a bucket of water (with bleach added) immediately after rinsing, then machine wash and double-rinse before drying (the double rinse removes the bleach, which also can be irritating).

- *Cradle cap.* Apply natural oil to the scalp before bed and leave it on all night. The scales can then be removed with a soft toothbrush and natural shampoo.

- *Heat rash.* The obvious solution is to cool off living areas and have the baby cozily but loosely dressed. Teach the mother to check the baby's temperature by feeling its hands and feet, which should be slightly cool to the touch.

- *Thrush.* This mild infection can be identified by a white coating on the baby's tongue. Because the same organism that causes vaginal yeast causes thrush, screen the mother and treat her if necessary. If she is infected, remind her to assiduously wash her hands after toileting or any contact with the vaginal area. The baby can be treated with topical applications of acidophilus solution, three times a day, by cotton swab.

Thrush may take several weeks to go away: be patient. If it is severe enough to interfere with nursing, the baby should see a physician.

In general, it is best to avoid synthetic, artificial substances for bathing and toileting. Baby powder may be blended with talc, a substance known to be dangerous to the lungs, and most baby oils are made with a base of mineral oil that leaches vitamins from the skin. Baby shampoos claim to be gentle, but most are complex chemical preparations rather than simple soaps. Many synthetic products also contain carcinogenic dyes, which can be absorbed through the skin. Suggest natural substances like olive or vitamin E oils and liquid castile soap (which can also be used as shampoo).

The Mother: Complications and Concerns

Minor Problems

- *Constipation.* This complaint commonly arises soon after the birth, particularly if labor has been prolonged. A daily serving of high-fiber bran cereal is probably the most effective and pleasant remedy. Prune juice, taken in moderation, can also be used for its softening effect. Adequate fluid intake is critical: most nursing mothers need about 3 qt. daily to meet their own needs and produce sufficient breast milk.

- *Hemorrhoids.* Most common immediately after delivery, these respond well to cool compresses and applications of witch hazel. If rupture and bleeding occur, aloe vera gel speeds healing. Both as a treatment and a preventive measure, follow the above recommendations for constipation.

- *Afterpains.* Occurring with a second or subsequent baby, these are generally experienced during nursing or immediately after. Some women say that these pains hurt more than labor. They are caused by loss of uterine tone with successive childbearing, so contractions prompting involution are more intense than usual. Herbs such as cotton root bark or cramp bark help by promoting uterine tone, and black haw tincture is particularly effective. It is also critical that the mother keep her bladder empty, or the uterus cannot fully contract. If the pain becomes debilitating, suggest she lie face down with a pillow beneath her lower abdomen to force the uterus firmly into place. Rarely, Motrin (ibuprofen) may be necessary for pain relief.

Postcesarean Concerns

Women who experience cesarean birth report higher levels of fatigue, breastfeeding problems, constipation, depression, anemia, headache, difficulty urinating, abnormal bleeding, urinary tract infection, abdominal pain, and vaginal discharge than women who have spontaneous vaginal birth.[6] They are also 80 percent more likely to be rehospitalized for wound complications, postpartum hemorrhage, uterine infection, cardiopulmonary and thromboembolic conditions, genitourinary tract disease, pelvic injury, gallbladder disease, or appendicitis.[7] These conditions impact not only the mother's recovery but also affect the physical and emotional health of baby and family. Every woman who has a cesarean should be aware of these risks.

Depression following a cesarean is in a class by itself. The mother may feel that she has failed her partner, the baby, and herself, particularly if she had general anesthesia and missed the actual moments of birth. This is especially difficult for the well-prepared mother who, aware of the importance of immediate bonding, may feel her relationship with the baby to be hopelessly damaged. Even if she has made peace with the cesarean, she may still have subconscious yearnings for the climax of birth and may dream vividly of vaginal delivery in the first few weeks postpartum. Acknowledge her loss, witness her feelings, and help her find a cesarean support group. If depression persists, refer her to counseling.

Hematoma

Hematoma is an asymmetrical and painful swelling in the perineal area. It is caused by soft tissue trauma and can occur with or without laceration and repair. If the perineum and vagina are intact, the hemorrhage almost always ceases spontaneously and the blood slowly reabsorbs. But if repair is done incorrectly—that is, homeostasis has not been achieved—bacteria may grow rapidly in the pooled blood, leading to infection. This can cause the repair to break down, because the edges will not adhere and close properly once sepsis develops. (Traction on the sutures from inflammation is another factor in repair dehiscence.)

If the mother has been repaired and develops a hematoma, immediately consult a physician so that antibiotic treatment can begin at once. To reduce swelling, have her alternate hot and cool soaks, which stimulate circulation and encourage reabsorption of pooled blood. Make sure she pours warm water with a bit of Betadine over the vaginal area each time she uses the toilet, and remind her to dry and air her perineum thoroughly afterward. If the repair does break down, reconstructive surgery may be necessary. Do your best to prevent this!

Uterine and Pelvic Infections

Symptoms of uterine infection—otherwise known as **puerperal infection or endometritis**—include fever over 101 degrees, elevated pulse, pelvic pain, malodorous lochia, and subinvolution of the uterus. Risk factors include anemia, a compromised immune system, prolonged rupture of the membranes (PROM), numerous vaginal exams in labor, manual rotation or other manipulations of the baby during labor, maternal exhaustion, delayed placental delivery, hemorrhage, uterine exploration (as for manual removal of the placenta or sequestered clots), postpartum dehydration, or improper perineal hygiene.

Another cause unaddressed in the literature is overactivity in the first few days postpartum. I have seen this twice in my practice; both women had other children to care for and resumed normal activities immediately after giving birth. Both had uncomplicated deliveries, with none of the precipitating factors cited above. One woman actually went to a swap meet the day after the birth, walking around in the heat and dust with nothing to drink for many hours! Take care to warn mothers who had easy deliveries that bed rest is essential postpartum, not only to aid recovery from birth *but also from the entire pregnancy*. Reiterate that adequate rest permits oxytocin to involute the uterus, tone the vagina, and facilitate breastfeeding, whereas stress or overactivity causes the countereffects of adrenaline to slow recuperation.

Sepsis may affect not only the uterus but also pelvic ligaments, connective tissue, and the peritoneal cavity, with symptoms of vomiting, chills, and extreme pain. Infection of these areas occurs only if uterine sepsis is untreated. Rarely, the tubes and ovaries may also be affected, usually by a preexisting gonorrhea infection that has flared up again.

Thrombophlebitis and Pulmonary Embolism

Thrombophlebitis is the inflammation of either a superficial or deep leg vein. Women with varicosities are particularly at risk. **Superficial thrombophlebitis** causes leg pain with heat, tenderness, and redness at the site of inflammation. To confirm, check for **Homan's sign** by having the mother sit up in bed with the leg extended, then gently press on her knee and dorsiflex her foot: if she has pain in her calf, the test is positive.

Deep thrombophlebitis is indicated by high fever, severe pain, edema, and tenderness along the entire length of the leg.

With either condition, contact a physician immediately. Meanwhile, have the mother stay in bed and keep the affected leg elevated. And tell her to keep her *hands off the leg*: if massaged, blood clots may loosen and enter her circulation. Should a clot lodge in her lungs, the life-threatening condition of **pulmonary embolism** will result, characterized by chest pain, shortness of breath, rapid respirations, and elevated pulse. If any of these develop, administer oxygen immediately and call the paramedics.

Difficulties with Breastfeeding

Problems with breastfeeding often spring from distraction. If a mother feels anxious about her primary relationship, worried about money matters, stressed over changes in her lifestyle, frustrated by lack of support, or impatient with her rate of recovery, she may find breastfeeding less than simple and fulfilling.

To address breastfeeding difficulties, we must first understand the physiology of lactation. Each breast has approximately twenty lobes, which consist of lobules divided into **alveoli** and **ducts**. The alveoli contain **acini cells**, which produce the milk, and **myoepithelial cells**, which contract and propel milk from the breast. **Lactiferous ducts** carry milk from the alveoli and empty into one large duct that widens to create a **lactiferous sinus** or **ampulla** near the nipple. **Lactiferous tubules** emerge at the surface of the nipple and release the milk from the breast. The nipple itself is comprised of erectile tissue, which contracts during nursing to control the flow of milk.

The baby's latch also determines how much milk it receives. For many years, standard advice was that it should take the areola symmetrically into its mouth, on the assumption that this would stimulate a complete release of milk. Now we know that an **asymmetric latch**—one with a greater portion of the areola taken in at the lower jaw than at the top of the mouth—positions the nipple more deeply so the sucking reflex can work most effectively (it also frees the baby's nose for easy breathing). Women who breastfed successfully discovered this more or less instinctively, although they may have worried from time to time that they weren't doing it exactly right.

Oxytocin stimulates letdown of the milk, but **prolactin** is responsible for milk production. Prolactin is inhibited during pregnancy by high levels of estrogen, which fall immediately after the birth to prompt lactation. Continued production of oxytocin and prolactin depends on frequent, long, and peaceful nursing sessions. The more relaxed the mother is when she nurses, the greater the release of these crucial hormones.

It is nature's design that by giving birth, a woman learns to let go of her inhibitions and trust her body. This is key to a successful breastfeeding experience. Nonetheless, disapproving relatives or unsolicited advice may largely negate maternal instincts. Breastfeeding is an intimate act between mother and baby that requires privacy, especially in the beginning. It is also a physically demanding activity and can be quite exhausting unless there is good physical and emotional support. If a mother is having breastfeeding problems unrelated to the mechanics of proper positioning, see that her needs for rest, good nutrition, privacy, and support are being met.

Orgasmic breastfeeding is more than just an intriguing concept; it is based in the physiology of the process. If oxytocin levels are high and the nursing mother is relaxed, she may experience orgasm. It is important that new mothers realize this so they will not worry if it occurs.

Breastfeeding can, in fact, have similar therapeutic value to sexual intimacy in affording a way for mother and baby to reaffirm their connection, stay close, and be of comfort to one another in times of change. It is a gift of tenderness and vitality, with the mother's urge to nurse the perfect complement to her baby's desire. Breastfeeding also provides an invaluable boon to infant/child maturation. In his excellent book, *Evolution's End*, Joseph Chilton Pearce explains that for optimal neurological development, the baby must have frequent face-to-face contact with its mother, and suggests that the relatively low protein content of breast milk prompts the newborn to nurse almost continuously so it can receive this crucial growth stimulus.[8] The more we learn about breastfeeding, the less we should be inclined to interfere with this highly personal and richly variegated intimacy between mother and child.

Physical complications of breastfeeding include **engorgement** and **mastitis**. Engorgement results from more milk than the baby immediately needs and may occur when the milk first comes in or when the baby gives up a feeding. Engorgement may be uncomfortable but will resolve spontaneously as supply adjusts to demand; it may be remedied by applying heat to the breast, massaging toward the nipple,

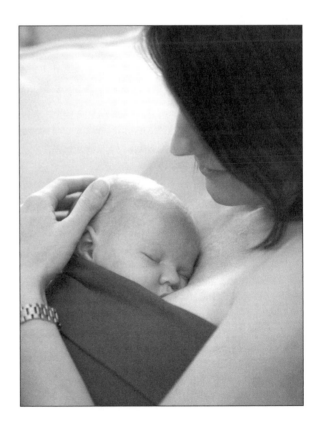

and then hand expressing milk to start it flowing. (See additional suggestions under "Day-Three Visit" on page 199 and in the "Herbs and Homeopathy Postpartum" sidebar on page 194.)

If milk is left pooled in the sacs (particularly a residual amount remaining time after time), it may become a breeding ground for bacteria entering through the nipple. This is how **mastitis** occurs. Personal cleanliness is important in preventing mastitis, as are proper positioning, proper latch, and relaxed and thorough nursing on demand. A healthy immune system, as maintained with adequate fluids, calories, and rest, is also critical. Mastitis is characterized by reddening of the breast (in lumpy areas or in streaks) and fever of 103 or 104 degrees. Borderline cases may be resolved with heat treatments, herbal or homeopathic remedies, and plenty of rest, but with high fever, antibiotics are necessary. Dycloxicillin is generally recommended because it does not destroy intestinal flora and will not hurt the baby, although the mother may experience indigestion. Timely treatment is critical to prevent an abscess from developing, which can further complicate breastfeeding.

Although it may be a long way off, some mothers want the facts about weaning right away. Recommend that the baby set the course if at all possible: its need for solid food will be indicated by interest in what others are eating (psychological readiness) and by teething (physiological readiness). If the baby is completely breastfed, solid foods are unnecessary for up to nine months, as it takes about this long for its digestive system to mature. A relaxed approach saves the mother a lot of trouble and allows the baby to follow its natural pace of development.

Postpartum Depression

Postpartum depression must be carefully differentiated from postpartum blues. Up to 70 percent of women experience the blues, which are associated with hormonal shifts, sleep deprivation, and impending lactation.[9] There is also evidence to suggest that the natural suppression of the maternal **hypothalamic-pituitary-adrenal axis (HPA)** in the immediate postpartum may cause emotional instability until full function resumes in about ten days.[10]

Ten Steps to Successful Breastfeeding

Excerpted from: *Protecting, Promoting, and Supporting Breastfeeding: The Special Role of Maternity Services* (A Joint WHO/UNICEF Statement, 1989, page iv)

1. Have a written breastfeeding policy that is routinely communicated to all health care staff.
2. Train all health care staff in skills necessary to implement this policy.
3. Inform all pregnant women about the benefits and management of breastfeeding.
4. Help mothers initiate breastfeeding within a half hour of birth.
5. Show mothers how to breastfeed and how to maintain lactation even if they should be separated from their infants.
6. Give newborn infants no food or drink other than breast milk, unless medically indicated.
7. Practice rooming-in—allow mothers and infants to remain together 24 hours a day.
8. Encourage breastfeeding on demand.
9. Give no artificial teats or pacifiers (also called dummies or soothers) to breastfeeding infants.
10. Foster the establishment of breastfeeding support groups and refer mothers to them on discharge from the hospital or clinic.

The blues are more likely to occur in women who are not physically up to par, particularly if the birth has been debilitating. A mother who hemorrhaged at birth might experience blues off and on for the first few weeks, due to anemia and exhaustion. If the mother has no history of emotional problems, look to her current health status. Check her hemoglobin, review her diet, and recommend supplements as indicated.

Even with no physical factors, the blues can affect any woman struggling with postpartum adjustments. As mentioned earlier, losses experienced at this time can be emotionally devastating: help the mother identify and articulate these.

Sometimes loss engenders grief; other times, anxiety. Here is one mother's description of her postpartum struggle:

> Postpartum blues? No, not me! The joy of long-awaited motherhood and the emotional stability I had achieved over the years disqualified me, I thought, as a candidate for the postpartum syndrome. But I was not immune! My "blues," however, did not fit the picture of what I had expected. In fact, I came to feel that nothing I'd read or heard had adequately prepared me since I was not depressed according to my usual definition.
>
> For me, the experience was one of drowning in a vacuum of mind, consumed with worry, anxiety, and uncertainty. The responsibility seemed overwhelming. In spite of reassurance from my midwives, doubts and questions plagued me. . . . Was my son becoming jaundiced? Was his cord healing properly? Why was his skin peeling? How would I bathe and groom him? I longed for the recommended rest and would be famished, yet could not seem to coordinate time for my own needs with that of caring for and feeding him every few hours. Trian was a good, quiet baby, but I didn't have a handle on my end at all. I felt like I was failing miserably at my goal of being a perfect mother.
>
> Trian was several days old when I suddenly realized while nursing him that I had not leisurely touched and explored his whole body. At this moment, I knew I had been in a vacuum for days, functioning but not fully aware.

> To my amazement, I just couldn't "organize" my newborn. Fifteen years of pride at being a successful organizer in my career now proved totally useless. I had to learn to simply flow with Trian, emotionally and psychically, and let go of intellectual anticipation, expectations, and planning.
>
> My love for Trian was the grounding cord that held me together as I floundered with anxiety at the enormous task before me. When I learned to recognize my signs of postpartum syndrome—irrational fears overtaking me, heart racing, nausea, excessive perspiration, and shallow breathing—I would relax, do the deep breathing I had been taught for the birth, and concentrate on how much I loved my baby. This allowed me to center myself and deal rationally with my fears so that I could carry on.

Having regular outings with family and friends—doing whatever it takes to get time away from home and the usual routine—is a powerful antidote for postpartum blues. Most babies will sleep contentedly during a long car ride, which provides a much-needed break for everyone. Frequently, what the mother needs most is physical and emotional space: a chance to get the baby off her body for a while. To make the most of this, she should use this time to recuperate, letting her mind and body rest completely. If she can get someone to watch the baby so she can be truly alone, she may enjoy a favorite leisure activity.

In contrast to the postpartum blues, postpartum depression develops at ten days after the birth or later, and tends to worsen with time. Occurrence is from 8 to 15 percent.[11] Depression not only affects mothers but also has been shown to negatively impact child development. Depressed mothers do less relating to their infants, who in turn show fewer positive facial expressions and have more eating and sleeping disorders.[12]

Occasionally, what appears to be postpartum depression may be caused by thyroid imbalance. Postpartum **thyroiditis** can lead to hypothyroidism, characterized by fatigue and depression. Thus

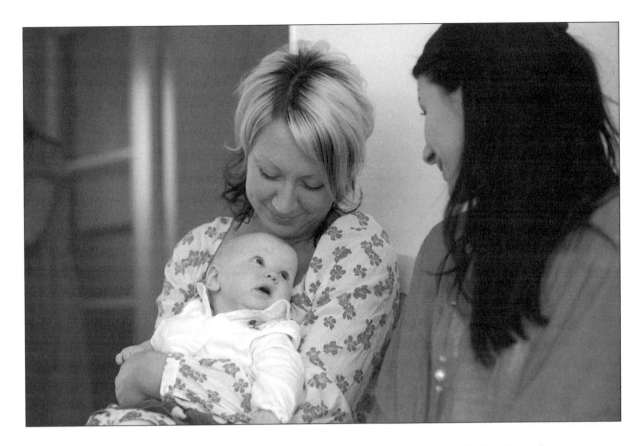

any new mother showing signs of depression should immediately be screened for thyroid problems.

Midwife Constance Sinclair has divided predisposing factors for postpartum depression into four categories:

1. *Psychiatric factors*, including negative birth experience, history of psychiatric disorder, low self-esteem, or stressful life events

2. *Demographic factors*, including age, marriage status, access to medical or social assistance, and economic difficulties

3. *Relationship factors*, including separation from parents in childhood; poor support in childhood; poor support in pregnancy; history of sexual, emotional, or physical abuse; or poor relationship with partner

4. *Cultural factors*, including lack of community support, spirituality, or clear role definition in culture[13]

Extensive research on postpartum depression by midwife Cheryl Tatano Beck resulted in the **Postpartum Depression Predictors Inventory (PDPI)**, with the following thirteen predictors:

1. Prenatal depression
2. Child care stress
3. Life stress
4. Lack of social support
5. Prenatal anxiety
6. Marital dissatisfaction
7. History of previous depression
8. Challenging infant temperament

9. Maternity blues

10. Low self-esteem

11. Low socioeconomic status

12. Unmarried

13. Unwanted or unplanned pregnancy[14]

One relationship dynamic particularly predisposes the mother to postpartum depression. If the father has been indifferent during the pregnancy but becomes compulsively bent on proving himself in the immediate postpartum, the mother may be more than a little disoriented and may have trouble trusting her instincts. Typically, she plays passive-dependent to his authoritarian role, and he responds to the demands of fatherhood with a strict set of rules regarding baby care, discipline, breast-feeding, housework, expenditures, sexuality, and so on. He may also use spiritual or political beliefs to judge the mother's performance. No wonder she gets depressed! I have had heated discussions with fathers of this temperament and find it does little good; if the mother has chosen this situation, what is an outsider to do? As a typical passive-dependent, she will ask continually for your advice but will seldom use it. Refer the mother to counseling and extract yourself from this configuration as soon as possible.

Postpartum depression resulting from a disappointing birth experience can be difficult to heal, particularly if pain medication was used and/or bonding was disrupted. Scars from these experiences run deep, and painful memories can be overwhelming in the early weeks when intensified by hormones and fatigue. Any mother who had to transport unexpectedly should be given repeated opportunities to go over the birth in detail and air all misgivings and regrets. At the root of her depression is grief, so support her in dealing with the loss of her birth dream by bearing witness. Let her define the issues and ask the questions she considers important when she is ready. If time goes by and she becomes increasingly depressed, refer her to counseling or hypnotherapy.

In contrast, a woman convinced that a "perfect" birth was her destiny may be embittered by transport and may have trouble caring for herself and the baby once out of the hospital. Keep a close eye on her. She desperately needs contact with more even-tempered, mature mothers, whose flexibility and receptivity she can emulate. Do what you can to facilitate this.

Besides counseling, treatments for postpartum depression include allopathic and natural remedies. It is important to understand the physiology of depression to appreciate the pros and cons of each. The current rise in depression in general mirrors increased levels of stress in our lives, estimated to be a hundred times greater than that faced by our grandparents. The more stressed we are, the more catecholamines (adrenalines) we produce. Serotonin balances the effects of these, but overproduction of catecholamines makes it hard for the body to make enough serotonin to keep up. Without adequate serotonin, we become anxious or depressed on an ongoing basis.

Drugs like Prozac (fluoxetine) and Zoloft (sertraline), which belong to a class known as **SSRIs** (or selective serotonin reuptake inhibitors), keep serotonin circulating in the body. But they *do not increase levels of serotonin*; instead, they cause the body to use up its reserves by pulling them into the nerve synapses. Adverse affects of violent outbursts and suicidal urges are now well publicized. Natural aids to serotonin production include the amino acid tryptophan (found in turkey breast, tamari soy sauce, raw crimini mushrooms, cod, snapper, halibut, chicken breast, shrimp, scallops, and tofu); omega fatty acids; vitamins B-6, B-2 (riboflavin), and B-3 (niacin); folic acid; and magnesium. Found in health-food stores, the supplement 5-HTP may be especially helpful, as tryptophan converts to this before converting to serotonin. Coffee, alcohol, chocolate, and cigarettes must be strictly avoided.[15]

On the other hand, the most extreme form of depression, **postpartum psychosis**, requires expert and immediate treatment. Characterized by manic or depressive episodes of confusion or disorientation,

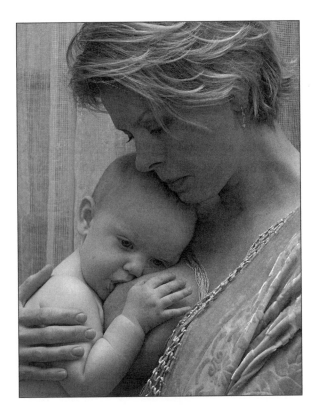

delusional thinking, and suicidal or infanticidal behaviors, this condition has been brought to the public eye with horrific cases of mothers harming or even killing their children. Mothers with a history of bipolar disorder are particularly at risk. The incidence of postpartum psychosis is 2 to 3 percent, or eighty thousand women in the United States annually.[16] If you are at all concerned that a mother in your care may be at risk for this, secure the advice and support of a family health agency before referring her to a psychiatrist.

Sexual Adjustment

Maintaining sexual communication after the birth can definitely help a couple surmount the stresses of this period. But if they are used to making love on the spur of the moment or taking their time, a newborn will undoubtedly get in the way. Like it or not, their intimate relationship must somehow incorporate the baby.

Put simply, love is the key to making this adjustment. If the mother and her partner consider the baby an extension of their love, they will find their way through the frustrations of this time. Their intimacy will deepen—although fatigue, tension, loss of privacy, and a sense of isolation can make getting together difficult.

Expectations run high at six weeks postpartum, as this is when the mother is supposed to be recovered and ready for sex again. But at this point, she is completely absorbed with her baby: they are virtually inseparable. They are also psychically attuned to the extent that the mother will wake seconds before her baby begins fussing to be fed, or the baby will wake crying when its mother has had a bad dream. These powerful bonds are important to the health of the family but may also cause sex to be pushed aside indefinitely.

Unsettling feelings of dependency can also dampen desire. As one mother bluntly put it, "I realized when I was pregnant that I really needed to depend on this guy. Now here I am with a little baby, and I feel so helpless. . . . What if he [partner] turns out to be a creep?" Our culture glorifies motherhood, but then again, we worship youth, the perfect body, and overt sexuality. No wonder new mothers may feel invisible as sexual beings.

The mother's partner has his or her own challenges to face. He or she may be more desirous of time with the baby than expected and so may resent having to work. If the mother clings for want of companionship and reassurance, her partner will feel torn in two, and she will in turn feel guilty and insecure. These stresses may push both of them to the breaking point. Although sex is a logical way to reunite diverging energies in a relationship, growing resentment can interfere.

The best solution is to have a grandmother, other female relative, or a trusted friend or sitter take the baby for an afternoon or evening so the couple can get away for some time alone (expressed milk can be frozen in a glass bottle and warmed in a bowl of water). Once in privacy, partners should take time to relax and talk before diving into sex with overloaded expectations. If getting away is impossible, the next best alternative is to have a weekly date night for dinner, a DVD, and lovemaking in some private part of the house. Older children can spend the night with friends or relatives. And even if the baby interrupts, at least the couple knows their next date is only a week away.

Although prolactin tends to repress desire, oxytocin serves to increase it. Oxytocin levels have been shown to be exceptionally high in women who nurse for long periods on demand. And if a couple can make it happen, the simple fact is that the more sex we have, the more we want. This is due to the action of dopamine, which counteracts prolactin and causes us to perceive and pursue pleasure. Thus sex itself may be a remedy for sexual disinterest. Masturbation works, too.

Couples must place a premium on keeping their rites of intimacy. If partners make a point of daily check-in with each other, they can certainly hold their ground and find new ways of being together. With time, and with intention, sex can become more meaningful, wild, and wonderful than ever before—*but it does take time.*

Contraception

Before sexual activity resumes after birth, heterosexual couples must address contraceptive issues. It feels strange to return to birth control after not having to bother for so long and, depending on the method used, may be just one more barrier to intimacy.

Birth control pills are not really suitable for breastfeeding mothers—estrogen suppresses milk production, and progesterone-only minipills are not as effective as the combination formulas. The

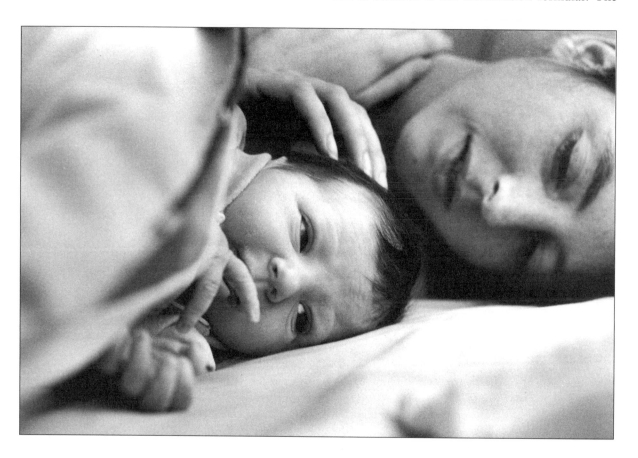

Copper 7 IUD is another option, but many women find this less than desirable due to side effects of chronic bleeding and low-grade infection. The fertility awareness method is difficult to implement postpartum, as the course of lactation causes erratic fluctuations in basal body temperature and cervical mucus. Norplant and Depo-Provera often cause heavy bleeding and delay menstruation when discontinued. This leaves the barrier methods: condom or diaphragm.

Apart from the difficulty of finding an appropriate birth control method is the difficulty of being diligent in its use. One of the more subtle conflicts affecting couples who have known the thrill of conscious conception and ecstatic childbirth is the desire for the no-barriers sexual intensity that accompanies these events, versus the desire to delay or forgo having more children. This conflict is usually unspoken, but after some time has passed and the family has stabilized, this psycho-erotic desire for conception can rise up and wreak havoc with future plans.

Coping with these feelings depends on acknowledgment and communication. A couple may succeed at preventing conception, but unless conflicts regarding the use of birth control are expressed, intimacy is at risk. Encourage them to consider contraception an open issue, one apt to arise repeatedly for review and worthy of sensitive and candid discussion.

Notes

1. Doña Queta Contreras and Doña Irene Sotelo, Midwifery Today conference notes, Oaxaca, Mexico, October, 2003.
2. Erica P. Gunderson, Sheryl L. Rifas-Shiman, Emily Oken, Janet W. Rich-Edwards, Ken P. Kleinman, Elsie M. Taveras, and Matthew W. Gillman, "Association of Fewer Hours of Sleep at 6 Months Postpartum with Substantial Weight Retention at 1 Year Postpartum," *American Journal of Epidemiology* 167, no. 2 (January 2008): 178–87.
3. Helena Goldani, Heloisa Bettiol, Marco A. Barbieri, Antonio Silva, Marilyn Agranonik, Mauro B. Morais, and Marcelo Z. Goldani, "Cesarean Delivery Is Associated with an Increased Risk of Obesity in Adulthood in a Brazilian Birth Cohort Study," *American Journal of Clinical Nutrition* 93 (June 2011): 1344–47.
4. P. Bager, M. Melbye, K. Rostgaard, C. Stabell Benn, and T. Westergaard, "Mode of Delivery and Risk of Allergic Rhinitis and Asthma," *Journal of Allergy Clinical Immunology* 111, no. 1 (January 2003): 51–56. L. Niers, R. Martin, G. Rijkers, F Sengers, H. Timmerman, N. van Uden, H. Smidt, J. Kimpen, and M. Hoekstra, "The Effects of Selected Probiotic Strains on the Development of Eczema," *Allergy* 64, no. 9 (September 2009): 1349–58.
5. M. Mylos and D. Macris, "Circumcision: Male—Effects upon Human Sexuality," in *Human Sexuality: An Encyclopedia*, ed. Vern Bullough and Bonnie Bullough (New York: Garland Publishers, 1994): 119–22.
6. C. Glazener, M. Abdalla, P. Stroud, S. Naji, A. Templeton, and I. T. Russell, "Postnatal Maternal Morbidity: Extent, Causes, Prevention and Treatment," *British Journal of Obstetrics and Gynecology* 102 (1995): 282–87. M. E. Hannah, W. J. Hannah, E. D. Hodnett, B. Chalmers, R. Kung, A. Willan et al., "Outcomes at 3 Months after Planned Cesarean vs. Planned Vaginal Delivery for Breech Presentation at Term: The International Randomized Term Breech Trial," *Journal of the American Medical Association* 287 (2002): 1822–31.
7. Glazener et al., "Postnatal Maternal Morbidity," 282–87. M. Lydon-Rochelle, V. L. Holt, D. P. Martin, and T. R. Easterling, "Association between Method of Delivery and Maternal Rehospitalization." *Journal of the American Medical Association* 283 (2000): 2411–16.
8. Joseph Chilton Pearce, *Evolution's End: Claiming the Potential of Our Intelligence* (San Francisco: Harper San Francisco, 1992).
9. F. G. Cunningham et al.,*Williams Obstetrics*, 20th ed. (Stamford, CT: Appleton and Lange, 1997).
10. M. A. Magiakou et al.,"Hypothalamic Corticotropin-Releasing Hormone Suppression during the Postpartum Period: Implications for the Increase of Psychiatric Manifestations at This Time," *Journal of Clinical Endocrinology and Metabolism* 81 (1996): 1912–17.
11. M. Righetti-Veltema et al., "Risk Factors and Predictive Signs of Postpartum Depression," *Journal of Affective Disorders* 49 (1998): 167–80.
12. L. Lamberg, "Safety of Antidepressant Use in Pregnant and Nursing Women," *Journal of the American Medical Association* 282 (1999): 222–23.
13. Constance Sinclair, *A Midwife's Handbook* (St. Louis, MO: Saunders, 2004), 239.
14. C. T. Beck, "Revision of the Postpartum Depression Predictors Inventory," *Journal of Obstetric, Gynecologic, and Neonatal Nursing* 31 (2002): 394–402.
15. Dean Rafflock and Virginia Rountree, *A Natural Guide to Pregnancy and Postpartum Health* (New York: Avery Penguin Putnam, 2002). George Mateljan Foundation, "World's Healthiest Foods Nutrient Rating System," www.whfoods.com.
16. Janet Balaskas, *Active Birth* (Boston, MA: The Harvard Common Press, 1992), 373.

CHAPTER 7

Becoming a Midwife

If you are considering becoming a midwife, this chapter is for you. However, know that the road to practice is seldom a straight one: educational pathways are often circuitous and require much determination and endurance. But what better introduction could there be to the dedication required by the work? Even as a student, you will know very long work hours, intense personal interactions, and repeated sacrifice of personal concerns. This is not for everyone, so it is best to begin by attending births as a doula to see if the path fits. Ultimately, midwifery must be less a career choice and more a calling.

If you decide to become a nurse-midwife, your course of study will be fairly well mapped out for you. See appendix N for a list of nurse-midwifery programs, or contact the American College of Nurse-Midwives (ACNM) for an update. For direct-entry programs, also see the list in appendix N.

The respective advantages and disadvantages of nurse- and direct-entry midwifery training have been partially articulated in chapter 1. To reiterate, a major advantage of being a nurse-midwife is legal practice throughout the United States, with reciprocity state to state. The political infrastructure of nursing has benefited nurse-midwifery, no doubt about it. But as HMOs seek to control costs by using nurse-midwives in high-volume clinics or labor units with little or no continuity of care, midwives are reduced to little more than obstetrical technicians. What's worse is that nurse-midwives are increasingly losing collective bargaining power as HMOs systematically fire them, only to rehire them for longer hours at less pay, often without benefits.

As for direct-entry midwifery, the fight for legitimacy continues. State by state, physician lobbies continue to throw up roadblocks so that midwives must repeatedly reorganize to meet new challenges to their right to practice. It all comes down to "pick your battleground"; only you can decide where you are most suited to struggle, for if you intend to practice full-scope, holistic midwifery, struggle you must.

Nonetheless, the way in which you are educated has everything to do with how you practice and how you define yourself professionally and politically. Nurse-midwifery programs are usually based in hospital: most are weighted toward theoretical instruction with minimal hands-on training, little continuity of care, and limited scope of practice.

Instructor and student alike are subject to highly restrictive practice protocols. Consequently, students may suffer overdevelopment of their analytical faculties at the expense of the intuitive, compassionate qualities so necessary for humane caregiving.

In my experience, the primary stumbling block for nurse-midwifery graduates is fear of the responsibility of private practice. All too often, graduates have done countless rotations in clinical settings but have never known primary responsibility for a single client from start to finish. When faced with life-threatening complications of shoulder dystocia or hemorrhage in a hospital setting, chain-of-command protocols required them to call for help and then step aside and watch. Predictably, they feel ill equipped to practice autonomously.

In contrast, the student in an apprenticeship (common in direct-entry training but also possible in some nurse-midwifery programs) is working one on one with clients throughout the perinatal cycle. She is also working one on one with her preceptor, requiring that she develop and refine not only technical skills, but also equally critical abilities to communicate assertively and listen effectively. Learning takes place in context, as the senior midwife (or clinical preceptor) debriefs the day's events. Students involved in cases from start to finish find it easier to track their technical and interpersonal skill development. Whatever your training route, look for a program that acknowledges students as adult learners with their own areas of expertise, and one that values personal growth and development.

Institutionally based programs may come and go, but apprenticeship will endure because it is community based, cost effective, and perfect for women with small children who require training within a flexible time frame. If you are considering the apprenticeship route, check first to see if your state has any provisions for qualifying midwives. Some states require academic programs in addition to apprenticeship; others have licensing or certifying mechanisms that are entirely competency based,

with the usual requisites of documented experience, skills verification, and comprehensive exam. Many states have incorporated NARM CPM requirements, and several use the CPM route exclusively. Consult www.narm.org for details. Consult www.meac.org for a list of accredited direct-entry programs. (Also see appendix N.)

If your state has no mechanism for regulating midwifery, you may wish to investigate the guidelines established by NARM for becoming a CPM and use these to create your own framework for learning. Once you know the core areas of knowledge and skill you need to demonstrate, and the amount of clinical experience needed to acquire this knowledge and skill, you will have some idea of how to proceed. Your initial efforts will most likely involve (1) studying midwifery texts, (2) participating in a midwifery study group, and (3) attending births as a doula or birth assistant.

For support in your learning process, I highly recommend that you join a student networking/advocacy group, such as the Student Section of MANA or the newly founded Future Midwives Alliance (http://futuremidwives.blogspot.com). The latter is working to develop a Students' Bill of Rights, which could greatly influence the quality of midwifery education. Get involved!

Textbooks and Other References

Aspiring midwives unable to be on call for births can begin with book study. To get your bearings on the various educational routes, read *Paths to Becoming a Midwife*, edited by *Midwifery Today* magazine. If you have already read extensively (on topics of childbirth politics, preparation, nutrition, breastfeeding, and parenting), concentrate on beginning midwifery texts. But if you have read very little, start with books that feature plenty of birth stories to help you glean the emotional and spiritual aspects of the childbearing experience.

Although there are many fine birth books available, some have become classics. Ina May Gaskin's *Spiritual Midwifery* features exceptional birth stories, as does her other text, *Ina May's Guide to Childbirth*. For the politics and anthropology of birth, don't miss Robbie Davis-Floyd's *Birth: An American Rite of Passage*. For a deeper understanding of physiologic birth, see my latest (with Debra Pascali-Bonaro) *Orgasmic Birth: Your Guide to a Safe, Satisfying, and Pleasurable Birth Experience*. Any book by Sheila Kitzinger is a pleasure to read; for a perceptive overview with extensive illustrations, try *The Complete Book of Pregnancy and Childbirth*. *The Labor Progress Handbook*, by Penny Simkin and Ruth Ancheta, is a remarkable little text loaded with illustrations that show how best to assist women in labor. Along these lines, also see *The Birth Partner*, by Penny Simkin, and for insight on prepared childbirth, try *Birthing from Within*, by Pam England and Rob Horowitz. These books can give the aspiring midwife a firm foundation from which to pursue other topics like breastfeeding and early parenting.

When ready to move on to midwifery or obstetrical texts, Harry Oxorn and William R. Foote's *Human Labor & Birth* gives basic pregnancy and birth information in a concise outline format perfect for beginners. Diagrams are abundant, clear, and easy to understand. The main drawback of this reference lies in its focus on obstetrical care: there are lengthy sections on the use of forceps and vacuum extraction, and nothing on routine prenatal assessment. Suggested management of complications is quite moderate, though, and the tone of the text is fairly respectful of mother and baby.

Another well-known text is *Myles Textbook for Midwives*, edited by Diane Fraser and Margaret Cooper (15th edition). This essential text for British midwives is detailed and complete, with a strong emphasis on caregiving. The format lends itself to study, with realistic and profuse diagrams. *Varney's*

Midwifery (4th edition), by Helen Varney, is the primary text for nurse-midwifery programs in the United States. An outstanding aspect of this book is its sections on clinical procedures like venipuncture, Pap smear, and IV infiltration, with instructions that are fully detailed and easy to understand.

A newer and very useful text is *A Midwife's Handbook*, by Constance Sinclair. Designed to slip into your birth bag, this quick reference consolidates key information for handling complications, including herbal and homeopathic approaches. This book bears the mark of the midwife: practical, diverse, and complete.

And then there are the thoroughly remarkable texts by Anne Frye, *Holistic Midwifery*, Volumes I and II. Frye is an independent midwife and it shows: her books are grounded in respect for physiology and feature a wide range of caregiving approaches and treatments for full-scope practice. Her philosophy of care is entirely woman centered; her presentation of cultural diversity is unmatched by any other text. Absolute beginners may find these books a bit overwhelming, but they are essential. Another excellent book by Frye is *Understanding Diagnostic Tests in the Childbearing Year* (now in its seventh edition).

Although these references are more than adequate for basic practice, you may want an obstetrics text from time to time for in-depth understanding of any pathological development or if only to be aware of the medical standard of care. *Williams Obstetrics* is notoriously challenging for beginners, due to its dry, scientific style. However, it has been said in terms of research that "all roads lead to *Williams*," as it is probably the most comprehensive text. Invest in a good medical dictionary, like *Tabers*, to help you wade through the terminology. A newer text used by many midwifery programs is *Obstetrics*, edited by Gabbe, Niebyl, and Simpson. If possible, compare the two and see which suits you best.

Another groundbreaking work, *Obstetric Myths versus Research Realities*, by Henci Goer, examines the research on such controversial subjects as gestational diabetes, episiotomy, cesarean delivery of the breech, postdatism, and induction of labor. Her latest book, *The Thinking Woman's Guide to a Better Birth*, is one of the best to recommend to anyone skeptical about out-of-hospital birth. Marsden Wagner's *Born in the U.S.A.* covers similar material but focuses primarily on the political underpinnings of the overuse of technology in the perinatal period.

Of course, the list goes on. *The Wise Woman Herbal for the Childbearing Year*, by Susun Weed, is a great resource for herbs, as is *The Natural Pregnancy Book*, by Aviva Jill Romm.

Other valuable sources of information include midwifery newsletters or journals. The *MANA News* focuses on political issues of midwives in the United States (www.mana.org). *The Journal of Nurse-Midwifery* (published by the ACNM) offers research, networking, and an open forum (www .acnm.org). *Birth: Issues in Perinatal Care* also publishes research, with a focus on humanizing obstetrics (http://blackwellpublishing.com/journal .asp?ref=0730-7659). *Midwifery Today*, an inspiring magazine for aspiring and experienced midwives alike, features research-based updates and articles on various themes (midwiferytoday.com); the organization also publishes a monthly e-zine and hosts conferences in the States and various international locations. And check out the new *Squat Birth Journal*, with its international focus on birth as a human rights issue (squatbirthjournal.blogspot.com).

Also see if your state midwifery association publishes a newsletter, or you may wish to subscribe to newsletters from other states. Contact MANA for more information.

Doula Work or Birth Assisting

Attending births as a doula is an important step in midwifery training. Absolute beginners benefit from discovering the extent to which birth is nonintellectual and transformative. Women who have already had children have an opportunity to refine their understanding of the adage, "It's not my birth," as they help those who need support have the best possible experience.

Aspiring midwives who have not had children may encounter skepticism regarding their suitability for this work or may wonder about this themselves. I must admit that I once thought it nearly impossible for anyone who had not given birth to be truly effective in this role. But through exposure to many exceptional students, I came to appreciate that the most important qualification is knowledge of one's inner resources gained by some experience of being on the edge, facing one's demons, or suffering grief through personal loss. Still, any aspiring midwife who has not given birth should attend births as early in training as possible so her text-acquired knowledge will not overwhelm her instinct, intuition, or common sense.

Whether assisting births at home or in a hospital, there is a lot to learn. If the mother's partner or other helpers are present, you must find ways to work respectfully within her intimate circle. As you respond to requests for comfort measures, demonstrate massage techniques, or suggest certain labor positions, you discover the effectiveness of these relative to the woman and her situation. If the mother is alone, you will soon begin to appreciate the devotion and endurance that will be required of you as a midwife. Most beginning birth assistants worry about making mistakes, saying or doing the wrong thing, or being rebuffed by the laboring woman. But rest assured: as long as you surrender your own fear of birth's intensity and keep pace with the mother's rhythms and needs, you will know what to do in the moment. Speaking and acting spontaneously may be unnerving at first, but every student midwife must find her own voice in order to encourage laboring women to express themselves freely.

Whatever your role, the first few births you attend will be profoundly affecting. Reverence for the power of birth, and willingness to feel it on a visceral level, are the best possible start for an aspiring midwife. As patterns of labor and the intensity of the process become familiar, turn your attention to the skills and style of the midwife or physician in attendance. It is easy to be critical at this stage, to focus on the flaws of more experienced practitioners rather than on their strengths. But keep these observations to yourself—there is no point in alienating those with whom you work, as you never know what favor you may require from them some time in the future. Keep the channels of communication open, and above all, learn from your seniors—don't merely react to them.

Assisting at Home

Most birth assistants work in the hospital, as that is where women are the least likely to have support. So if you have an opportunity to attend a homebirth, count your blessings! Homebirths generally involve minimal intervention and provide opportunities to experience spontaneous, physiologic birth. Clear your mind of prejudice and observe; notice how different women respond to labor, which positions work best for each, which breathing patterns seem most effective, and how best to involve and integrate the rest of the family.

The latter—wisely assessing how to focus the efforts of everyone on the birth team—is one of the subtler aspects of effective assisting. A competent doula discreetly directs the mother's supporters to effective participation based on what each can handle. Primary relationships can be greatly strengthened in labor; old wounds can be healed and new patterns set. Thus the birth assistant's primary task is to inspire enough self-confidence in the mother that she can let go and enjoy intimacy with her partner and other supporters if she so desires. This contributes to bonding among all involved, which in turn can ease challenging postpartum adjustments.

Sometimes a midwife will use the doula's "extra pair of hands" for some routine task and, sensing

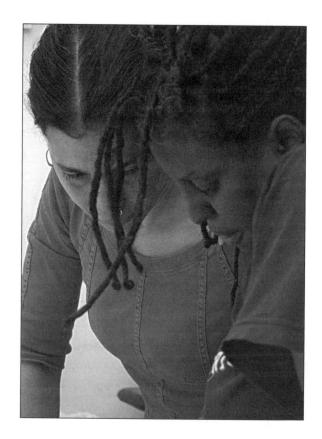

enthusiasm, will do a bit of teaching. I recall one midwife calling me to attention while she was suturing, telling me to "watch and learn." The labor had been difficult, and I had been holding a flashlight at the perineum for what seemed like forever: my arm was aching and my interest was wavering. But because of what I saw, I acquired a better understanding of the repair process. Never pass up an opportunity to assist a primary care provider, especially at homebirths, where there is more time to ask questions and opportunity to follow up later.

Assisting in Hospital

Hospital doula work affords the opportunity to serve a diverse group of women while learning about current obstetrical practice. It also provides a potentially shocking introduction to the political aspects of medicalized childbirth. Thus some beginners shun birth attendance in hospital, believing their personal discomfort level to indicate that homebirth assistance is their destiny. This may result in a very long wait to attend births—a very long wait indeed.

Apart from all that is offensive about hospital births, they definitely provide opportunities to see complications that seldom occur at home and to observe medical management of preexisting pathology. A student seeking apprenticeship or other clinical training may find that potential preceptors appreciate this experience, as it demonstrates that she can handle being on call and will support women in labor no matter what the circumstances.

Early in my apprenticeship, I began doing hospital doula work to augment sporadic homebirth attendance. I registered as a volunteer at the local general hospital and was well received because of problems with understaffing. I agreed to be available several nights a week, and over a ten-month period, attended nearly sixty births. On-the-spot assisting is a boon to mothers unprepared for labor and definitely tests the mettle of the aspiring midwife.

One very unappealing aspect of working in hospital is the environment: hospital rooms are typically overheated, lack adequate ventilation, and have harsh, overly bright lighting. A former student confided that she takes nice pieces of fabric; strings of battery-operated lights, flowers, or greenery; and small birthing goddess statues with her to births and, with the mother's consent, transforms the hospital room as best she can. Despite this, interventions of continuous fetal monitoring, IV, and repeated vaginal exams may end in the use of pain medication and Pitocin, with resulting fetal distress and cesarean birth. To witness this scenario repeatedly can be deeply disturbing, especially for a doula who has seen the alternative in homebirth. Just as the mother can be undermined by tension, so may the birth assistant, who must address her own stress levels before she can hope to reassure her client.

When doing on-the-spot assisting, always remember that an unprepared mother must contend

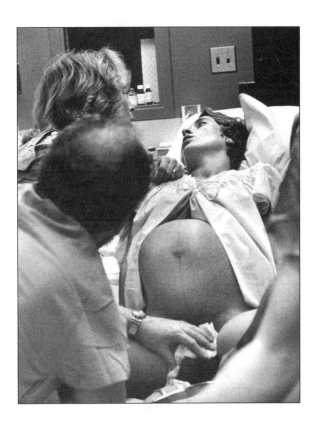

not only with pain, but also with fear. If confronted with a woman who is writhing or screaming, first calm yourself, then make eye contact and explain that you are there to help. Women terrified by their sensations often breathe too rapidly, resulting in hyperventilation. Avoid this by having her breathe lightly, or better yet, by slowing her breathing down. Start by breathing at her rhythm, and then ask her to breathe with you as you make each breath a fraction slower and deeper than the one before. Place a hand on her belly and as you look into her eyes, suggest that she bring her breath down to the baby. It may take some time to win her trust, but don't give up!

Once the mother's breathing is regular, relaxation can be initiated by touch, massage, and verbal encouragement. Ask between contractions if you can rub her back, whether she would like to sit up or lean forward, and so on. If she is tightening her hips or legs, a foot massage may help her let go. She may also respond to phrases like, "Let your legs feel heavy" or "Let your bottom melt into the bed." The most important thing you can do at any birth is to run oxytocin, expressing warmth and love in all you do, so that the mother's adrenaline levels will diminish and her oxytocin levels will rise.

Still, unprepared mothers often progress very slowly, trying your patience. To stay calm and present, you must validate your own physical and emotional needs. If the mother you are assisting is alone, perhaps you can invite another doula to work with you so you have someone to spell you. If this is not possible, find the staff coffee room, and while a nurse is checking on the mother, you may be able to take a quick break. Because hospital rooms are often overheated, wear something light, cool, and loose, and bring an extra change of clothes in case you are in the way when the mother vomits or her waters release. As a precaution against blood-borne diseases, you may wish to wear protective eyeglasses, and you should bring your own gloves for handling underpads and so on. Wash your hands frequently, as hospital rooms are dirty and germ ridden. Bring lip balm and lozenges to keep your mouth moist, as breathing with the mother may chap you. Also bring enough food and bottled water to see you through twenty-four hours.

A major challenge in assisting mothers in hospital is discontinuity of care. Even if the mother has a private physician, her labor may be managed by nurses or residents she has never met, and then, as shifts change, new faces appear. Thus a doula must repeatedly navigate the practice style and beliefs of new staff, and if the mother is a private client, she must continue to reassert the mother's wishes.

Do not think for a minute, though, that your work in hospital is futile. Women never forget an act of kindness in labor, whether a simple touch, encouraging word, or compassionate look. I know this from my own first birth in 1972. Overwhelmed by a Pitocin-induced labor of only two-and-a-half hours, my Lamaze preparation was useless; the contractions peaked immediately and I never had more than ten seconds' rest between them. Basically, I screamed my way through labor, and the nurses shunned me because I wanted a natural birth. But then, one came in and sat at the edge of my bed, touched my thigh and said quietly, "Let's just try to slow your breathing down a little," showing me what to do, and letting me squeeze her arm so hard I am sure she had fingernail marks the next day. I can't say she made everything better, but I will never forget her sweet face, her kind intent, and her caring spirit.

Remember what was said earlier about brainwave frequencies in labor. Birthing women are highly aware of what those around them are feeling: what they believe and what they fear. You can't hide anything from a laboring woman, so don't bother to try. By the same token, whatever you give from the heart will be remembered. You are part of the birth story, a story that woman will never forget.

It should be obvious by now that getting to know mothers in advance of labor (either as private clients or through a service that matches doulas and mothers prenatally) is beneficial. Schedule as many meetings as needed to go over birth preparations, birth team relationships, her expectations of you and yours of her. Of course, you will be on call for these births: good preparation for the midwifery lifestyle. To compensate for your abrupt and frequently prolonged absences, you will learn to give intimate relationships special attention before leaving for a birth and as much energy as you can muster upon your return. Particularly if you are out-of-pocket for gas and other expenses, you will come to know the frustrations of doing hard work for minimal compensation. As you realize the time and energy commitment involved in midwifery, you will understand the support you will need in your personal life to make the work sustainable.

What are some other ways to keep up your birth attendance? If you have birth experience, with techniques and insights to share, teaching childbirth preparation classes may be the answer. Depending on where you live, you may or may not need certification to do this. Register your course at a local resource center, where you might also volunteer in order to gain exposure and make contacts. Or perhaps you can offer prenatal exercise or yoga classes. Educators are often asked to births as support persons, thus teaching is a potent avenue into the birthing community.

Midwifery Study Groups

Participating in a midwifery study group can be an exciting and integrating learning experience. Even if you are enrolled in a program with classroom instruction, you can still benefit from the support and insight that being with other students can provide. If you are organizing a study group on your own, you may want to invite experts in your locale to come and teach on certain subjects. Listening to experienced practitioners discuss case histories is a practical education that can't be beat.

I participated in a study group for more than a year, and during that period went from student to primary caregiver. Each time we met, we discussed recent experiences at births, which often determined our next study topic. Two midwives, an obstetrician, and a pediatrician also participated, teaching us skills and adding insight. During the course of our time together, we worked in teams as doulas or at prenatals, births, and postpartum visits under the guidance of our midwife instructors. These liaisons later blossomed into midwifery partnerships.

Apprenticeship

Ideally, networking and volunteering in your birth community will allow you to meet a number of senior midwives, and you will find one with whom you can establish a healthy working relationship. Students often worry about finding an apprenticeship, and it is true that political and legal difficulties have caused the number of practicing midwives to be somewhat erratic. Nevertheless, maintaining a high profile among local midwives is always a step in the right direction. Attend any meetings where they are likely to gather and without pressuring anyone, get to know as many as possible. If you start to feel desperate, remember that for the apprenticeship to work, it must feel right not only to the midwife, but also to you: don't settle for anything less than a good match!

How will a student know when she is ready to apprentice? After mastering core midwifery knowledge and attending a number of births, she will feel confident in a way that prompts her to move ahead. Her personal life and finances must (I repeat, must) be sufficiently in order to take the responsibility of being on call. She must understand that she is making a *long-term commitment* to the midwife who trains her, who will count on her to provide as much assistance as possible in exchange for her training. She should be eager to learn and able to humble herself to the wisdom of the midwife from whom she is soliciting instruction. This does not preclude asserting her own ideas at appropriate moments and in a respectful way, but she must have the interpersonal skills to do so.

Apprenticeship usually begins with assisting at prenatals and acquiring rudimentary skills of uterine palpation, fundal height assessment, fetal heart auscultation, and maternal blood pressure assessment. With time, the apprentice will not only assist at births but will also share the weighty responsibility of comanaging (and debriefing) emergency complications and transports. Depending on the size of the practice, apprenticeship can last for several years or more.

How can an apprentice best contribute to the midwife's practice? She can assist with housekeeping, bookkeeping, filing, copying, ordering and stocking supplies, errand running, and public relations. She can provide emotional support to clients at births when the midwife is occupied with technical duties or is tired from another birth. She can field

Core Areas of Study: General Subjects

- Aseptic Technique
- Human Reproduction and Sexuality
- Anatomy of Pregnancy, Birth, and Postpartum
- Physiology of Pregnancy, Birth, and Postpartum
- Applied Microbiology of Pregnancy, Birth, and Postpartum
- Embryology/Fetal Growth and Development
- Pharmacology of Pregnancy, Birth, and Postpartum
- Nutrition for Pregnancy, Birth, and Lactation
- Obstetrical Procedures for Complicated Pregnancy and Birth
- Well-Woman Gynecology and Contraceptive Care
- Childbirth Education, Theory
- Childbirth Education, Instruction
- Infant and Child Development
- Provision of Care: Prenatal Period
- Risk Assessment
- Comprehensive Prenatal Care
- Communication and Counseling Techniques
- Common Complaints in Pregnancy
- Charting
- Interpretation of Medical History, Lab Work, and Diagnostic Testing
- Complications of Pregnancy
- Contraindications for Out-of-Hospital Birth
- Provision of Care: Intrapartum Period
- Assisting at Normal Labor and Birth
- Complications of Labor and Birth
- Emergency Care
- Immediate Care of Mother and Newborn
- Assessment of Lacerations and Appropriate Response
- Newborn Exam
- Provision of Care: Postpartum Period
- Lactation Physiology and Support
- Newborn Care
- Common Postpartum Problems
- Newborn Complications and Appropriate Response
- Maternal Complications and Appropriate Response

the basic concerns and questions of new mothers and offer breastfeeding support.

Students sometimes have difficulty forging agreements with their senior midwife regarding the rate at which they will acquire skills and primary care experiences. In this respect, participation in a formal program can provide some structure to apprenticeship.

In my school, the National Midwifery Institute, Inc. (codirected with Shannon Anton), the apprentice and senior midwife (preceptor) sign a detailed agreement outlining their respective duties and obligations and are periodically required to give written feedback to each other and the program on how the agreement is working out. Accountability of preceptor to student (and vice versa) is further assured by MEAC accreditation standards for ethical and fiscal integrity. For a complete listing of midwifery programs, including those that are MEAC accredited, see appendix N.

In self-directed training, the backbone of apprenticeship is skills acquisition and verification. In 1995, NARM conducted a survey of midwives to determine entry-level skills for direct-entry practice. The resulting practical skills list is utilized by NARM in the CPM certification process. Sharon

Evans and Pam Weaver outline these skills step by step in the handbook, *Practical Skills Guide for Midwifery*.[1] Using the list and the handbook, an apprentice and her senior midwife can formulate a plan so that the skills and experience necessary for certification or licensure are acquired in a reasonable amount of time.

What about educational costs? Apprenticeship is traditionally a relationship of exchange, whereby a master of a given trade exchanges knowledge for labor. But when apprenticeship is housed in a formal program leading directly to licensure or certification, the student should expect to pay for it. This brings up a major concern: with the demands of being on call 24/7, how will the apprentice be able to work and train at the same time? Flexible, part-time work is the ticket, be it data entry or processing, web design, other online business, teaching childbirth classes (participants will be understanding if you are called to a birth), or doula work (in partnership, so one can take over if the other cannot be present at a birth). Yet another idea is to **share an apprenticeship**, with each student assigned certain weekdays for being on call and doing prenatal or postpartum visits. Occasionally, a midwife will pay her apprentice a nominal sum for transportation and child care and, if she intends to incorporate her as a partner, may gradually increase her pay to partnership level.

How will the apprentice know when she is ready to practice independently? Meeting state or national standards for skills, experience, and knowledge is but one aspect of preparedness. Some students are by nature overeager and need extra time to integrate the finer aspects of caregiving; others are timid and must be challenged with unexpected responsibilities to help them realize their competence. Some students need to work with a second midwife or in a different setting, perhaps at a high-volume clinic or birth center, before feeling ready to strike out on their own.

Other Direct-Entry Options

The best way to explore formal schooling options is to contact MEAC for a list of accredited programs. Some offer distance learning, while others are entirely on-site. Some offer a bachelor or master's degree, while others are three-year vocational programs. Many allow training internationally. To decide if a program is right for you, study its philosophy and purpose statement to see if it aligns with your own as you consider the curriculum's structure and content. Also ask to speak to former or current students. Imagine what your experience of student life will be like, and ask yourself whether it is sustainable, particularly if you have small children or other family obligations.

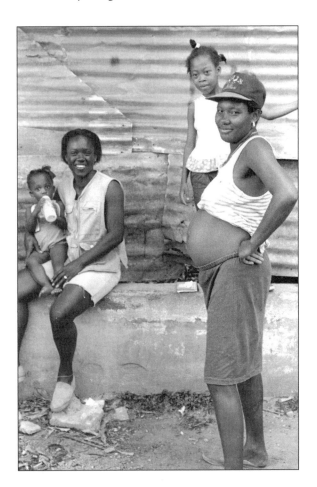

If you are unsure of what kind of program to choose, consider your learning style. Do you need formal structure to master academic material, that is, a classroom setting with quizzes, tests, and assignment due dates? If so, look for an on-site program. Are you a self-starter who enjoys working autonomously or needs time flexibility? If so, look for a distance program. In general, the best programs offer opportunities to integrate theory and practice right from the start.

Nurse-Midwifery Programs

Nurse-midwifery programs vary greatly in terms of prerequisites. Some require a BSN; others, an RN certificate only. Several master's programs incorporate nursing into midwifery training and accept students with BA or BS degrees in any subject: in three years, the student earns an RN, MSN, and CNM.

To more realistically assess what a program has to offer, consider the clinical settings involved. If most or all of these are tertiary, high-tech medical centers, you will practice active management rather than woman-centered care. Programs with training in birth centers or hospitals known for expectant management teach more of the art of midwifery.

Frontier Nursing University's Community-Based Nurse-Midwifery Education Program (CNEP) and the Midwifery Institute at Philadelphia University are unique in that most course work and clinical practice occur at a distance. When applying to a distance program, ask to speak to current students or recent graduates to get a better sense of what your educational experience will be like.

If you are planning on the nursing route to practice, check out the Bridge Club. This organization works in conjunction with both the ACNM and MANA and represents midwives striving to practice autonomous, woman-centered care, many of them doing out-of-hospital birth.

The best advice for nurse-midwifery students is to be realistic about how training is likely to affect them. Most CNM programs are hospital based, and with the U.S. cesarean rate at 33 percent, it is easy to see how mistrust of the birth process and fear of the responsibility of primary care could creep into a student's psyche. You must be proactive to counteract this: for example, by taking a diametrically opposed training on intuition, shamanic studies, or dream work—anything to keep the nonlinear aspects of your mind active. Good nutrition, regular exercise, and stress management are also essential.

Note

1. Sharon Evans and Pam Weaver, *Practical Skills Guide for Midwifery*, 2nd ed. (Bend, OR: Morningstar Publishing, 1999).

CHAPTER 8

The Midwife's Practice

As a midwife's status changes from apprentice to primary caregiver, her focus shifts from the thrill of assisting births to her burgeoning professional responsibilities. To practice effectively, she must successfully combine the demands of work with those of her personal life. Putting together a cohesive and comfortable practice can be quite challenging for a beginner.

The best way to start is to clearly articulate your philosophy of care. This is the linchpin on which many of your practice decisions will be based. Your philosophy should incorporate your beliefs regarding optimal care and responsibility in childbearing. If your philosophy is clearly stated, it will define your purpose. For example, if your philosophy states that midwifery should serve the needs and desires of childbearing women, your purpose would be to support women in choosing how they wish to give birth. From this point forward, the structure of your practice should at all times and in all ways uphold your philosophy and express your purpose.

It might seem that all midwives share the same philosophy of care. But one has only to look at the services and clientele of several different practices to see that this is not the case. If you are unclear on your philosophy, you may wish to try this simple exercise:

1. Choose *one* of the following statements:
   a. "The most important thing a pregnant woman can do is . . ."
   b. "A pregnant woman should never . . ."
   c. "A pregnant woman's partner's role is to . . ."
   d. "A pregnant woman's partner should never . . ."
   e. "A new mother should definitely . . ."
   f. "The role of the mother's partner postpartum is to . . ."

2. Using the statement you selected, complete the sentence spontaneously and as exhaustively as possible, not censoring anything but jotting down whatever comes to you. You may have quite a list when you finish, but you will probably find that one "should" or "shouldn't" stands out and is highly charged.

3. Take that highly charged "should" or "shouldn't" and in the same spontaneous way as before, write down why this matters so much

to you—why is this such a big deal? You are not defending or rationalizing here, but rather, exploring what happened in your personal life that led you to feel this so strongly.

4. To conclude, recognize this "should" or "shouldn't" for the bias it is and look closely at how it might impact a mother or partner's experience of receiving care from you.

Were you to do this exercise in a group, you might be surprised to find a few participants holding biases in direct contrast to yours. The same is true of midwives: we all have our biases and, on that basis, decide which clients we take into our practices. If we are smart, we refer mothers who activate our biases to midwives who might better care for them. The point is that our biases determine, to large extent, our motivation for, and philosophy of, caregiving.

As regards getting your practice to match your philosophy of care, there is much to consider. You must figure out backup arrangements, define your working relationship with partners or other assistants, choose an office location, name your business, establish a financial structure, create promotional materials and marketing strategies, and so on, all based on your purpose and the anticipated needs and desires of your clientele.

It may be difficult to find your footing in the beginning, particularly in terms of finances. Will your client volume be adequate to pay the bills? Would it be better to have an office in your home to keep overhead low until your practice gets going? Is your personal life stable enough to withstand these start-up stresses, and if not, what must you do to make it so? Keep an eye on the bottom line but stay positive. If need be, supplement your income with the suggestions for apprentices, above.

Especially in the beginning, your clients will take much of your energy as you struggle to make the best impression and agonize over every detail. Your personal life may begin to show some strain, and that puts an extra burden on you. Just remember to take one challenge (and one day) at a time

and do step back periodically to reflect on your progress. Experienced midwives typically meet with their associates weekly to go over client issues, attend to business matters, and to otherwise clear the air. Especially in the beginning, consider having these meetings in casual or retreat settings, which are more conducive to the visioning needed to get your practice flourishing.

Location: Urban or Rural Practice?

Urban Practice

Urban practice has benefits in the ready availability of medical facilities, support from other midwives, and access to consultation. However, close contact with the medical community demands good working relationships.

Ease of urban practice depends largely on your legal status. If you are practicing illegally or in a hostile environment, you will eventually be in the untenable position of having to transport and face the consequences of inadequate or nonexistent backup. Upholding the safety of mother and baby may require you to relay details of the case that could incriminate you. Thus you must be discreet, get support from your peers, and gain clear agreements with your clients as to your limits.

If political oppression is not an issue, an urban lifestyle may impact your clients and affect your practice. It is not easy to persuade a busy mother that she needs to slow down and let the pregnancy determine her lifestyle rather than the other way around. And too, the stresses of noise, air pollution, and harried pace are hardly conducive to good health.

Making time to really get to know your clients is another issue. Visits during daytime hours are standard, but the mother's or partner's work schedule may interfere. She may request evening appointments, but you must make time for yourself and your family. You may be able to see the mother during the day but may not spend much time with her partner. To compensate for this, home visits may be necessary.

Sometimes an urban location has several midwifery practices, and competition becomes an issue. In my area, a new model of care has emerged, known as the Bay Area Homebirth Collective. This involves the practices of five midwives who support each other in many ways, while their clients reap the benefits of a large pool of homebirth parents with whom they can socialize and share resources. The midwives back each other up at births but, in the role of assistant, their only obligations are to (1) meet the mother once prior to the birth, (2) attend when she is close to delivery, and (3) stay briefly postpartum (barring emergencies). For this, the assistant receives a fee of $600, allowing the primary midwife to retain the rest of the money the client pays, rather than having to split 50/50 with a partner. The collective also organizes events for the general public, and the feeling of camaraderie is strong indeed.

Although urban midwifery has its challenges, opportunities for personal and professional growth are tremendous. Working in this setting takes a midwife across class and cultural boundaries, fostering flexibility and insight.

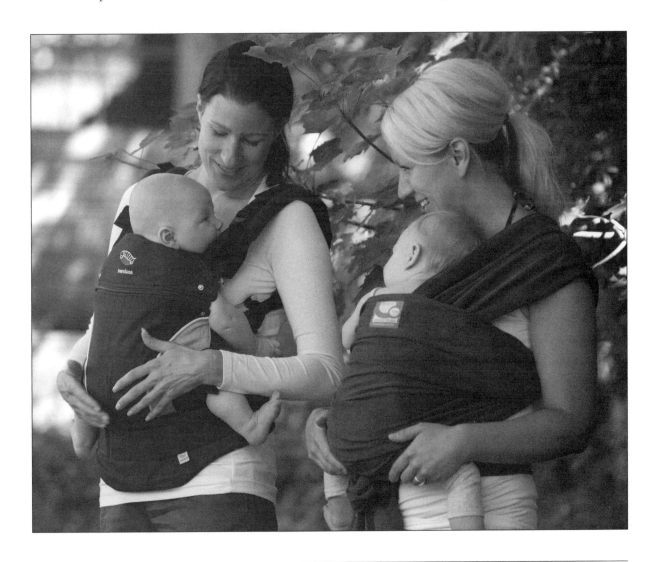

Rural Practice

As regards rural practice, open space, clean air, and a relaxed lifestyle are perks for the midwife and her clientele. Living with awareness of nature can be strengthening and relaxing for mothers, and they may find support more easily in a small community. Birth in a rural setting may also be an extended family event, in contrast to the couple-only style of birthing emblematic of urban woman's social isolation.

Problems may result from a large practice radius. In urban practice, it makes sense to do prenatals on certain days at a central location, but this may not be workable in the country. For example, if mothers are already en route for prenatals and you must rush to a birth, they may be quite unhappy to have driven long distances only to have to turn around and go home. Rural midwives end up doing a lot of care at their clients' homes, unless they have a skilled assistant or backup from other midwives. In this respect, the collective model cited above can work for rural midwives, too: even if only two participate, it will still save each a good bit of time and energy.

Along these lines, what rural midwives often miss is contact with others in practice. Midwives need regular opportunities to share experiences in peer review or with continuing education. If these opportunities are not available locally, the rural midwife may have to travel to an urban location to have this kind of contact.

Medical backup and consultation may also be limited in rural areas: it may be very difficult to get a second or third opinion. And transport time may be considerable. Thus any midwife practicing more than half an hour from the nearest hospital will need advanced skills and equipment.

Equipment

It is usually best to purchase equipment slowly, using the apprenticeship period to try out various brands to see which suit you best. Slow acquisition is also easier on the pocketbook. A complete midwife's kit, including birth bag and resuscitation equipment, can easily run around $4,000. See appendix M for a list of necessities, and appendix B for birthing-supply companies. Certain basics like urine sticks, nonsterile exam gloves, Betadine or Hibiclens antiseptic, lubricating jelly, sterile gauze pads, underpads, paper cups (for urine testing), bulb syringe, and heating pad can be purchased at your local drugstore.

When students ask me what equipment to purchase first, I suggest a **fetascope**. This tool for taking fetal heart tones can be your ticket to interact with pregnant women and will give you the opportunity to develop a trained ear before you begin primary care. Doula clients or mothers in childbirth classes are usually happy to have you listen to the baby and may also want you to palpate for position, size, and so on. The best fetascope currently available is the Allen Series 10, which features an amplification unit in the horn (avoid Allen-type economy models). If you elect to purchase a Doppler, the most popular model is the Huntleigh, available in audio-only or with audio-plus-digital display. Both come with water and shockproof 2 MHz probes and cost around $600.

Other items, like your **sphygmomanometer** (blood pressure cuff), should be purchased by comparison shopping, your goal being quality without tinsel: blood pressure cuffs are sporting some stylish colors of late, but apart from looks, the most important component is the gauge. The cuff, bladder, and tubing are readily and cheaply replaced, but the gauge should be built to last. Make sure it is constructed without an automatic pin stop, which keeps the gauge at zero even if it needs adjustment. The unit should come with a warranty of at least three years, and the gauge should be certified (you can see a registered number stamped on the face of any decent gauge).

Although your lab will supply everything you need for doing blood draws, consider purchasing a **hemoglobinometer** for office use. These currently run from $250 to $400—much less expensive than a centrifuge.

Beyond what your lab provides, you should stock disposable items for urinalysis and pregnancy testing; collection devices, fixative, and long-handled sterile cotton swabs for Pap smears; lancets, cotton balls, and Band-Aids for venipuncture; and glucose-testing strips. You will also need a **hanging scale** to weigh the newborn: the digital model runs around $155 and the mechanical model, $85 (prices include flannel sling).

Your **resuscitation equipment** should include DeLee suction devices, adult and newborn pocket masks, adult oxygen mask, oxygen tanks and regulator, and a bag-mask unit for the baby. The Mercury Disposable Infant Resuscitator costs around $45 and may be a wise choice for the midwife with a small practice. For a more permanent investment, both the Hudson Lifesaver Infant Resuscitator ($210) and the Ambu Mark IV Baby Resuscitator ($270) are excellent choices; the latter meets and exceeds all standards for neonatal resuscitation.

Make sure your **hand instruments** are 100 percent stainless steel. It is particularly important that your blunt scissors be top quality as you will use them repeatedly for cord cutting. It is also wise to get at least one good needle holder as the precision work of suturing is best accomplished with a quality tool: the finest are made in Germany by Medline and Miltex and are lifetime guaranteed. A less expensive grade is entirely adequate for instruments like ring forceps or mosquito forceps that you will rarely use.

Last but not least are the restricted items: **suture material** and **syringes**. If you have authorization to purchase these items in your state, no problem; otherwise, you may be able to enlist the help of a colleague with the proper credentials. The same goes for **oxytocic drugs** and other medications; if you are legally authorized to order these, count your blessings. Otherwise, if you must rely on a sympathetic physician or other midwives, stock up whenever you have the opportunity.

Setup and Administration

In terms of physical setup, you have a number of choices. You can see clients in your home, using a bedroom for exams and your living room for waiting. You can see clients in their homes (some midwives do this exclusively). If you elect to rent an office, you will need to find a facility with a room for exams, waiting area, restroom, and storage area. If you set up a freestanding birth center, all of the above plus birth rooms should be housed together.

Prenatal care by home visit is undoubtedly the first choice for most mothers. Midwives who offer this report fewer transports in labor, and for the most part, feel the driving is worth it. Being in a mother's home repeatedly can shed light on household and relationship dynamics that might not otherwise be discovered until labor. Visits are more leisurely and often involve sharing meals: all in all, a more intimate caregiving experience.

Next to this, clients would probably prefer to see you in your home rather than in an office. The obvious drawback is that you must keep everything neat and clean on a regular basis. This can be especially challenging if you have just come in from a birth at 3 a.m., and appointments start in a few hours. Lack of privacy for family members is yet another issue: there may be strenuous objections from your partner if he or she needs extra sleep or solitude. If the cost of renting an office is prohibitive, consider sharing office space with other midwives or health providers in your area.

Whatever you decide, your exam room should be arranged for comfort and efficiency. Most women prefer to be examined on a bed rather than an exam table. Choose a firm mattress, large enough for you and your assistant to sit comfortably on either side of the mother. Another possibility is either a chaise lounge (if not too low) or antique "fainting sofa," with chairs on either side. Use a closet for storage, a corner of the room for lab equipment, and your exam room is ready to go.

In the waiting area, you need adequate seating, a water cooler, toys for small children, birth pictures (or art) on the wall, birth and parenting periodicals on end tables, and a bookcase with lending library. Also post important documents, such as the Patient's Bill of Rights in your state of practice, the WHO/ UNICEF Breastfeeding Resolution, the WHO Resolution on Midwifery, and so on.

In terms of clinic supplies, what will you need, and how much should you keep in stock? Besides your equipment, see the list in the previous section for disposable items to have on hand. Take inventory of cleaning products, hand soap, toilet paper, tissues, and paper towels weekly. Keep tabs on your stock of forms and make sure you have the necessary supplies for filing, bookkeeping, and correspondence. Have backup cartridges for your printer, CDs for your computer, and so on. It never hurts to post a running list of needs, with highlighted priorities. No matter what your level of practice, keep it organized.

How much time should you set aside for initial, follow-up, and routine visits? That depends on your style and volume of practice. If you assist four to six births per month, you can probably limit yourself to two clinic days per week. Allow two hours for the initial visit and one-and-a-half hours for the visit immediately following, as medical history intake and review, consent to care, nutritional counseling, physical assessment, and/or pelvimetry take some time. For routine checkups, an hour should be sufficient, with twenty-five minutes for physical assessment and the rest for discussion.

If physical findings are questionable or topics of conversation result in controversy or upset, a visit may run over. With the latter, know when it is time to stop: you can always follow up later by phone.

You may want to schedule mothers due at the same time so their appointments overlap, giving them a chance to connect. This brings up another option in caregiving: **group prenatal care**. This requires a large block of time (perhaps an entire day)

when all your mothers (and their partners, if available) come together for discussion and prenatals. As the conversation rages, you pull women aside one by one for their clinical evaluations. Depending on your practice volume, you may need an assistant to facilitate the discussion or help with exams. Women love this opportunity to socialize and may choose to share in one another's prenatals. New mothers may come back with their babies and birth stories. Beloved California midwife June Whitson (who died of breast cancer in 2002) introduced this system as the best possible way to help new mothers find support and autonomy (it is now known as **village pregnancy** or **centering pregnancy**).

Apart from prenatals, schedule weekly business meetings with your colleagues to go over finances, marketing, special events, and so on. This is also a good time to discuss purchasing new reference books, equipment, or furnishings for your facility. Consider dividing weekly meetings into two segments: the first for business and the second for airing interpersonal concerns. The latter is critical to the psychological health of your practice. Occasionally, or perhaps initially, an outside facilitator may be helpful. Make separate time for case review.

Schedule a comprehensive annual review of all aspects of your business: forms, facilities, organization, location, image, competition, finances, marketing strategies, and professional relationships. Use this time to create long-term goals for your practice, in contrast to the short-term, problem-solving focus of weekly meetings. Review your philosophy of care and purpose statements: is your work still in keeping with these? If not, make the necessary revisions.

Be sure your filing system is at all times in order. Although laws vary from state to state, medical records must be kept for many years (for example, twenty-one years in California). Closed cases should be filed by year and kept in a fireproof container (for more on this, see the section on HIPAA guidelines later in this chapter). You may also need to hire an accountant or consult an expert on tax laws and organizational options relevant to small-business owners. Good references on this subject are *Small Time Operator*, by Bernard Kamoroff, and *Business Mastery*, by Cherie Sohnen-Moe.

Regarding the legal aspects of midwifery practice, I highly recommend the book, *Law and Professional Issues in Midwifery: Transforming Midwifery Practice*, by Richard Griffith, Cassam Tengnah, and Chantal Patel. Although it is written primarily for the European market, it is full of case histories that make vividly clear the various ethical and legal dilemmas of our work today.

General Presentability and Personal Hygiene

Most professional women carefully plan their wardrobes for a variety of occasions, and there is no reason a midwife should not do the same. Clothes to wear to births should be readily washable; dark-colored pants are most practical. Tops should be layered, as the amount of warmth required upon arrival will be way too much once the birth room is adequately heated for delivery. Some midwives prefer to wear waterproof aprons in the final stages of labor. Apron or not, you should definitely have a change of clothes with you at all times.

One of the reasons there is less infection with homebirth is that the mother has resistance to microorganisms in her environment. However, she may not have resistance to what you bring in from outside. This is why your clothes should be completely clean and why you always wash your hands upon arrival. This is important with postpartum home visits as well: wash your hands before examining the mother and again before handling the baby.

When doing prenatals in your office or home, observe proper aseptic technique and always wash your hands before and after each client. Clean, fresh-smelling clothes make a good impression. (In fact, pregnant women are exceedingly sensitive to smell, which is why you should avoid wearing perfume or cologne.)

To return to wardrobe, consider several highly presentable outfits for greeting the public. Midwives are increasingly called to political work in the legislature or the public arena, and for that you will need a suit, heels, the whole bit. Don't be put off by the notion of dressing to fit the part. If life is a stage, then it pays to have your costumes in order.

Fees

A midwife's fee should be fair and affordable for her clientele. Beyond that, a sliding-scale policy makes way for exceptions. Many midwives have great success with this and find most of their clients more than willing to pay the full amount. Politically speaking, it's best to charge what other midwives in your area are charging: resist the temptation to underbid your "competitors" to get clients.

The services your fee includes and how you would like it to be paid should be detailed in your Professional Disclosure form. If you expect a payment at every visit, make sure this is realistic given your client's work and pay schedule. If and when you make exceptions, be sure they are not more than you can personally bear. Negotiations around money can strengthen a relationship or undermine it dramatically. If you individualize payment plans, they must be consistently enforced.

If the mother is behind on her balance at twenty-eight weeks, firm up future payments more precisely. Most midwives ask to be paid in full by thirty-six weeks. In terms of taking health insurance, some PPOs cover midwifery care but billing is tricky: ask experienced midwives in your community for tips. Many midwives prefer to have their clients file for reimbursement rather than having to do it themselves.

Public Relations and Education

The first step in public relations is to make your practice visible. Begin with the obvious and list your services with birth-related resource centers or online networks in your area. If you feel comfortable doing so, advertise in the Yellow Pages. Then contact prominent, alternative health care providers who might be willing to refer clients to you (homeopaths, acupuncturists, naturopaths, massage therapists, herbal practitioners, or therapists). As you may be asked to provide feedback on your care, offer your clients a form for this purpose in the postpartum period. Also keep up with any online reviews of your practice: check out your Yelp ratings from time to time.

Regardless of topic, use any public-speaking opportunity to introduce your services: have business cards or brochures ready for the taking. Consider hosting a video and information night for the general public. Even small, informal video showings with clients and their friends will keep your name circulating and bring you business by word-of-mouth.

Larger events such as workshops, forums, or panel discussions take some effort to coordinate and require plenty of advance publicity to assure good attendance. These may or may not be profit generating, but their main function is to expose a large, diverse audience to the benefits of midwifery and, more specifically, to your services.

You might also consider renting a table at local music festivals or other outdoor events. Stock your table with DVDs and books, T-shirts, birth art, and bumper stickers. Of course you will have brochures on your services prominently displayed, but general information on midwifery, such as that featured in the pamphlet, *The Midwifery Model of Care* (available from MANA), should also be available.

Television and radio appearances can boost public awareness of birth options and your practice, but you must be prepared. Anticipate questions you are likely to be asked, and know your statistics. And remember that you can always respond to an unappealing question with one you would rather answer, as the media savvy do. For example, if your interviewer asks, "Is homebirth safe?" you might respond with, "Well, who says hospital birth is all that safe?" and launch into a discussion of the "cascade of interventions" or the side effects of cesarean birth. If you are badgered, don't get flustered: calmly return to your key position statement, pose another question, or raise a new issue more to your liking. If your interview is being taped, stick to simple statements less likely to be distorted by editing. The same goes for statements you make to journalists.

Midwife Diane Barnes claims that the remarkable success of her freestanding birth center was largely due to advertising spots on cable TV networks. She warns that results take time: in her case, calls started to pour in after six months or so. The obvious advantage of paying for advertising is that you get to say, and portray, exactly what you want the public to know about you and your services.

Whenever you go public for midwifery, know that your words and appearance reflect on the entire profession. Prepare carefully, dress the part, and ask your colleagues for feedback on your performance.

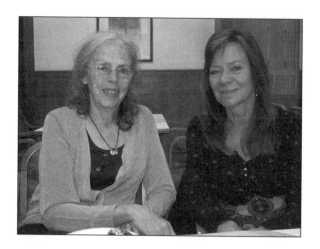

Medical Backup and Consultation

By grace, faith, or the law of averages, a midwife's first births usually go well. But with time, the unusual and unexpected begin to manifest along with a desire for more in-depth medical consultation and assistance.

In areas where midwifery is illegal, a new midwife may be hesitant to seek out medical backup. But if transport becomes necessary, she must have a good relationship with the local hospital if she hopes to safeguard her client's well-being. Long before we became midwives, my first partner and I began working on getting backup at a hospital where we already worked as doulas. We used the "iron fist in a velvet glove" approach, maintaining a low profile while persistently advocating our clients' wishes. We won the confidence of staff by being clearheaded and articulate and by presenting complete, well-organized client records. After several drop-in transports, the head obstetrician called and asked if we would like his assistance on a continuing basis, and we formalized our backup relationship.

If you must transport to a hospital where you do not have backup, maintain an open, adaptable, friendly attitude. The staff may be suspicious at first but might become accommodating if you act responsibly and present the details of your case intelligently. Although some physicians may remain hostile, others will be curious to learn just what midwives do and so may give you opportunities to demonstrate your skills and knowledge.

Particularly if you do not have backup at your local hospital, it is crucial that you understand the psychology of labor and delivery personnel. The nursing staff is generally overworked, underpaid, and underacknowledged, so why not offer assistance? Although nurses are legally responsible for routine assessments, you can certainly fetch drinking water, help your client to the bathroom, and change bedding. When the birth is over and you are preparing to leave, go out of your way to personally thank every nurse who participated.

If the hospital trains residents, your situation is challenging but promising. Fresh out of school, heads crammed with information, residents are primed to answer questions. In fact, speculative discourse is their forte and your key to forging a connection. If you acknowledge the resident's authority in the realm of information as you project authority in action, you will be perfect complements. Pose a question on episiotomy, for example, and the resident may be only too happy to discuss the data as you provide perineal support. Suddenly, the baby is crowning, and you are catching it together.

Understand that residents are generally overworked and exhausted. By way of acknowledging this, a former apprentice of mine made a point of offering candy or gum to the resident on duty, followed by a vigorous shoulder rub as I went ahead and attended our client. Before you leave, be generous with gratitude and praise, as an appreciative colleague.

In contrast, the attending obstetrician may be in and out of the room before you have a chance to say a word. If so, immediately step out in the hall to converse. Establish your authority by asking whether he or she has reviewed the chart or would like to see it, and ask his or her opinion on the case. Listen respectfully, chime in with agreement whenever you can, but assume a collegial air as you discuss your client in as technical terms as possible. If the physician suggests a course of action with which you do not agree, never confront him or her directly. Reiterate his or her recommendation so it is clear that you understand, and then offer to present it to the mother. Once alone with her, let her know her options. You will, of course, express your opinion if requested. When she has decided what she wants to do, present her decision to the physician. Thus you avoid confrontation while upholding principles of woman-centered care. Even if the physician is entirely disinterested in your ideas, fear of liability will prompt him or her to at least consider the mother's wishes.

If you are in very good standing at a particular hospital, you may link up with several doctors, and if problems arise in the future you can choose your consult at will. But in the early stages of establishing backup, consider distributing your clients among various practitioners so as not to overwhelm any one of them. Decide on whom to consult according to what is required. For example, if you need an ultrasound for suspected twins (and you do not assist twins at home), order it through an obstetrician likely to support vaginal twin birth. You need not be picky with an ultrasound for third-trimester bleeding. But if you are trying to establish dates on a latecomer with uncertain menstrual history, you might have a general practitioner do the authorization to avoid involving an obstetrician in what might later be construed as a postdates pregnancy.

If you are licensed or certified to practice in your state, backup requirements are probably spelled out in your law. Some midwives must have backup with a particular physician, who may have a cap on how many midwives he or she may assist. Sometimes midwife and backup physician are required to work under written practice guidelines, which, due to malpractice concerns, can make formal backup almost impossible to obtain. If so, a progressive local hospital may be receptive to your transports.

Another approach is to have mothers find their own backup. This may be your only option if you practice in a conservative area. In other words, a physician unwilling to back you personally might feel more comfortable backing your client as his or her private patient. Advantages of this arrangement are (1) the midwife is free to practice according to midwifery guidelines, (2) the mother is free to choose her own physician, and (3) liability for the physician, professionally and politically, is reduced. This is in keeping with the original *MANA Standards and Qualifications for the Art and Practice of Midwifery* statement, which states that requiring the midwife to have a relationship with a particular physician is at odds with a mother's right to self-determination.

In areas where the political climate is very oppressive and the "old boys" are out to get you, finding backup may seem impossible. Nevertheless, explore each and every inroad. If you can't find a sympathetic doctor, perhaps you can find a progressive labor and delivery nurse who might be willing to give you advice from time to time or even put in a good word for you with hospital staff. This takes time and is more than a little humiliating, but you owe it to your clients. The ideal is to have backup at every hospital where client insurance might necessitate transport.

Here is a story (from the days when midwifery was illegal in California) of acquiring backup on the spot. This was a first birth, and after many hours of active but ineffective labor resulting in maternal exhaustion, we all agreed on transport. Our usual backup doctor was not available, so we were forced to take "OB potluck." As the mother curled up contentedly on her hospital bed, we could see that she had wanted to be in the hospital all along. But after forty-eight sleepless hours, my partner and I felt only relief. Our rapport with the nurses had always been great, and that night, even the head nurse (who was usually a bit disapproving) seemed sympathetic and supportive.

Progress with Pitocin was much more rapid than anyone expected. Braving disapproval, my partner donned a glove and checked the mother, who was fully dilated. By the time the head nurse came back, the head was showing and I was giving perineal support. She paused and took it all in before going to get the doctor. As the doctor came in and the nurses gathered around, the head was close to crowning. My partner took heart tones as I continued perineal support. When a nurse brought the instrument tray and asked the doctor where she wanted it, she said, motioning to us, "Ask them; I don't have anything to do with it." The tray was placed at the end of the bed, and after an awkward moment, someone unwrapped it for us. Good thing, too, for just then, a lovely baby girl was born. The doctor stepped up to help me check for tears:

the perineum was intact but there was an internal muscle split. "She may need a few stitches there," she commented.

"No," I said, "just press down with some gauze, and it will stop bleeding." She did so and watched, waited a moment, and concurred as I told her, "Those little tears heal fine all by themselves . . . ."

After some time had passed, she motioned me to step outside the room. "Uh oh," I thought, "This is it. I'm busted." Instead, she held up the birth certificate and asked me uncertainly, "Do you sign this, or should I?"

In my amazement, I uttered, "I consider it a privilege to be able to work here, so just do whatever works best for you."

"Okay, I'll sign it," she said. "You know, this is the first time I've ever done this." Then came a marvelous exchange of warmth and appreciation, with good feelings all around.

Whatever the genesis of your consulting relationship, continue to cultivate it. Periodic chart review, and disclosure of major revisions in your protocol, are critical to maintaining a solid working relationship. Friendly lunch dates are a good idea, too. Trust and openness between you and your backup associates make all the difference in crisis situations.

Medical Records

As her training nears completion, the apprentice should begin collecting forms from various midwives so she can begin designing her own. Please consider the forms in the appendix not as models but as samples you should adapt to your own practice needs. Plan to revise your forms periodically, perhaps with your annual review of practice.

Charting

A medical chart is a *legal document*, thus the importance of complete and accurate charting cannot be overemphasized. In the event of a civil or malpractice suit, your chart may be your only witness to quality care. For this reason, assiduously record every assessment and recommendation you make, as well as all discussions between you and (1) the mother, (2) other health care providers, (3) your backup physician(s), and (4) hospital staff.

Certain styles of charting are considered the most legally defensible. Apart from your boxed page of vital assessments, notes and commentary should be on lined paper, and writing should be continuous, broken only by your initials and the date and time of each assessment. *Do not leave any part of a line blank*: start your next entry mid-line if need be. If your forms have areas left partially empty, a court could find your entire chart invalid because you could easily go back and add to your notes at any time. Also, take care not to cross out information so it is unintelligible: put a straight line through it, write "error" above it, and date and initial it (no white-out either). Occasionally, you will need to end an entry with both your initials and the mother's, for example, in the event she declines a routine procedure.

You might also consider charting electronically, as is now standard in hospital. Look online for "midwifery charting software." As for making your notes amendment proof, your software should have a time and content locking function that prevents later revision, although some programs, such as that offered by GetPrivatePractice.com, feature a fifteen-minute edit function, showing both the original note and the changed version. This program also offers a client-sharing feature, which allows clients to log in and see their records.

A standard format for note taking in the health professions is **SOAP charting**. These initials stand for *subjective* (the mother's report), *objective* (your clinical evaluations), *assessment* (your preliminary or defininitive diagnosis), and *plan* (tests and evaluations yet to be performed, guidelines for the mother, and follow up plan), all of which are crucial aspects of caregiving that must be documented. For example, say your client at twenty-six weeks complains of middle back pain. You would write or type:

- **S:** Mother complains of middle back pain, pain and urgency with urination.

- **O:** CVAT present, temp 101.6, pulse 80 (8 points above baseline), urine dipstick showed trace leucocytes and blood, performed cultures for BV, chlamydia, GC to rule out vaginal or cervical infections, collected urine sample for lab urinalysis.

- **A:** Possible kidney infection.

- **P:** Consult with backup physician or clinic (name), mother to increase fluids (including unsweetened cranberry juice), eliminate sugar and caffeine, suspend sexual activity pending lab results, take her temperature every four hours and report any elevation or change in symptoms, follow-up visit or instructions to be based on lab work and consult with physician or clinic (name).

Informed Choice

And yet, SOAP charting does not cover everything. Make note of every discussion relevant to the situation, as cited in the first paragraph of the "Charting" section. Include not only personal interactions, but also phone or email consultations (the latter should be printed out and placed in the chart). Note the mother's response to recommended tests or procedures, along with information provided on respective benefits and risks. California legal code is very specific on this point; patients have the right to

receive as much information about any proposed treatment or procedure as the patient may need in order to give informed consent or to refuse this course of treatment. Except in emergencies, this information shall include a description of the procedure or treatment, the medically significant risks involved in this treatment, alternate courses of treatment or non-treatment and the risks involved in each.[1]

To cover this detail, controversial tests or procedures such as GBS or postdates screening require separate **informed choice documents**. Besides the above inclusions, there must be a place for the mother's response and signature (with her initials on every page). These documents can be lengthy: for example, a GBS screening document might include current CDC guidelines, articles on pros and cons of antibiotic treatment, and alternatives such as Hibiclens washes or herbal formulas with their respective pros and cons.

If you remain unconvinced that this is necessary, imagine yourself in court, facing the parents of a stillborn, postdates baby who claim, "She told us we needed a nonstress test, but she didn't tell us what could happen if we said no." Of course, none of us want to think that we might be sued. We tell ourselves that we screen more carefully or maintain higher standards for communication and caregiving than the "average" midwife. But I know of several experienced, dedicated, and competent midwives who have been sued, and the effects, both professionally and personally, have been devastating.

However, lest we dismiss midwifery wisdom entirely, cultivating the best possible relationships with our clients does make a difference, especially if we put them in charge of decision making right from the start. Although most hospitals still have patients sign a blanket consent form (rather than individual forms, as above), medical textbooks increasingly allude to the importance of good practitioner-patient relations in avoiding litigation.

A Few More Tips

When doing prenatals, make notes during rather than after the visit. Yes, this can be distracting in the midst of a passionate discussion, but unless you stop and make notes in the moment, you may forget important details later on. During labor this becomes more difficult, especially during second stage. Midwife Tish Demmin suggests putting strips of masking tape on your pants, jotting notes there, and transferring them to the chart as soon as possible. It is particularly important to note both time and results of all fetal heart rate assessments.

In the event of transport, update the chart completely before arriving at the hospital; it will be scrutinized (and may be photocopied). Note when you first contacted the hospital, the name of the person you spoke to, and what they recommended. Continue to make notes once you arrive: you cannot assume the hospital's charting system to be unbiased or as complete as your own. This is for your protection, though it will also be important to the mother later for purposes of debriefing her experience.

The statute of limitations runs three years for criminal charges, much longer for civil and malpractice suits (up to thirty years), so keep your charts or electronic backup locked in a fireproof safe, and be sure your family members know of their location.

Client Confidentiality and HIPAA Guidelines

Another critical principle of practice is upholding **client confidentiality** at all times. This can be challenging if one of your clients hears that another had a difficult birth and asks you about it. Particularly if there is some question of why you handled the case as you did, the temptation to explain or defend your actions may be very strong. But the only ethical response is to refer the curious client directly to the mother, who can tell her whatever she chooses.

Midwifery students or other associates in the practice must be in agreement on this issue. Legal strictures in this regard are detailed in the **Health Insurance Portability and Accountability Act (HIPAA)**. The HIPAA guidelines apply specifically to health practitioners that bill insurance, although midwives now use them as a matter of course. For details and updates, see the website of the administrative agency, U.S. Department of Health and Human Services, at www.hhs.gov/ocr/hipaa.

HIPAA guidelines mandate that client records must be secure at all times. For example, if you are doing a home visit, you cannot bring other clients' charts into the house with you, although they may be locked, out of view, in your car. Similarly, your file cabinet containing charts must be locked unless under your direct supervision. All inactive files must be stored in locked, fireproof containers. See appendix O for a summary of the guidelines.

Partnership, Collective, or Group Practice

No matter where you are located, working in some form of partnership is the safest way to practice. Midwives who work alone are rare, as a second pair of skilled hands is important in the event of emergency and essential if both mother and newborn need help. Long or difficult labors often produce a depressed baby and tired uterus apt to hemorrhage. How can a solitary midwife deal with these complications simultaneously? How can she possibly resuscitate the baby and do bimanual compression on the mother at the same time?

As mentioned earlier, in the collective model, a second midwife meets the mother in advance, attends the birth when it is imminent, and receives a flat fee. But by the usual definition, partnership is comprised of two midwives sharing equally the responsibilities and income of a practice. This may be the best way for a new midwife to practice as she gets adjusted to the rigors of the work. Working with a partner can give her confidence in her abilities as she identifies areas where she needs to advance her knowledge or skill.

Practically speaking, partners can spell one another at births, fill in emotionally or physically for each other in times of personal crisis, and rotate

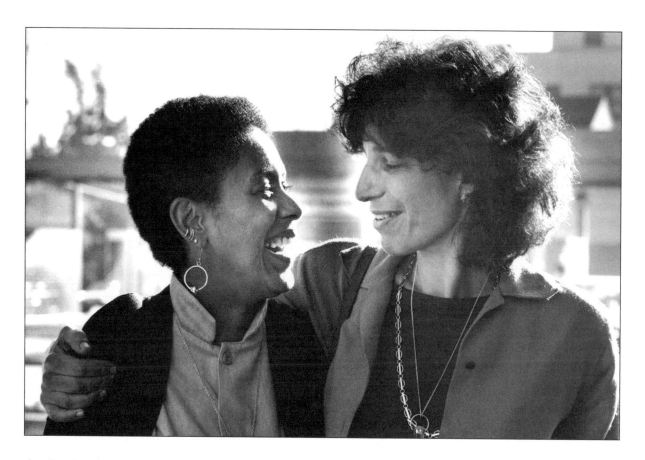

days/weeks of prenatal or postpartum visits. Ironing out disagreements can reveal blind spots and keep humility a constant for both. Jointly evolving creative responses to problematic situations is one of the highlights of partnership. As partners learn to respect one another's intimacies with various clients, they learn to take pleasure in high- and low-profile roles. In a successful partnership, midwives truly enjoy one another's company, not unlike a successful marriage.

Group practice is another option, in which several midwives rotate being on call for a shared clientele. The advantages and disadvantages are obvious: time off call is a huge perk, but lack of continuity of caregiver argues strongly against this model unless the midwife participants are very experienced and have excellent communication skills. Group practice also calls for in-depth weekly meetings to go over developments at prenatals of a more personal nature that might not be captured in charting.

Training the Student or Apprentice

Why bother with the added responsibility of training an apprentice? There are several reasons, the most obvious being help with the work. An apprentice can save you time and energy by monitoring early labor, assisting at prenatals, running errands, doing bookkeeping and filing, and keeping the office clean and tidy. With studies fresh in mind, she can offer new, interesting bits of information to you and your clients. When you are tired or worn thin, she can lend you some of her beginner's stamina and passion. With just a little guidance on your part, her enthusiasm can revitalize your practice.

Other benefits are less tangible but more personally affecting. Deep satisfaction can be found in transmitting knowledge, and it can be exciting to tailor information to a student's degree of readiness as you observe her growth. Interdependency of teacher and student fosters an intimacy that can be a great pleasure. Those trained by apprenticeship recognize its advantages over other educational models: the learning process is integrated and thus more complete, and if the apprentice trains in a community where she will one day practice, she is well prepared to field the health needs and issues of her future clientele.

Although training an apprentice allows you to play a pivotal role in preserving this traditional entry route to our profession, it can also be a challenge. It requires top-notch communication and a clear understanding of normal stages in the process. Not to condescend, but the stages of parent-child relationship are remarkably similar to those of the midwife-apprentice configuration. They are (1) infancy—the time of being one, (2) childhood—the time of being together, (3) adolescence—the time of breaking away and being separate, and (4) adulthood—the time of being together again. For the apprentice, the stages of falling in love are also relevant: (1) infatuation, (2) disillusionment and struggle, (3) communication and compromise, and (4) mature love.

In the beginning, both teacher and student are generally pleased with the promise and excitement of their new relationship. But gradually, differences arise. The apprentice may be disappointed that her teacher does not seem open to experimentation or willing to give her as much responsibility as she thinks she can handle. The senior midwife may feel that her student lacks humility, expects too much too soon, or has lost interest in basic tasks she did so willingly in the beginning.

These power struggles herald the adolescent phase of the relationship. The apprentice may openly contradict her teacher, and if the midwife responds by limiting privileges, the apprentice may threaten to leave. But if the two can hold to their original commitment while articulating their expectations and needs, the relationship can mature into mutual respect and understanding. Many a former apprentice has phoned me in the early months of practice to say that she finally understood the degree of responsibility I carried and why I was so conservative at times. At this point, teacher and student begin a new relationship as equals.

Unfortunately, many apprenticeships do not survive the adolescent phase and reach maturity. As a mother of teens, I realized that no matter how defiant or insulting they became, I needed to do everything in my power to keep communication channels open. I also learned how important it is to help adolescents find appropriate outlets for their fulminating energies. When your apprentice reaches this stage, inspire her to work harder and come to terms with her limits by giving her responsibilities at the edge of her grasp.

At the same time, you might consider taking a junior apprentice. The senior apprentice can teach the junior what she has learned and so test her wings while still being supervised. The dynamics of this arrangement work quite well: the senior midwife is in charge, with the senior apprentice directing the junior in basic responsibilities and tasks. As the senior apprentice begins doing catches under supervision, the junior can assist, giving the midwife a brief but well-deserved rest.

This break is unfortunately short lived, as the junior apprentice must advance in her training. Once the senior apprentice has fulfilled licensing/certification requirements, you may need to set a graduation date to encourage her to get out on her own. Celebrate when she passes her licensing/certification exam. And once she is in practice, refer a few clients to her to help her get started. Or, if she decides to relocate, recommend her to other midwives in her new locale.

Growing pains are part of the apprenticeship process, but if conflicts become disruptive, create more structure. The National Midwifery Institute, Inc. (of which I am codirector) offers a blueprint to help midwife and apprentice develop realistic timelines for skills and knowledge acquisition, with guidelines for communication and feedback. The NARM Certified Professional Midwife (CPM) process also provides a blueprint for learning. If your apprentice is not enrolled in a program, give her reading and research assignments relevant to the NARM process. Have her write up analyses of particularly difficult cases. Test her by oral or practical examination. Your student must have ample opportunity to demonstrate her learning, and you, a chance to evaluate the effectiveness of your teaching methods.

In the document *Qualifications and Competencies of Midwifery Teachers*, the International Confederation of Midwives (ICM) states that the competencies of midwifery educators include the following:

1. Knowledge of theories of adult learning.

2. The ability to use a variety of competency-based teaching methods to facilitate learning, given the range of human behavior among students.

3. A solid foundation in organizing, implementing, and evaluating the effectiveness of the midwifery curriculum, in keeping with local, country, and regional needs.

And midwifery teachers should do the following:

1. Maintain an up-to-date knowledge base in midwifery theory and practice, and promote evidence-based practice at all times.

2. Understand their own values and biases related to teaching and learning.

3. Provide an environment for values clarification among learners related to working a variety of clients (provision of culturally relevant care).

4. Promote the professional/ethical aspects of midwifery care in keeping with the ICM International Code of Ethics for Midwives.

5. Create a learning environment based on mutual respect and trust.

6. Be guardians of safe, competent, respectful midwifery care. Collaborate with other professionals as members of the health care team.

7. Maintain current clinical practice.

Regarding this list of competencies, every midwifery instructor should be familiar with various learning styles and types of intelligences she may encounter in her students. As author Howard Gardner reveals in his book *Frames of Mind*, we tend to approach learning by employing one or more of seven intelligences:

1. **Verbal/linguistic.** Learning through written and spoken language

2. **Logical/mathematical.** Learning by deductive reason, recognition of abstract patterns

3. **Intrapersonal.** Learning based on self-awareness, metacognition, intuition

4. **Interpersonal.** Learning in relationship to others, based on communication

5. **Musical/rhythmical.** Learning based on sound, tonal patterns, rhythm

6. **Body/kinesthetic.** Body-based knowing and learning through movement

7. **Visual/spatial.** Learning based on sight, and an ability to visualize[2]

With this in mind, present information in a variety of ways. For example, when teaching fetal heart tone patterns that might occur in labor, provide written information, use diagrams to illustrate, sound out various rhythms, and suggest that students tap along to the beat while you do so. Interpersonal learning is facilitated by discussion with other students (in person or online), while intrapersonal learning is prompted by assignments involving self-reflection. To help your apprentice better understand the roles of reason, intuition, and compassion in midwifery work, have her read *Emotional Intelligence*, by Daniel Goleman.[3]

Considering the weighty responsibilities of midwifery practice, instruction should be as student centered as possible. From the beginning, put your apprentice in charge of her learning process. Ask her how she learns best, and whether she needs more or less structure to meet her learning objectives. Continually give her opportunities for self-evaluation. And get her hands-on experience as soon as possible. Remember that she is there to learn, not to practice. Her responsibilities should change continuously so she can achieve proficiency in all areas.

Thoroughly debrief your apprentice after births by asking for her experience of the event: was there anything that occurred that she didn't understand or that she felt should have been handled differently? Challenge her to think as an equal (this may greatly abbreviate the adolescent phase) and take the time to provide both factual information and context for her learning.

As mentioned earlier, the structure of a practice impacts the learning dynamic. There are a variety of possible practice arrangements; here is a sampling, with pros and cons of each:

- *One midwife, one apprentice.* It is undeniably cost saving for a midwife to practice solo, counting on an apprentice for assistance and paying her a nominal sum concomitant to her level of responsibility. But this arrangement is quite stressful in the early stages, especially if the apprentice is inexperienced.

- *One midwife and two apprentices (one senior and one junior).* This has been discussed already as per its value in helping the senior apprentice consolidate her learning by teaching the junior. The downside is that the two may, on occasion, conspire against the midwife. Training two students at once is more work and more responsibility than training just one, even though there is also more opportunity to receive assistance.

- *Two midwives and one apprentice.* This can be a confusing arrangement if the midwives have significant differences in how they work.

Then again, the contrast can be instructive for the apprentice and may keep her from getting stuck in one way of thinking or practicing. A distinct benefit of this setup is that the apprentice is strictly a student: the midwives have the support of one another and need not saddle her with responsibilities she may not be ready to handle. By the same token, they must be careful to see she has ample opportunity to demonstrate her learning and to advance at a reasonable pace.

- *Two midwives and two apprentices.* This arrangement is optimal in several respects: the apprentices not only have opportunity to observe different styles of practice but also to compare notes on their experiences. As there are two of them, they have a stronger voice in the practice. The midwives also benefit from the opportunity to compare notes and double-check their evaluations of their students. The main drawback is the complex interpersonal dynamic inherent in a practice this size. It may be best for each midwife to take primary responsibility for one apprentice.

If you have a solo practice, you might enhance your apprentice's experience by asking another midwife to take her to a few births. This is particularly appropriate if you have a small practice. Once arranged, the three of you should periodically discuss the apprentice's goals and accomplishments, so everyone is on the same page.

Training an apprentice is a lot of work but well worth it. Once you experience the joy of teaching this way, you will probably want to continue. In so doing, you will make an invaluable contribution to the international effort to keep community-based learning alive and growing.

Peer Review

Peer review provides a mechanism for midwives to jointly review their work. In a larger sense, peer review promotes quality assurance by encouraging safe and responsible care. Exposure to the practices of others motivates midwives to continually upgrade their knowledge and skill. They thus become accountable to one another, and ultimately to the profession at large.

Peer review is also known as **chart review** because it features discussion of challenging cases. Besides debriefing less-than-optimal outcomes, cases in progress are also discussed. In the event of a tragic occurrence like neonatal death, emergency peer review may serve to forestall litigation and keep rumors from spreading throughout the community.

All it takes to begin peer review is a group of midwives committed to meeting every six to eight weeks. Three participants minimum, ten maximum, is ideal. Here is a description of how each midwife participates:

- She states the number of normal births attended since the last meeting.

- She reports fully on any births with complications, including her assessment of what might have been done differently.

- She presents all prenatal cases with risk factors, including those referred to another provider.

- She takes feedback from the group.

Since quality assurance is a major goal of peer review, continuing education might occur as follow-up.

Perhaps the greatest benefit of peer review is that it promotes midwifery as an autonomous and self-regulating profession. It is a required part of the CPM process, and many states offering midwifery licensing or certification either require or recommend peer review on an ongoing basis. Peer review has become increasingly popular with physician groups, in response to the malpractice crisis. It is one way to weed out incompetent or irresponsible providers.

Peer review may also help defend a midwife who has been unjustly accused of wrongdoing. My local group once called an emergency meeting to address a case with dissatisfied parents threatening to sue. After a review of written testimony from both sides, we found in favor of the midwife, at the same time making recommendations to help her avoid a similar situation in the future. We made a statement supporting her management of the case, and the parents took no further action. This process is particularly efficacious if dissatisfied clients are talking around town.

On the other hand, lack of consumer participation in peer review is fundamentally at odds with the principles of holistic caregiving. New Zealand midwife Joan Donnely was the first to espouse the merits of involving consumers in virtually every aspect of midwifery's regulation, including annual review of standards, peer review, conflict resolution, and disciplinary proceedings. She claimed this was essential to counteract the historical tendency of professions that self-regulate to become self-serving and elitist.

It takes some courage to participate in peer review at first, especially if you have been isolated in your work. It is normal to fear that no other midwife thinks or does as you do, when in fact most midwives operate from a common base of knowledge and experience. Peer review will improve your practice, your communication with other midwives, and your confidence in your work.

Notes

1. California Code of Regulations Title 22, section 70707. For a brief overview of this code, see "California Patient's Rights Administrative Code 70707," 2005, www.obfocus.com/prenatal/Cborenglish.html (accessed March 6, 2012).

2. Howard Gardner, *Frames of Mind: The Theory of Multiple Intelligences* (New York: Basic Books, 1993).

3. Daniel Goleman, *Emotional Intelligence: Why It Can Matter More Than IQ* (New York: Bantam Books, 1997).

CHAPTER 9

The Long Run

This final chapter focuses on the midwife again, this time in terms of the many adaptations involved in continued practice. No doubt about it, midwifery is a way of life, both grueling and transformative. The intense and unpredictable nature of this work soon persuades the novice that midwifery is much more than the joy of assisting births. It works a woman on all levels, either disintegrating her or bringing her to essence.

In optimal caregiving, the midwife is not the only one making assessments. Before entrusting herself to care, the mother will scrutinize the midwife carefully: her appearance, personality, and character. At the same time, the midwife encourages this by being candid and forthcoming. Thus each prenatal visit provides an opportunity to deepen communication and develop trust. But this does not afford the midwife much privacy and so can be draining at times.

On the other hand, beginning midwives may get so carried away by the thrill of practice that they overwhelm clients with their enthusiasm. This contradicts the model of woman-centered care, based on receptivity and discretion. To be truly of service, the midwife must be sensitive enough to pick up her cues and respond without ego. This brings up the critical difference between making assessments and passing judgment. We can easily pass judgment at the threshold of our limitations, particularly on someone who inadvertently reveals these limitations by leaving our expectations unmet. In contrast, the ability to make assessments has no strings attached and is the key to a sane and enduring practice.

Most beginners fail to realize the extent to which midwifery will affect their personal lives. There may be upheavals in love, especially if the imperative for deep communication is threatening to the midwife's significant other. Men in particular may feel this as pressure to be more than they are. Some partners feel jealous or insecure if their way of making a living seems less principled or dynamic. This may necessitate a candid review of personal and professional goals, both long and short term. It has been said that midwifery is the acid test of a relationship, which is absolutely true.

Conversely, it is important that the midwife acknowledge the demands her work may place on

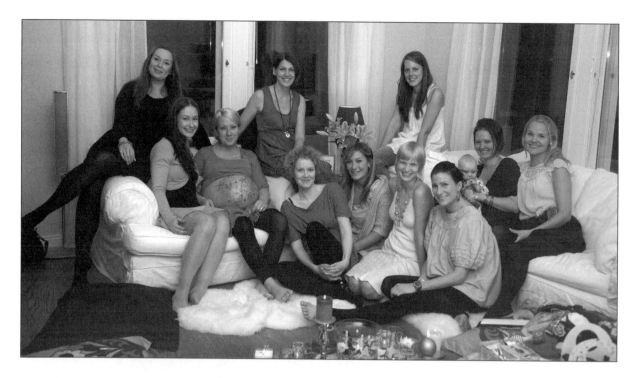

her intimate relationships. Abruptly running off to births can be hard on small children and really rough on a nursing baby. Not to mention the obvious: more than once I have been interrupted by "the call" in the middle of lovemaking. Occasionally, I've thought as I answered my phone, "Don't let this be a heavy one" or even, "I hope no one's in labor." Usually this was because my children or partner needed attention; I had shopping, cleaning, or pressing paperwork to do, or I desperately needed to relax without interruptions. Being on call means keeping one's self, home, and family in a constant state of readiness. Consider getting help with this if necessary. And keep your practice at a workable level: if doing homebirths, this is around four to six births a month, which generally allows time to process and integrate your experiences, catch up on sleep, get the rest of your life back in order, and rejuvenate before going on.

Here are some beliefs about caregiving (provided by Anne Frye) that could negatively impact a midwife's work and health:

- A competent midwife can handle anything.
- A competent midwife always knows what is going on.
- A competent midwife can always trust her judgment.
- A compassionate midwife always acquiesces to the mother's wishes.
- A competent midwife never transports.
- A competent midwife transports at the first hint of a problem.
- A competent midwife never has a mother or baby die under her care.

And here are some healthier possibilities:

- As a midwife, I support each woman to have the most healthy and healing birth experience possible.
- As a midwife, I must remember that what is most healthy and healing is different for every woman and may differ from what might be so for me.

- As a midwife, I need to recognize complications that require care I cannot provide and deal with them appropriately.

- As a midwife, I understand that birth, by its very nature, cannot be completely understood or predicted.

- As a midwife, I need appropriate and healthy professional limitations and boundaries regarding the types of situations I am willing and competent to handle.

- As a midwife, I cannot control whether someone lives or dies. I can control only how I prepare myself to take on the responsibility of being a primary attendant and how I respond to the situation in the moment.[1]

Every midwife must be able to get help when she is floundering. This means learning to take as well as give, humbling herself to wise counsel, being receptive to her intimates, and listening well to the experience of other midwives. In short, she needs to access her recuperative powers. Intrinsic to this is development of her intuition. At first, she may feel somewhat uncomfortable as hunches and precognitions play themselves out in her work and life. But this is part of a long tradition of women's ways of knowing, and it is crucial for handling the challenges of comprehensive and safe care.

Part of the task of nurturing psychic faculties and protecting the delicacy in oneself as these emerge is to take reflective time each day. This can be difficult with young children but easier to manage if incorporated from the beginning. Along these lines, a student of mine recalled that her mother routinely sent her and her sister for naps every day after lunch. They never slept, and she eventually realized her mother knew this and didn't care. But with regular time out, she learned to treasure her privacy while her mother was reading, relaxing, and otherwise taking care of herself.

In the same vein, midwifery practice requires the art of energy conservation. You cannot afford situations where the appropriate course of action is perfectly clear, but you lack the strength to carry it out. Yaqui shaman Don Juan says that for all humans, power is a natural enemy; in midwifery practice, it is power derived from increasing clarity that may lead us beyond our capacity.[2] Overextension, even when the calling is clear, leads to burnout. To avoid this, delegate responsibility to your supporters or associates. Know when to say no, and be aware that this may change daily. Develop the necessary skills (psychological and/or spiritual) to clear others' energies from your system so your personal boundaries are continually reset.

It is interesting to note how lessons inherent in birthing apply to the midwife's practice. The frustration and strain of trying to make labor fit a preconceived pattern is similar to what she may experience if she tries to grow her practice too quickly or keep it at a certain size. And just as there comes a time in second stage when the mother must stop bearing down in order to ease her baby out, the midwife must also know when to ease up and let go. By all means, pass clients on whenever you feel yourself at capacity: the number you can handle will fluctuate according to other obligations in your personal life. Learn to recognize signs of burnout, such as faulty communication, distraction or absent-mindedness, or in progressed cases, hysteria. Without exception, midwives need regular vacations. Anticipate this, and create a support system strong enough to allow for your absence. Working collectively or in a group practice might help you more readily realize this goal.

Speaking of which, midwives often forget to apply their knowledge of health promotion to their own lives. Nutrition should be optimal on clinic days or in the midst of a long labor. Mental deliberations concerning a complicated pregnancy or pending labor may take so much energy that extra sleep is required.

Stress-reduction techniques, such as herbal remedies for relaxation, massage therapy, hot baths, and regular exercise, all have an important place in the midwife's daily life. The bottom line is nourishment: figure out what you need and make sure to get it.

In the same vein, the demands of the work may interfere with personal development. Some midwives feel guilty making time for this, but a certain degree of narcissism is healthy, especially in such a strenuous profession. Pursuing personal passions and interests apart from the work can counterbalance the selflessness it often requires. One of the midwife's most important gifts to her clients is the ability to think creatively, and to keep this alive it must be nourished. Finding pleasure in many things, expanding her horizons on a regular basis, she is not just the changer, but also the changed.

She should also nurture her professional identity by participating in local, state, and national midwifery organizations. Especially if she works in a hostile community, contact with a larger circle of midwives can help her rise above these concerns and recall her original dedication to this work. I still remember my first MANA conference: what a powerful awakening of identity and purpose! These continuing-education opportunities also keep the midwife current on the latest research, which can inspire her to try new approaches in practice.

As you become seasoned in the work, take care not to become jaded. Just when you think you have seen it all, some new configuration sets you back on your heels and teaches you humility once again. Tune up your sensitivities so intuitive directives keep coming through, and be grateful for higher intelligence.

In the end, what is at the heart of our work? What makes the difference in crisis? What keeps us coming back for more? Pure and simple, it is the transformative power of love. No matter where midwifery takes you, do not forget this. Be who you are, and do what you can to keep your love alive.

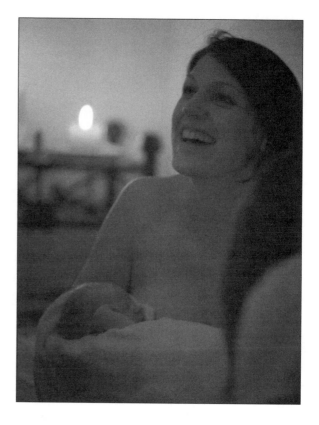

Notes

1. Anne Frye, *Holistic Midwifery*, vol. 2 (Portland, OR, Labrys Press, 2004).
2. Carlos Casteneda, *The Teachings of Don Juan* (New York: Pocket Books, 1968), 82–87.

For Parents: Support Your Local Midwife!

Here are some suggestions for keeping midwifery alive in your community:

1. Because the midwife's fee is usually modest, give her a bonus if you can possibly afford it. Consider the astronomical amount charged by physicians; particularly if your midwife assisted you above and beyond her usual duties, pay her accordingly.

2. If you cannot afford more than the basic fee, perhaps you can help with clerical work or child care. In the past, midwives were fully supported by their communities, all their personal and material needs completely met. Traditionally, midwives have been older women, past childbearing and unburdened with family responsibilities. But today, due to the practice's recent resurgence, this has changed: midwives are coming from the younger generations. This is why help with child care is so important: even if you are only able to volunteer once, it will be greatly appreciated.

3. Understand that in many states, midwives are under fire politically and may need support for legislative efforts. Contact your local or state midwifery association to see how you can help. Perhaps you can send a letter or email to your legislator or the editor of your local newspaper, make a donation, or help organize a public event. Let everyone know how much having a midwife meant to you!

4. Tell your friends all about midwifery and out-of-hospital birth. Refer them to books, videos, or articles. Solicit their questions and inspire them with your passion. Move them to investigate alternatives and make informed decisions. With your help, midwifery will not only survive but also flourish!

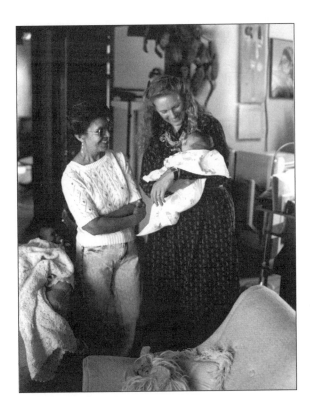

Appendix A

MANA STATEMENT OF VALUES AND ETHICS

Approved by the MANA Board and Membership, August 2010

STATEMENT OF VALUES

The Statement of Values and Ethics of the Midwives Alliance of North America (MANA) is a critical reflection of moral issues as they pertain to maternal and child health. It is intended to provide guidance for professional conduct in the practice of midwifery, as well as influence MANA's organizational policies, thereby promoting high-quality care for childbearing families.

Since what we value infuses and informs our ethical decisions and actions, the Midwives Alliance of North America affirms:

I. **Woman As a Unique Individual:**
   A. We value each woman as a strong, creative, unique individual with life-giving powers.
   B. We value each woman's right to a supportive caregiver appropriate to her needs and respectful of her belief system.
   C. We value a woman's right to access resources in order to achieve health, happiness and personal growth according to her needs, perceptions and goals.
   D. We value a woman as autonomous and competent to make decisions regarding all aspects of her life.
   E. We value the empowerment of a woman during the processes of pregnancy, birth, breastfeeding, mother–infant attachment and parenting.

II. **Mother and Baby as Whole:**
   A. We value the mother and her baby as an inseparable and interdependent whole and acknowledge that each woman and baby have parameters of well-being unique to themselves.
   B. We value the physical, psychosocial and spiritual health, well-being and safety of every mother and baby.
   C. We value the mother as the direct care provider for her unborn child.
   D. We value the process of labor and birth as a rite of passage with mother and baby as equal participants.
   E. We value the sentient and sensitive nature of the newborn and affirm every baby's right to a caring and loving birth without separation from mother and family.
   F. We value breastfeeding as the ideal way to nourish and nurture the newborn.

III. **The Nature of Birth:**
   A. We value the essential mystery of birth.
   B. We value pregnancy and birth as natural, physiologic and holistic processes that technology will never supplant.
   C. We value the integrity of a woman's body, the inherent rhythm of each woman's labor and the right of each mother and baby to be supported in their efforts to achieve a natural, spontaneous vaginal birth.
   D. We value birth as a personal, intimate, internal, sexual and social experience to be shared in the environment and with the attendants a woman chooses.
   E. We value the right of a woman and her partner to determine the most healing course of action when difficult situations arise.
   F. We value the art of letting go and acknowledge death and loss as possible outcomes of pregnancy and birth.

IV. **The Art of Midwifery:**
   A. We value our right to practice the art of midwifery, an ancient vocation of women.
   B. We value multiple routes of midwifery education and the essential importance of apprenticeship training.
   C. We value the wisdom of midwifery, an expertise that incorporates theoretical and embodied knowledge, clinical skills, deep listening, intuitive judgment, spiritual awareness and personal experience.
   D. We value the art of nurturing the inherent normalcy of pregnancy and birth as expressions of wellness in a healthy woman.
   E. We value continuity of care throughout the childbearing year.
   F. We value birth with a midwife in any setting that a woman chooses.
   G. We value homebirth with a midwife as a wise and safe choice for healthy families.
   H. We value caring for a woman to the best of our ability without prejudice with regards to age, race, ethnicity, religion, education, culture, sexual orientation, gender identification, physical abilities or socioeconomic background.
   I. We value the art of empowering women, supporting each to birth unhindered and confident in her natural abilities.
   J. We value the acquisition and use of skills that identify and guide a complicated pregnancy or birth to move toward greater well-being and be brought to the most healing conclusion possible.
   K. We value standing up for what we believe in the face of social pressure and political oppression.

V. **Woman as Mother:**
   A. We value a mother's intuitive knowledge and innate ability to nurture herself, her unborn baby and her newborn baby.
   B. We value the power and beauty of a woman's body as it grows in pregnancy and a woman's strength in labor and birth.
   C. We value pregnancy and birth as processes that have lifelong impact on a woman's self-esteem, her health, her ability to nurture and her personal growth.
   D. We value the capacity of partners, family and community to support a woman in all aspects of pregnancy, birth and mothering and to provide a safe environment for mother and baby.

VI. The Nature of Relationship:

A. We value an egalitarian relationship between a woman and her midwife.

B. We value the quality, integrity and uniqueness of our interactions, which inform our choices and decisions.

C. We value mutual trust, honesty and respect.

D. We value a woman's right to privacy, and we honor the confidentiality of all personal interactions and health records.

E. We value direct access to information that is readily understood by all.

F. We value personal responsibility and the right of a woman to make decisions regarding what she deems best for herself, her baby and her family, using both informed consent and informed refusal.

G. We value our relationship to a process that is larger than ourselves, recognizing that birth is something we can seek to learn from and to know, but cannot control.

H. We value humility and the recognition of our own limitations.

I. We value sharing information and understanding about birth experiences, skills and knowledge.

J. We value a supportive midwifery community as an essential place of learning.

K. We value diversity among midwives that broadens our collective resources and challenges us to work toward greater understanding.

L. We value collaboration between a midwife and other health-care practitioners as essential to providing a family with resources to make responsible and informed choices.

M. We value the right and responsibility of both a midwife and a woman to discontinue care when insurmountable obstacles develop that compromise communication, mutual trust or joint decision-making.

N. We value the responsibility of a midwife to consult with other health-care practitioners when appropriate and refer or transfer care when necessary.

VII. Cultural Sensitivity, Competency and Humility

A. We value cultural sensitivity, competency and humility as critical skills for the midwife to master in an increasingly multicultural society.

B. We value cultural sensitivity—a midwife's awareness of and ability to honor differences between people and the cultural values of the women she serves.

C. We value the importance of cultural competency in addressing the social and economic barriers to access to care for vulnerable, underserved and marginalized women, thereby improving maternal and infant health and the well-being of families.

D. We value cultural humility as a lifelong process of self-reflection and self-critique in order to develop a respectful partnership with each woman.*

*Section VII is derived from Melanie Tervalon and Jann Murray-Garcia, "Cultural Humility versus Cultural Competency: A Critical Distinction in Defining Physician Training Outcomes in Multicultural Education," *Journal of Health Care for the Poor and Underserved* 9 (May 1998): 117–25.

STATEMENT OF ETHICS

Our values inform and inspire midwifery practice in our hearts and minds. Acting ethically is an expression of our values within the context of our individual, geographic, religious, cultural, ethnic, political, educational and personal backgrounds and in our relationships with others. As we seek to respond in the moment to each situation we face, we call upon ethical principles of human interaction as follows:

- Beneficence—to act so as to benefit others
- Nonmaleficence—to avoid causing harm
- Confidentiality—to honor others' privacy and keep personal interactions confidential
- Justice—to treat people respectfully and equitably
- Autonomy—to respect an individual's rights to self-determination and freedom to make decisions that affect his or her life

The equality and mutuality of the relationship between midwife and client create a foundation uniquely suited to integrate these principles. As midwives, we seek to benefit women and babies in our care. Mutual trust and respect are critical to the success of a relationship that requires joint decision-making at every level. Moral integrity, truthfulness and adequate information enable all participants to judge together the best course of action in varied situations.

Judgments are fundamentally based on awareness and understanding of ourselves and others. They grow out of our own sense of moral integrity, which is born within the heart of each individual. Becoming self-aware and increasing understanding are ongoing processes that must be nurtured as a function of personal and professional growth. MANA's affirmation of individual moral integrity and recognition of the complexity of life events bring us to an understanding that there cannot possibly be one right answer for all situations. Since the outcome of pregnancy is ultimately unknown and is always unknowable, it is inevitable that in certain circumstances our best decisions in the moment will lead to consequences we could not foresee.

We recognize the limitations of traditional codes of ethics that present a list of rules to be followed. Therefore, a midwife must develop a moral compass to guide practice in diverse situations that arise from the uniqueness of pregnancy and birth as well as the relationship between midwives and birthing women. This approach affirms the mystery and potential for transformation present in every experience and fosters truly diverse practice. Midwifery care is woman-led care with informed choice and a clear set of values at its core. Decision making is a shared responsibility with the goals of healthy women and babies and of gentle, empowering births with a focus on individual and family needs and concerns. Ultimately, it is at the heart of midwifery practice to honor and respect the decisions women make about their pregnancies and births based on their knowledge and belief about what is best for themselves and their babies.

There are both individual and social implications to any decision-making process. Our decisions may be impacted by the oppressive rules and practices of a society that is often hostile to homebirth, midwives and midwifery clients. Our actual choices may be limited by the medical, legal, political, economic, cultural or social climate in which we function. The more our values conflict with those of the dominant culture, the greater the threat to the integrity of our own values, and the greater the risk that our actions may lead to professional repercussions or legal reprisal. In such conditions we may be unable to make peace with any course of action or may feel conflicted about a choice already made. The community of women, both midwives and those we serve, may provide a fruitful resource for continued moral support and guidance.

In summary, acting ethically requires us to define our values, respond to the communities of families, midwives and cultures in which we find ourselves, act in accord with our values to the best of our ability as the situation demands, and engage in ongoing self-examination, evaluation, peer review and professional growth. By carefully describing the multifaceted aspects of what we value and defining the elements of moral integrity and decision making, we have created a framework for ethical behavior in midwifery practice. We welcome an open and ongoing articulation of values and ethics and the evolution of this document.

MANA CORE COMPETENCIES FOR MIDWIFERY PRACTICE

Approved by the MANA Board, August 2011

I. General Knowledge and Skills

The midwife's knowledge and skills include but are not limited to:

- A. communication, counseling and education before pregnancy and during the childbearing year;
- B. human anatomy and physiology, especially as relevant to childbearing;
- C. human sexuality;
- D. various therapeutic health care modalities for treating body, mind and spirit;
- E. community health care, wellness and social service resources;
- F. nutritional needs of the mother and baby during the childbearing year;
- G. diversity awareness and competency as it relates to childbearing.

The midwife maintains professional standards of practice including but not limited to:

- A. principles of informed consent and refusal and shared decision making;
- B. critical evaluation of evidence-based research findings and application to best practices;
- C. documentation of care throughout the childbearing cycle;
- D. ethical considerations relevant to reproductive health;
- E. cultural sensitivity and competency;
- F. use of common medical terms;
- G. implementation of individualized plans for woman-centered midwifery care that support the relationship between the mother, the baby and their larger support community;
- H. judicious use of technology;
- I. self-assessment and acknowledgement of personal and professional limitations.

II. Care During Pregnancy

The midwife provides care, support and information to women throughout pregnancy and determines the need for consultation, referral or transfer of care as appropriate. The midwife has knowledge and skills to provide care that include but are not limited to:

- A. identification, evaluation and support of mother and baby well-being throughout the process of pregnancy;
- B. education and counseling during the childbearing cycle;
- C. identification of pre-existing conditions and preventive or supportive measures to enhance client well-being during pregnancy;
- D. nutritional requirements of pregnant women and methods of nutritional assessment and counseling;
- E. emotional, psychosocial and sexual variations that may occur during pregnancy;
- F. environmental and occupational hazards for pregnant women;
- G. methods of diagnosing pregnancy;
- H. the growth and development of the unborn baby;
- I. genetic factors that may indicate the need for counseling, testing or referral;

J. indications for and risks and benefits of biotechnical screening methods and diagnostic tests used during pregnancy;

K. anatomy, physiology and evaluation of the soft and bony structures of the pelvis;

L. palpation skills for evaluation of the baby and the uterus;

M. the causes, assessment and treatment of the common discomforts of pregnancy;

N. identification, implications and appropriate treatment of various infections, disease conditions and other problems that may affect pregnancy;

O. management and care of the Rh-negative woman;

P. counseling to the woman and her family to plan for a safe, appropriate place for birth.

III. Care During Labor, Birth and Immediately Thereafter

The midwife provides care, support and information to women throughout labor, birth and the hours immediately thereafter. The midwife determines the need for consultation, referral or transfer of care as appropriate. The midwife has knowledge and skills to provide care that include but are not limited to:

A. the processes of labor and birth;

B. parameters and methods, including relevant health history, for evaluating the well-being of mother and baby during labor, birth and immediately thereafter;

C. assessment of the birthing environment to assure that it is clean, safe and supportive and that appropriate equipment and supplies are on hand;

D. maternal emotional responses and their impact during labor, birth and immediately thereafter;

E. comfort and support measures during labor, birth and immediately thereafter;

F. fetal and maternal anatomy and their interrelationship as relevant to assessing the baby's position and the progress of labor;

G. techniques to assist and support the spontaneous vaginal birth of the baby and placenta;

H. fluid and nutritional requirements during labor, birth and immediately thereafter;

I. maternal rest and sleep as appropriate during the process of labor, birth and immediately thereafter;

J. treatment for variations that can occur during the course of labor, birth and immediately thereafter, including prevention and treatment of maternal hemorrhage;

K. emergency measures and transport for critical problems arising during labor, birth or immediately thereafter;

L. appropriate support for the newborn's natural physiologic transition during the first minutes and hours following birth, including practices to enhance mother–baby attachment and family bonding;

M. current biotechnical interventions and technologies that may be commonly used in a medical setting;

N. care and repair of the perineum and surrounding tissues;

O. third-stage management, including assessment of the placenta, membranes and umbilical cord;

P. breastfeeding and lactation;

Q. identification of pre-existing conditions and implementation of preventive or supportive measures to enhance client well-being during labor, birth, the immediate postpartum and breastfeeding.

IV. Postpartum Care

The midwife provides care, support and information to women throughout the postpartum period and determines the need for consultation, referral or transfer of care as appropriate. The midwife has knowledge and skills to provide care that include but are not limited to:

    A. anatomy and physiology of the mother;

    B. lactation support and appropriate breast care including treatments for problems with nursing;

    C. support of maternal well-being and mother–baby attachment;

    D. treatment for maternal discomforts;

    E. emotional, psychosocial, mental and sexual variations;

    F. maternal nutritional needs during the postpartum period and lactation;

    G. current treatments for problems such as postpartum depression and mental illness;

    H. grief counseling and support when necessary;

    I. family-planning methods, as the individual woman desires.

V. Newborn Care

The midwife provides care to the newborn during the postpartum period, as well as support and information to parents regarding newborn care and informed decision making, and determines the need for consultation, referral or transfer of care as appropriate. The midwife's assessment, care and shared information include but are not limited to:

    A. anatomy, physiology and support of the newborn's adjustment during the first days and weeks of life;

    B. newborn wellness, including relevant historical data and gestational age;

    C. nutritional needs of the newborn;

    D. benefits of breastfeeding and lactation support;

    E. laws and regulations regarding prophylactic biotechnical treatments and screening tests commonly used during the neonatal period;

    F. neonatal problems and abnormalities, including referral as appropriate;

    G. newborn growth, development, behavior, nutrition, feeding and care;

    H. immunizations, circumcision and safety needs of the newborn.

VI. Women's Health Care and Family Planning

The midwife provides care, support and information to women regarding their reproductive health and determines the need for consultation or referral by using a foundation of knowledge and skills that include but are not limited to:

    A. reproductive health care across the lifespan;

    B. evaluation of the woman's well-being, including relevant health history;

    C. anatomy and physiology of the female reproductive system and breasts;

    D. family planning and methods of contraception;

    E. decision making regarding timing of pregnancies and resources for counseling and referral;

    F. preconception and interconceptual care;

    G. well-woman gynecology as authorized by jurisdictional regulations.

VII. Professional, Legal and Other Aspects of Midwifery Care

The midwife assumes responsibility for practicing in accordance with the principles and competencies outlined in this document. The midwife uses a foundation of theoretical knowledge, clinical assessment, critical-thinking skills and shared decision making that are based on:

A. MANA's Essential Documents concerning the art and practice of midwifery,

B. the purpose and goals of MANA and local (state or provincial) midwifery associations,

C. principles and practice of data collection as relevant to midwifery practice,

D. ongoing education,

E. critical review of evidence-based research findings in midwifery practice and application as appropriate,

F. jurisdictional laws and regulations governing the practice of midwifery,

G. basic knowledge of community maternal and child health care delivery systems,

H. skills in entrepreneurship and midwifery business management.

MANA STANDARDS AND QUALIFICATIONS FOR THE ART AND PRACTICE OF MIDWIFERY

Revised & Approved October 2005

The midwife practices in accord with the *MANA Standards and Qualifications for the Art and Practice of Midwifery* and the *MANA Statement of Values and Ethics*, and demonstrates the clinical skills and judgments described in the *MANA Core Competencies for Midwifery Practice*.

1. **Skills:** Necessary skills of a practicing midwife include the ability to:
   - Provide continuity of care to the woman and her newborn during the maternity cycle. Care may continue throughout the woman's entire life cycle. The midwife recognizes that childbearing is a woman's experience and encourages the active involvement of her self-defined family system.
   - Identify, assess and provide care during the antepartal, intrapartal, postpartal and newborn periods. She may also provide well woman and newborn care.
   - Maintain proficiency in life-saving measures by regular review and practice
   - Deal with emergency situations appropriately
   - Use judgment, skill and intuition in competent assessment and response.

2. **Appropriate equipment and treatment:** Midwives carry and maintain equipment to assess and provide care for the well-woman, the mother, the fetus, and the newborn; to maintain clean and/or aseptic technique; and to treat conditions including, but not limited to, hemorrhage, lacerations, and cardio-respiratory distress. This may include the use of non-pharmaceutical agents, pharmaceutical agents, and equipment for suturing and intravenous therapy.

3. **Records:** Midwives keep accurate records of care for each woman and newborn in their practice. Records shall reflect current standards in midwifery charting, and shall be held confidential (except as legally required). Records shall be provided to the woman on request. The midwife maintains confidentiality in all verbal and written communications regarding women in her care.

4. **Data Collection:** It is highly recommended that midwives collect data for their practice on a regular basis and that this be done prospectively, following the protocol developed by the MANA Division of Research. Data collected by the midwife shall be used to inform and improve her practice.

5. **Compliance:** Midwives will inform and assist parents regarding public health requirements of the jurisdiction in which the midwifery service is provided.

6. **Medical Consultation, Collaboration, and Referral:** All midwives recognize that there are certain conditions for which medical consultations are advisable. The midwife shall make a reasonable attempt to assure that her client has access to consultation, collaboration, and/or referral to a medical care system when indicated.

7. **Screening:** Midwives respect the woman's right to self-determination. Midwives assess and inform each woman regarding her health and wellbeing relevant to the appropriateness of midwifery services. It is the right and responsibility of the midwife to refuse or discontinue services in certain circumstances. Appropriate referrals are made in the interest of the mother or baby's wellbeing or when the required or requested care is outside the midwife's personal scope of practice as described in her practice guidelines.

8. **Informed Choice:** Each midwife will present accurate information about herself and her services, including but not limited to:
   - her education in midwifery
   - her experience level in midwifery
   - her practice guidelines
   - her financial charges for services
   - the services she does and does not provide
   - her expectations of the pregnant woman and the woman's self-defined family system.

     The midwife recognizes that the woman is the primary decision maker in all matters regarding her own health care and that of her infant.

     The midwife respects the woman's right to decline treatments or procedures, and properly documents these choices. The midwife clearly states and documents when a woman's choices fall outside the midwife's practice guidelines.

9. **Continuing Education:** Midwives will update their knowledge and skills on a regular basis.

10. **Peer Review:** Midwifery practice includes an on-going process of case review with peers.

11. **Practice Guidelines:** Each midwife will develop practice guidelines for her services that are in agreement with the *MANA Standards and Qualifications for the Art and Practice of Midwifery*, the *MANA Statement of Values and Ethics*, and the *MANA Core Competencies for Midwifery Practice*, in keeping with her level of expertise.

12. **Expanded scope of practice:** The midwife may expand her scope of practice beyond the MANA Core Competencies to incorporate new procedures that improve care for women and babies consistent with the midwifery model of care. Her practice must reflect knowledge of the new procedure, including risks, benefits, screening criteria, and identification and management of potential complications.

The following sources were utilized for reference: Essential documents of the National Association of Certified Professional Midwives 2004, American College of Nurse-Midwives documents and standards for the Practice of Midwifery revised March 2003; ICM membership and joint study on maternity; FIGO, WHO, etc. revised 1972; New Mexico regulations for the practice of lay midwifery, revised 1982; North West Coalition of Midwives Standards for Safety and Competency in Midwifery; Varney, Helen, *Nurse-Midwifery*, Blackwell Scientific Pub., Boston, MA 1980.

Appendix B

RESOURCES

Alliance for Transforming the Lives of Children
901 Preston Avenue, Suite 400
Charlottesville, VA 22903-4491
www.atlc.org

American Association of Birth Centers (AABC)
3123 Gottschall Road
Perkiomenville, PA 18074
(866) 542-4784
www.birthcenters.org

American College of Nurse-Midwives (ACNM)
8403 Colesville Road, Suite 1550
Silver Spring, MD 20910
(240) 485-1800
www.acnm.org

Association for Pre- and Perinatal Psychology
and Health
PO Box 1398
Forestville, CA 95436
(707) 887-2838
www.birthpsychology.com

Association of Radical Midwives (ARM)
62 Greetby Hill
Ormskirk, Lancashire, L39 2DT
United Kingdom
www.midwifery.org.uk

Baby, Birth and Beyond (supplies)
1076 W. Hayden
Hayden, ID 83825
(888) 683-2678
www.babybirthandbeyond.com

The Big Push for Midwives (consumer arm for CPMs)
www.pushformidwives.org

The Birth Facts
www.thebirthfacts.com

Birthing From Within
PO Box 60259
Santa Barbara, CA 93160
(805) 964-6611
www.birthingfromwithin.com

Birth with Love Midwifery Supplies
Ollie Anne Hamilton
513 27th Street N.
Great Falls, MT 59401
(800) 434-4915
www.birthwithlove.com

Birth Works International
PO Box 2045
Medford, NJ 08055
(888) 862-4784
www.birthworks.com

BOLD
A Global Movement to Make Maternity Care
Mother-Friendly
PO Box 42292
Washington, DC 20015
www.boldaction.org

The Bradley Method
PO Box 5224
Sherman Oaks, CA 91413-5224
(818) 788-6662; (800) 4-A-BIRTH
www.bradleybirth.com

Calm Birth
233 5th Street, Suite B
Ashland, OR 97520
www.calmbirth.org

Canadian Association of Midwives
59 Riverview
Montréal, Québec H8R 3R9
Canada
(514) 807-3668
www.canadianmidwives.org

Cascade Health Care Products, Inc.
1826 NW 18th Avenue
Portland, OR 97209
(503) 595-1720; (800) 443-9942
www.1cascade.com

Childbirth Connection
260 Madison Avenue, 8th Floor
New York, NY 10016
(212) 777-5000
www.childbirthconnection.org

Childbirth Graphics (supplies)
5045 Franklin Avenue
Waco, TX 76710
(800) 299-3366 ext. 287
www.childbirthgraphics.com

Citizens for Midwifery (CFM)
PO Box 82227
Athens, GA 30608-2227
(888) 236-4880
www.cfmidwifery.org

Coalition for Improving Maternity Services (CIMS)
1500 Sunday Drive, Suite 102
Raleigh, NC 27607
(866) 424-3635
www.motherfriendly.org

The Compleat Mother (magazine)
PO Box 209
Minot, ND 58702
(701) 852-2822
www.compleatmother.com

DONA International
1582 S. Parker Road, Suite 201
Denver, CO 80231
(888) 788-DONA
www.dona.org

Doula World
Ori Eisen
6214 E. Hillery Drive
Scottsdale, AZ 85254-2568
www.doulaworld.com

Everything Birth (supplies)
PO Box 66781
Falmouth, ME 04105
(800) 370-1683
www.midwifesupplies.com

The Foundation for the Advancement of Midwifery
PO Box 320667
Boston, MA 02132
www.formidwifery.org

Future Midwives Alliance
www.futuremidwives.blogspot.com

Gentlebirth.org (research)
Ronnie Falcao, LM, MS, CPM
www.gentlebirth.org

HypnoBirthing Institute
PO Box 810
Epsom, NH 03234
(603) 798-4781; (603) 798-3286
www.hypnobirthing.com

In His Hands Birth Supplies
PO Box 467
Liberty Hill, TX 78642
(800) 247-4045
www.homebirthsupplies.com

International Association of Infant Massage (IAIM)
PO Box 6370
Ventura, CA 93006
(805) 644-8524
www.iaim-us.com

International Birth and Wellness Project
12 Batchelder Street, Suite 2
Boston, MA 02125-2653
(887) 334-4297
www.alace.org

International Center for Traditional Childbearing
(ICTC)
PO Box 11923
Portland, OR 97211
(503) 460-9324
www.ictcmidwives.org

International Cesarean Awareness Network, Inc.
(ICAN)
PO Box 98
Savage, MN 55378
(800) 686-ICAN
www.ican-online.org

International Childbirth Educators Association (ICEA)
PO Box 20048
Minneapolis, MN 55420
(952) 854-8660
www.icea.org

International Confederation of Midwives (ICM)
Laan van Meerdervoort 70
2517 AN The Hague
The Netherlands
www.internationalmidwives.org

International MotherBaby Childbirth Organization
(IMBCO)
PO Box 2346
Ponte Vedra Beach, FL 32004
rae@imbci.org
Skype: raedavies (Ponte Vedra Beach, FL)
(904) 285-0028
www.imbci.org

La Leche League International (LLLI)
PO Box 4079
Schaumburg, IL 60168-4079
(847) 519-7730
www.lalecheleague.org

Lamaze International
2025 M Street NW, Suite 800
Washington, DC 20036-3309
(202) 367-1128; (800) 368-4404
www.lamaze.org

MIDIRS (Midwives Information and Resource Service)
9 Elmdale Road
Clifton, Bristol BS8 1SL
United Kingdom
www.midirs.org

Midwifery Education Accreditation Council (MEAC)
PO Box 984
La Conner, WA 98257
(360) 466-2080
www.meacschools.org

Midwifery Today, Inc.
PO Box 2672
Eugene, OR 97402-0223
(800) 743-0974
www.midwiferytoday.com

Midwives Alliance of North America (MANA)
611 Pennsylvania Avenue SE, #1700
Washington, DC 20003-4303
(888) 923-MANA (6262)
www.mana.org

Midwives Model of Care
www.midwivesmodelofcare.org

MoonDragon Birthing
Salem, MA 01970
(978) 744-5583
www.moondragon.org

Mothering (magazine)
PO Box 1690
Santa Fe, NM 87504
(505) 983-8040
www.mothering.com

Mothers Naturally (consumer group through MANA)
www.mothersnaturally.org

National Organization of Circumcision Information
Resource Centers (NOCIRC)
PO Box 2512
San Anselmo, CA 94979
(415) 488-9883
www.nocirc.org

National Organization of Mothers of Twins Club, Inc.
(NOMOTC)
2000 Mallory Lane, Suite 130-600
Franklin, TN 37067-8231
(248) 231-4480
www.nomotc.org

North American Registry of Midwives (NARM)
Applications
Sharon Wells
PO Box 420
Summertown, TN 38483
(888) 426-1280
www.narm.org

Perinatal Education Associates, Inc. (supplies)
8235 Old Troy Pike, Suite 280
Dayton, OH 45424
(866) 88-BIRTH
www.birthsource.com

Postpartum Support International
6706 SW 54th Avenue
Portland, OR 97219
Office: (503) 894-9453
Support Helpline: (800) 944-4773
www.postpartum.net

The Safe Motherhood Quilt Project
149 Apple Orchard Lane
Summertown, TN 38483
InaMayGaskin@gmail.com
www.rememberthemothers.org

SLC Birth Supplies
PO Box 1225
Oakhurst, CA 93644
(888) 683-2678
www.birthsupplies.com

Squat Birth Journal
squattingbirth@gmail.com
www.squatbirthjournal.blogspot.com

United States Breastfeeding Committee (USBC)
2025 M Street NW, Suite 800
Washington, DC 20036-3309
(202) 367-1132
www.usbreastfeeding.org

Waterbirth International
PO Box 5578
Lighthouse Point, FL 33074
(954) 821-9125
www.waterbirth.org

World Alliance for Breastfeeding Action (WABA)
PO Box 1200
10850 Penang
Malaysia
+011-60-604-6584816
www.waba.org.my

World Health Organization (WHO)
Avenue Appia 20
1211 Geneva 27
Switzerland
www.who.int/topics/midwifery

Your Water Birth.com (water birth supplies)
Better Choices LLC
110 W. 6th Avenue, #191
Ellensburg, WA 98926
(509) 962-8630
www.yourwaterbirth.com

MEDICAL/HEALTH HISTORY

Please fill out this medical and personal history very carefully. When you come for your next visit, we will go over the history together and discuss any questions that you might have. Just leave blank any technical terms or questions with which you are not familiar.

Personal Information

Name _____ Date_____

Maiden name (or any name that might have been used on previous medical records) _____

Address _____ Phone_____

Email address _____

Date of birth _____ Height _____ Usual weight_____

Occupation _____

Partner's name (if applicable) _____

If partnered, how long have you been together? Are you married? _____

Partner's address and phone _____

Emergency contact person and relation _____ Phone _____

Who referred you to me? _____

Insurance (or do you need assistance with information on insurance?) _____

Pediatrician _____

Do you have any drug allergies or sensitivities? _____

Menstrual History

When do you think you may have conceived? _____

Are your cycles regular? _____

Do you have pain with menstruation? _____

LMP—last menstrual period _____

   ◯ Yes ◯ No   Was it normal in length and heaviness of flow?

   ◯ Yes ◯ No   Did you have a pregnancy test?

   ◯ Yes ◯ No   Was this a planned pregnancy?

PMP—previous menstrual period _____

Were you using birth control when you conceived?

   ◯ Yes ◯ No   What kind? _____

Any complications after abortion or miscarriage?

   ◯ Pain ◯ Infection ◯ Incomplete ◯ Emotional distress ◯ Excessive bleeding

If Rh−, did you receive RhoGAM? ◯ Yes ◯ No

Obstetrical History

Total pregnancies: _____

Full term: _____

Premature: _____

Abortion: _____

Ectopic: _____

Miscarriage: _____

Twins: _____

Living children: _____

Cesarean section: _____

VBAC: _____

Please list information about your previous births:

Date Mo./Yr.	# of Weeks	Length of Labor	Sex M/F	Place of Birth	Comments/Complications	Breastfed

Medical History

Please check if you have had any of the following conditions. In the space below, record date, treatment, and any follow-up you received. Also feel free to list any other important conditions or concerns.

○ Kidney disease
○ Diabetes
○ Hypertension
○ Epilepsy
○ Heart disease
○ Thyroid problems
○ Blood-clotting problems
○ Asthma
○ Hepatitis
○ Liver problems

○ Tuberculosis
○ Cancer
○ Autoimmune disorder (Lupus, MS, HIV/AIDS)
○ Fibromyalgia
○ Pelvic/back injuries
○ Stomach problems
○ Bowel problems
○ Skin problems
○ Bladder infection

○ Anemia
○ Hospitalizations
○ Seizures
○ Surgeries
○ Hemorrhage
○ Allergies (including to food)
○ Severe headaches
○ Dental problems
○ Phlebitis/varicosities
○ Hemorrhoids

_____
_____
_____
_____

Is there any hereditary disease or condition in your family such as diabetes, cancer, heart defect, heart disease, hypertension? (List and indicate which relative has the disease or condition.) _____

_____
_____
_____

○ Yes   ○ No   Have you ever had a blood transfusion? Year _____ Location (country) _____

○ Yes   ○ No   Have you, the father, or biological donor of your baby ever had a baby with a birth defect or mental retardation?

○ Yes   ○ No   Do you, the father, or biological donor of your baby have any family members with birth defects or conditions diagnosed as genetic or inherited?

○ Yes   ○ No   Are you, the father, or biological donor of your baby, related by blood (e.g., cousins)?

Certain genetic problems may occur in the following ethnic/racial groups. Are you, the father, or biological donor of your baby:

○ Creole or French Canadian   ○ Jewish   ○ Black/African   ○ Asian   ○ Northern European   ○ Mediterranean

How many times was your mother pregnant? _____

How many children did she have? _____

Did she have any miscarriages? _____

How long were her labors? _____

Were there any complications in her pregnancies? _____

_____

How much did you weigh at birth? _____

What did your mother tell you about your birth? _____

_____

What did she say about birth in general? _____

_____

What have girlfriends or female relatives told you about birth? _____

_____

_____

Gynecological and Contraceptive History

When and where was your last Pap smear? _____

Have your last three Pap smears been normal? _____

If you ever had an abnormal Pap, give date and describe how it was resolved. _____

_____

Do you do self-exam of your breasts, and if so, how often? _____

Please check if you've ever had any of the following:

○ Yeast infection
○ Bacterial vaginosis
○ Syphilis
○ Genital herpes
○ Cervicitis
○ Ovarian cyst
○ Abnormal bleeding
○ Breast surgery
○ Trichomonas
○ Chlamydia
○ PID

○ Oral herpes
○ LEEP
○ Cervical cauterization or cryosurgery
○ Cone biopsy
○ Cerclage
○ Fibroids
○ Uterine surgery
○ Urinary tract surgery
○ Infertility
○ Gardnerella

○ Gonorrhea
○ Vaginal surgery
○ Genital sores
○ Condyloma (warts)
○ HPV (human papilloma virus)
○ Cervical polyp
○ Endometriosis
○ Breast lumps
○ Other reproductive problems/conditions

○ Yes   ○ No   Have you ever used birth control? If so, what kind? Problems or complications? _____

_____

Current Pregnancy

What prenatal care have you had up to the present? List all care providers, clinics, and hospitals where you have had care and also list what was done, especially any lab work, special testing, or ultrasounds. **We will need copies of all your records, so please have them sent ASAP!** _____

_____

_____

Please check if you've had any of the following problems **during this pregnancy**, and explain below:

- ○ Nausea
- ○ Headache
- ○ Leg cramps
- ○ Swelling
- ○ Urinary problems
- ○ Vaginal discharge
- ○ Indigestion
- ○ Vomiting
- ○ Dizziness

- ○ Fever
- ○ Rash
- ○ Bleeding gums
- ○ Constipation
- ○ Hemorrhoids
- ○ Abdominal/pelvic pain
- ○ Vaginal bleeding/spotting
- ○ Varicose veins
- ○ Backache

- ○ Diarrhea
- ○ Family problems
- ○ Loneliness
- ○ Relationship problems
- ○ Depression
- ○ Insomnia
- ○ Work problems

_____
_____
_____
_____

Have you used or been exposed to any of the following in this pregnancy?

- ○ Tobacco
- ○ Caffeine
- ○ Alcohol
- ○ Viruses
- ○ Measles
- ○ Cats

- ○ Vaccinations (please list below)
- ○ Ultrasound
- ○ X-rays
- ○ Herbs
- ○ Vitamins (please list below)
- ○ Nonprescription drugs (please list below)

- ○ Prescription drugs (please list below)
- ○ Fumes/sprays (please list below)
- ○ Other environmental hazards (please list below)

_____
_____
_____
_____

○ Yes   ○ No   Do you have any questions regarding exposures to substances not listed above? _____

What do you do for work and for how many hours per week? Are you sedentary or active on the job? _____

What does your partner (if applicable) do for work and for how many hours per week? _____

How would you describe your usual diet? _____

What do you do for exercise? _____
Do you feel you get enough rest? How many hours of sleep per night? _____

How do you feel about this pregnancy? _____
_____
_____

How does your partner (if applicable) feel about this pregnancy? _____
_____

○ Yes   ○ No   If you have noticed changes in your sexual relationship since becoming pregnant, would you like
                  an opportunity to discuss this ? _____

Do you plan to breastfeed this baby? If so, for how long do you think you'll nurse? _____
_____

Are there any particular ethnic, cultural, or religious preferences for your care that you'd like to discuss? _____
_____
_____

Do you feel you have adequate resources, that is, food, shelter, and money, for this pregnancy? _____
_____
_____

Do you have a car seat for the baby? _____

Please list the people you plan to invite to your birth. _____
_____

Have you faced any opposition to your plans for homebirth? _____
_____

What factors, if any, cause stress in your life, and how do you cope? _____
_____
_____

How do you cope with pain? _____
_____

What do you like to do to relax? _____
_____

Please give some thought to the following questions and write your ideas. If you and your partner are together, each
of you must answer. Read all questions before answering.

Why do you want to have this baby at home? _____
_____
_____
_____
_____

Partner: _____
_____
_____
_____
_____

What do you see as the duties or responsibilities of your midwife? _____
_____
_____
_____
_____

Partner: _____
_____
_____
_____

There are some things that can go wrong without prior warning during labor, birth, and postpartum. Some of these complications will probably never be eradicated no matter what our state of technology. There are certain risks involved in having your baby in a hospital as well as at home. If you are healthy, the chances of unpredictable complications are low. However, if such complications occur, you or your baby might be at greater risk because of being at home. If you opt for the risks involved in birthing at home, you need to find out what they are and how they can be dealt with. Please comment on what you know about risks and complications and how you feel about them: _____
_____
_____
_____
_____
_____

Partner: _____
_____
_____
_____
_____

How do you feel about going to the hospital to deliver if your midwife feels that complications are arising? _____
_____
_____
_____
_____

Partner: _____
_____
_____
_____
_____

How do you think you might deal with the problem of a baby or mother who suffered permanent injury or died at home? _____
_____
_____
_____
_____

Partner: _____
_____
_____
_____
_____

What do you think are the benefits of having your baby at home? _____
_____
_____
_____
_____

Partner: _____
_____
_____
_____
_____

Please add any comments or thoughts that you think might be important for your midwife to know about you: ____
_____
_____
_____
_____

MOTHER'S CONFIDENTIAL WORKSHEET

Thank you for taking the time to fill out this worksheet. *It will not become part of your chart: I will return it to you after review.* I realize that completing it may bring up unpleasant memories, and for that, I apologize. It is my hope that your pregnancy, birth, and postpartum will be as joyous and fulfilling as possible, and sometimes, unresolved traumas can interfere with this.

We will discuss these issues only as much as is comfortable for you. If you want more help than I can provide, I am happy to recommend compassionate practitioners who specialize in working with pregnant women.

Please answer these questions as honestly as possible:

○ Yes   ○ No   Do you suffer from recurrent anxiety or depression?

What have you done to address this? _____

_____

What is your situation now? _____

_____

○ Yes   ○ No   Do you have any other psychological diagnosis? If so, please list and explain how you were or are being treated. _____

_____

_____

○ Yes   ○ No   Have you ever attempted suicide? When? _____

_____

Does attempted suicide continue to be an issue? _____

_____

○ Yes   ○ No   Have you ever had anorexia, bulimia, or eating problems? _____

What have you done to address this? _____

_____

What is your situation now? _____

_____

○ Yes   ○ No   Did you suffer physical or emotional neglect as a child? _____

What have you done to address this? _____

_____

How does this affect you now? _____

_____

○ Yes   ○ No   Have you suffered physical or emotional neglect as an adult? _____

What have you done to address this? _____

What is your situation now? _____

_____

○ Yes   ○ No   Have you ever been in an abusive relationship (physically and/or emotionally intimidated, beaten, or injured)? _____

_____

What have you done to address this? _____

_____

What is your situation now? _____

_____

◯ Yes ◯ No Have you ever been molested or had nonconsensual sex with a partner, relative,
              or acquaintance? _____
What have you done to address this? _____

_____

What is your situation now? _____

_____

◯ Yes ◯ No Have you ever been raped? _____
What have you done to address this? _____

_____

How does this affect you now? _____

_____

◯ Yes ◯ No Have ever been subject to gynecological or obstetrical abuse? _____
What have you done to address this? _____

_____

How does this affect you now? _____

_____

◯ Yes ◯ No Do you think, or has anyone ever told you, that you have used alcohol or recreational drugs
              excessively? _____
What have you done to address this? _____

_____

Does this continue to be an issue? _____

_____

◯ Yes ◯ No Are you currently using any recreational drugs ? If so, what kind, and how recently? _____

_____

◯ Yes ◯ No Are you currently drinking alcohol? If so, how much? _____

_____

◯ Yes ◯ No Are you currently using tobacco? If so, how much? (If you once smoked and quit, give date.) _____

_____

◯ Yes ◯ No Have you ever used any drug intravenously (IV)?
◯ Yes ◯ No Do you think you are at increased risk for HIV/AIDS?
◯ Yes ◯ No Do you want information about safer sex practices?

The following is a list of stressors that can have an impact on your pregnancy, birth, or postpartum, as consequences of these can cause trauma that may remain deeply rooted. On a scale of one to ten (with ten being the greatest intensity), how high was your stress level in response to these occurrences?

_____ Serious money problems (date) _____
_____ A caregiver to someone ill or impaired (date) _____
_____ Sudden death of a loved one (date) _____
_____ Parents separated/divorced (date) _____
_____ Separated/divorced (date) _____

_____ Witnessed domestic violence (date) _____

_____ Family member jailed (date) _____

_____ Jailed (date) _____

_____ Lived in war zone (date) _____

_____ Sexually harassed (date)_____

_____ Saw robbery or attack (date) _____

_____ Robbed/attacked (date) _____

_____ Painful medical procedure (date) _____

_____ Saw accident (date) _____

_____ Had accident (date) _____

_____ Was in serious disaster (date/location)_____

_____ Had a hard time with elective abortion or miscarriage (date) _____

If you have experienced any other significant stressors, please indicate, rate, and date below: _____

_____

_____

_____

Again, thanks for completing this worksheet!

(Regarding the stress index, acknowledgments go to Mickey Sperlich for her excellent article in *Midwifery Today*, "Survivor Moms: Multiple Trauma Exposures and the Development of Post Traumatic Stress Disorder," Summer 2009.)

PRENATAL CARE RECORD

Name _____ Phone _____

LMP _____ EDD _____

Visit	Date	Weeks Gestation	Urine	Weight	Pulse/ BP	FHR	Presentation/ Position	Fundal Height	Internal Exam	Next Appt.	Provider (Initials)

PRENATAL CARE PROGRESS NOTES

Name _____ EDD _____

LABOR RECORD

Name _____ Date _____

Labor onset: Latent _____ Active _____

Baby's position _____ EDD _____

Membranes _____ Usual FHT _____

Concerns _____ Midwife _____

Observations on arrival _____

Time	BP/Pulse	Fetal Heart Tones	Urinalysis	Contractions	Internal Exam

LABOR CARE PROGRESS NOTES

Name _____ Date _____

_____
_____
_____
_____
_____
_____
_____
_____
_____
_____
_____
_____
_____
_____
_____
_____
_____
_____
_____
_____
_____
_____
_____
_____
_____
_____
_____
_____
_____
_____
_____
_____
_____
_____
_____

Appendix G

TRANSPORT RECORD FROM HOME DELIVERY

Midwife _____ Date/time _____

Mother's name _____ Partner's name _____

Address _____

EDD _____ Mother's age _____ Gravida _____ Para _____

Prenatal History

Gestational age 1st visit _____ Weight gain _____ Usual BP _____

Urine _____ Edema _____ Pelvimetry _____ Fundus _____

HCT/HGB _____ ABO & Rh _____ GBS _____ at _____ weeks HBsAg _____

Comments _____

_____

Labor History

Began labor _____ Initial events _____ Midwife arrived at _____

General observations _____ Vaginal exam _____

Comments _____

_____

Course of Labor

Inactive labor _____ Active labor _____ Pushing _____

Ruptured membranes _____ How? _____ Meconium? _____

Fetal response to labor _____

_____

Comments _____

_____

Reasons for transport _____

_____

_____

_____

_____

_____

_____

_____

_____

_____

BIRTH RECORD: MOTHER

Name _____ Date of birth _____
Phone (home) _____ (work) _____ Age _____
Address _____
Gravida _____ Para _____ EDD _____ Date of birth _____ Time _____
GBS _____ at _____ weeks

Labor Summary
Latent _____ hrs.
1st stage _____ hrs.   2nd stage _____ mins.   3rd stage _____ mins.
Membranes ruptured at _____ Spontaneously _____ Surgically _____ Clear _____ Stained _____
Estimated blood loss _____ Treatment _____
Comments/problems _____

Placenta
Size _____ Adherent clot _____
Method of delivery _____ Missing cotyledons _____
Infarcts _____ Calcifications _____ Succenturiate lobe _____
Time cord cut _____ Number of vessels in cord _____

Perineum
Lacerations _____ Repairs _____

Immediate Postpartum
BP _____ Pulse _____ Fundus _____
Shower _____ Urination _____ Food/drink _____
Stable at _____

BIRTH RECORD: BABY

Name _____ Sex _____ Weight _____ Length _____ Chest _____ Head _____
Apgar: 1 minute _____ 5 minutes _____ Suctioning _____
Resuscitation _____
Molding, Caput, Hematoma _____ Eye medication _____ Vitamin K _____
Nursing _____
Unusual behavior problems or abnormalities _____
_____
_____

If problems develop and you call in, give time of birth, sex, weight, Apgar, respirations per minute, temperature, and heart rate and describe symptoms.

Appendix I

NEWBORN EXAMINATION

DATE_____
APGARS (1 minute _____)
        (5 minutes _____)
SEX _____ WEIGHT _____
AXILLARY TEMPERATURE _____
TOTAL LENGTH _____
HEAD (O.F.) _____
CHEST _____

APGAR	0	1	2
Heart rate	Absent	Under 100	Over 100
Respirations	Absent	Slow (Irr.)	Good (cry)
Muscle tone	Limp	Some flexion	Active
Color	Blue/white	Blue hands or feet	Pink totally
Response to nasal catheter	None	Grimaces	Sneeze or cough

1. GENERAL APPEARANCE _____
   (Activity, tone, cry)
2. SKIN _____
   (Polycythemia, jaundice, desquamation, lanugo, vernix, birth marks)
3. HEAD, NECK _____
   (Molding, caput, bruising, cephalhematoma, fontanelles)
4. EYES _____
   (Red spots, jaundice, pupils, tracking, medication instilled)
5. ENT _____
   (Ear shape, ear placement, reactivity to sound, lips, palate, frenulum)
6. THORAX _____
   (Retractions)
7. ABDOMEN _____
   (Cord, masses, bowel sounds)
8. HEART _____
   (Heart rate, femoral pulses)
9. GENITALS _____
   (Testes descended, edema, clitoris)
10. REFLEXES _____
   (Sucking, swallowing, palmar, Moro, Babinkski, plantar, step)
11. SPINE/ANUS _____
   (Sinuses, anus patent)
12. LUNGS _____
   (Respirations, all quadrants clear)
13. EXTREMITIES _____
   (Fingers, toes, clavicles, hip creases or abduction)

COMMENTS _____
_____
_____

CLINICAL ESTIMATION OF GESTATIONAL AGE

CLINICAL ESTIMATION OF GESTATIONAL AGE
An Approximation Based on Published Data*

PATIENT'S NAME _____

⬆ **Examination First Hours**

WEEKS GESTATION

PHYSICAL FINDINGS	20	21	22	23	24	25	26	27	28	29	30	31	32	33	34	35	36	37	38	39	40	41	42	43	44	45	46	47	48
VERNIX	APPEARS					COVERS BODY, THICK LAYER																SCANT, IN CREASES			NO VERNIX				
BREAST TISSUE AND AREOLA	AREOLA & NIPPLE BARELY VISIBLE NO PALPABLE BREAST TISSUE														AREOLA RAISED		1-2 MM NODULE		3-5 MM	5-6 MM		7-10 MM			7-12 MM				
EAR — FORM				FLAT, SHAPELESS												BEGINNING INCURVING SUPERIOR		INCURVING UPPER 2/3 PINNAE			WELL-DEFINED INCURVING TO LOBE								
CARTILAGE					PINNA SOFT, STAYS FOLDED										CARTILAGE SCANT RETURNS SLOWLY FROM FOLDING			THIN CARTILAGE SPRINGS BACK FROM FOLDING						PINNA FIRM, REMAINS ERECT FROM HEAD						
SOLE CREASES						SMOOTH SOLES 1 CREASES								1-2 ANTERIOR CREASES		2-3 ANTERIOR CREASES	CREASES ANTERIOR 2/3 SOLE			CREASES INVOLVING HEEL				DEEPER CREASES OVER ENTIRE SOLE					
SKIN — THICKNESS & APPEARANCE	THIN, TRANSLUCENT SKIN, PLETHORIC, VENULES OVER ABDOMEN EDEMA													SMOOTH THICKER NO EDEMA					PINK	FEW VESSELS	SOME DES-QUAMATION PALE PINK		THICK, PALE, DESQUAMATION OVER ENTIRE BODY						
NAIL PLATES	AP-PEAR											NAILS TO FINGER TIPS											NAILS EXTEND WELL BEYOND FINGER TIPS						
HAIR	APPEARS ON HEAD			EYE BROWS & LASHES				FINE, WOOLLY, BUNCHES OUT FROM HEAD											SILKY, SINGLE STRANDS LAYS FLAT					RECEDING HAIRLINE OR LOSS OF BABY HAIR SHORT, FINE UNDERNEATH						
LANUGO	AP-PEARS				COVERS ENTIRE BODY										VANISHES FROM FACE			PRESENT ON SHOULDERS					NO LANUGO						
GENITALIA — TESTES									TESTES PALPABLE IN INGUINAL CANAL								IN UPPER SCROTUM					IN LOWER SCROTUM						
SCROTUM									FEW RUGAE								RUGAE, ANTERIOR PORTION				RUGAE COVER		PENDULOUS						
LABIA & CLITORIS									PROMINENT CLITORIS LABIA MAJORA SMALL WIDELY SEPARATED								LABIA MAJORA LARGER NEARLY COVERED CLITORIS						LABIA MINORA & CLITORIS COVERED						
SKULL FIRMNESS			BONES ARE SOFT					SOFT TO 1" FROM ANTERIOR FONTANELLE									SPONGY AT EDGES OF FON-TANELLE CENTER FIRM		BONES HARD SUTURES EASILY DISPLACED					BONES HARD, CANNOT BE DISPLACED						
POSTURE — RESTING	HYPOTONIC LATERAL DECUBITUS							HYPOTONIC			BEGINNING FLEXION THIGH		STRONGER HIP FLEXION		FROG-LIKE		FLEXION ALL LIMBS		HYPERTONIC					VERY HYPERTONIC					
RECOIL - LEG				NO RECOIL				NO RECOIL								PARTIAL RECOIL			BEGIN FLEXION NO RE-COIL				PROMPT RECOIL						
ARM						NO RECOIL													PROMPT RECOIL MAY BE INHIBITED					PROMPT RECOIL AFTER 30° INHIBITION						

| 20 | 21 | 22 | 23 | 24 | 25 | 26 | 27 | 28 | 29 | 30 | 31 | 32 | 33 | 34 | 35 | 36 | 37 | 38 | 39 | 40 | 41 | 42 | 43 | 44 | 45 | 46 | 47 | 48 |

POSTPARTUM CARE

Mother _____ Baby _____ Phone _____

Date	Temp/ Pulse	BP	Nipples/ Breastfeeding	Uterus	Lochia	Perineum	Baby's Cord	Baby's Color/ Behavior

Date	Uterus	Lochia	Breastfeeding	Cervix	Vaginal/Abdominal Tone	Parenting
3 weeks						
6 weeks						

POSTPARTUM CARE PROGRESS NOTES

Mother _____ Baby _____

Appendix L

POSTPARTUM INSTRUCTIONS

1. Let us know if you soak more than one pad in 20 minutes—massage your uterus firmly to re-contract it, and if bleeding doesn't stop, contact us at once or seek emergency care.

2. Change your pad with each trip to the bathroom, and rinse perineum with warm water.

3. Check your uterus for firmness and/or tenderness several times a day, for three days at least.

4. Notice if your flow has any bad odor (it should smell like your menses)—and report to us.

5. Take your temperature twice daily for at least four days.

6. Drink lots of water (about three quarts daily to establish milk flow) and make one quart of that a mixture of shepherd's purse and comfrey tea (for healing and bleeding control).

7. If you've had stitches, soak them in (or use compresses of) warm water or ginger tea—three or four times daily. Air-dry immediately after, in sunlight if possible. Report any pain.

8. If your baby's cord has been cut, clean the stump carefully with hydrogen peroxide or alcohol every few hours (or at each diaper change). Pay special attention to the folds where the cord joins the skin.

9. Nurse as much as the baby wants (usually every 2 to 3 hours; do not go more than 4 hours without nursing).

10. If the baby begins to look yellow within the first 24 hours, call us immediately.

11. Don't hesitate to call us if the baby seems disinterested in nursing, listless, or irritable.

12. Get lots of rest, sleep when the baby sleeps, eat lots of good food with plenty of iron to replenish lost blood, and ask visitors for real help—like doing your dishes or laundry. Work into activity slowly, and you won't have any sudden breakdowns later.

13. Try to take the parenting one day at a time—call if you feel upset, sad, or depressed.

14. Special instructions: _____

_____

_____

_____

_____

_____

_____

_____

_____

_____

_____

_____

THE MIDWIFE'S KIT

fetascope

Doppler (optional)

watch, with second hand

blood pressure cuff

stethoscope

three curved hemostats (Rochester-Pean)

one pair blunt scissors with blunt points

one pair sharp scissors with sharp points

one pair umbilical scissors

one Averbach cord bander

two needle holders (or substitute a Russian forceps for
    one needle holder)

three mosquito forceps

one ring forceps

stainless-steel cord clamps (Hazeltine)

stainless-steel instrument tray with cover

sterile gloves (elbow-length and wrist-length)

regular exam gloves

vinyl gloves (for use with oil or for women with
    latex allergy)

disposable underpads

lubricating jelly

5 cc syringes

3 cc syringes

1.5-inch, 21-gauge needles (injections)

0.5-inch, 23-gauge needles (suturing)

suture material (3-0 chromic)

lidocaine anesthetic

Pitocin

Methergine

erythromycin eye ointment

vitamin K for baby

lancets for newborn heel sticks

nitrazine paper

urine testing sticks

glucose testing strips

pregnancy tests

plastic disposable amnihooks

DeLee mucus traps

cord blood tubes

bulb syringe

Betadine solution

Hibiclens solution

alcohol prep pads

4 x 4 sterile gauze pads, or topper sponges

water bottle

heating pad

stamp pad

light (and extension cord if needed) for suturing

plasticized or fiberglass tape measure

infant scale

oxygen system with infant resuscitation unit
    (Mercury Disposable Infant Resuscitator, the
    Hudson Lifesaver Infant Resuscitator, or the Ambu
    Mark IV Baby Resuscitator)

pocket masks for resuscitation (newborn and adult)

IV equipment (optional)

blood draw equipment (optional)

hemoglobinometer and lancets

blood glucose monitor and lancets

Pap smear supplies not provided by lab

herbs and tinctures

homeopathic remedies

CARE AND PREPARATION OF INSTRUMENTS

Most of the instruments require no special care, except for those that must be scrubbed and sterilized repeatedly. Careful cleansing immediately after use is a good idea as dried blood cakes up the hinges and is difficult to remove. Use scouring pads to clean blood from the grooved blades of the forceps and needle holder.

The first method for sterilizing your instruments is by boiling. Boil instruments and instrument tray in a large pot of water for twenty-five minutes. Remember to sterilize the tongs that you will use for removing instruments from the water, and be sure to place them in the water with handles up. Once the twenty-five minutes have passed, let the pot cool off a bit and then remove the tray with your tongs. Open some packets of sterile gauze, put on a sterile glove, and line your tray with the gauze. Then use the tongs once again to place the instruments in the tray, and cover (either drip-dry the cover as it is removed or blot with sterile gauze). Place in a doubled paper bag, wrap it up snugly, tape, and date it.

A simpler method is by baking. All you have to do is bake your double-wrapped package of tray, liner, and tools for one hour in a 250-degree oven. Be sure to add a pan of water so the bag doesn't scorch. Simply remove, cool, tape, date, and store.

Repeat sterilization every two weeks.

PARENT'S SUPPLY LIST

Betadine or Hibiclens solution
olive oil
bulb syringe (rubber ear type, 3 oz.)
4 x 4 sterile gauze pads (two dozen)
cotton balls
hydrogen peroxide
oral/axillary thermometer
bendable straws
hot and cold packs
plastic mattress protector
plastic drop cloth
bleach
flashlight with extra batteries

plastic trash bags
disposable underpads (at least twenty)
sanitary napkins (heavy and minipads) plus belt
four sheets, cases for all pillows, four washcloths, four towels, eight receiving blankets—all dried in a hot dryer for ten extra minutes and bagged in plastic, then taped shut
cotton newborn cap
herbs: shepherd's purse, comfrey, ginger root, and so on
plastic eye dropper
water birth tub (rent or purchase) if water birth desired
sitz bath unit

MIDWIFERY PROGRAMS AND INSTITUTIONS

MEAC-Approved Direct-Entry Programs

Bastyr University Department of Midwifery
14500 Juanita Drive NE
Kenmore, WA 98028-4966
(425) 602-3380
Midwifery Program Supervisor: Mary Yglesia
myglesia@bastyr.edu; mwadvise@bastyr.edu
www.bastyr.edu/academics/areas-study/
midwifery-degree-programs

Birthingway College of Midwifery
12113 SE Foster Road
Portland, OR 97266
(503) 760-3131
President: Holly Scholles
info@birthingway.edu
www.birthingway.edu

Birthwise Midwifery School
24 S. High Street
Bridgton, ME 04009
(207) 647-5968
Executive Director: Heidi Filmore-Patrick
heidi@birthwisemidwifery.edu
www.birthwisemidwifery.edu

Florida School of Traditional Midwifery
810 E. University Avenue
Gainesville, FL 32601
(352) 338-0766; Fax: (352) 338-2013
Executive Director: Heart Phoenix
info@midwiferyschool.org
www.midwiferyschool.org

Maternidad La Luz
1308 Magoffin Street
El Paso, TX 79901
(915) 532-5895; Fax: (915) 532-7127
Director: Deborah Kaley
academic@maternidadlaluz.com
www.maternidadlaluz.com

Midwives College of Utah
(formerly Utah College of Midwifery)
1174 E. Graystone Way, Suite 2
Salt Lake City, UT 84106-2671
(866) 680-2756; Fax: (866) 207-2024
Director: Kristi Ridd-Young
office@midwifery.edu
www.midwifery.edu

National College of Midwifery
209 State Road 240
Taos, NM 87571
(575) 758-8914; Fax: (575) 758-0302
Acting President: Jenny West
info@midwiferycollege.org
www.midwiferycollege.org

National Midwifery Institute
PO Box 128
Bristol, VT 05443-0128
(802) 453-3332
Administrator and Codirector: Shannon Anton
Codirector: Elizabeth Davis
santon@nationalmidwiferyinstitute.com
www.nationalmidwiferyinstitute.com

Nizhoni Institute of Midwifery
3802 Alameda Way
Bonita, CA 91902
(619) 713-2892
Codirectors: Marla Hicks and Gerri Ryan
nizhonimidwives@gmail.com
www.midwiferyatnizhoni.com

Nonaccredited Direct-Entry Programs (may be state recognized)

Ancient Arts Midwifery Institute
(918) 720-2717 (cell)
ancientartmail@gmail.com
www.ancientartmidwifery.com
Director: Carla Hartley

Arkansas Midwives School and Services
4528 Huntsville Road
Fayetteville, AR 72701
(501) 571-2229
midwives@dicksonstreet.com
Director of Education: Teresa Elder, LM

The Farm Midwifery Workshops
42 The Farm
Summertown, TN 38483
(931) 964-2472
www.midwiferyworkshops.org

The Matrona
(828) 242-2188
www.thematrona.com
Diane Bartlett

Michigan School of Traditional Midwifery
PO Box 162
Mikado, MI 48745
(989) 736-6583
www.traditionalmidwife.com

Newlife School of Midwifery International
Davao City, Philippines
director@midwifeschool.org

ACNM-Approved Postbaccalaureate Programs

Case Western Reserve University
Frances Payne Bolton School of Nursing
Nurse-Midwifery Program
10900 Euclid Avenue
Cleveland, OH 44106-1712
(216) 368-2529
www.fpb.case.edu/MSN/midwifery.shtm
Director: Gretchen G. Mettler

Columbia University
School of Nursing
CUMSPH/ICAP
722 W. 168th Street, 7th Floor
New York, NY 10032-3703
(212) 305-5236
http://nursing.columbia.edu
Director: Laura Zeidenstein
BA/BS to RN/CNM/Graduate Option

East Carolina University
College of Nursing
Nurse-Midwifery Program
Health Science Building
Greenville, NC 27858
(252) 744-6402
www.ecumidwifery.net
Director: Rebecca Bagley
BA/BS to RN/CNM/Graduate Option
Fully Distance

Emory University
Nell Hodgson Woodruff School of Nursing
Nurse-Midwifery Specialty
1520 Clifton Road NE
Atlanta, GA 30322-0001
(404) 727-6961
http://nursing.emory.edu/index.html
Director: Jane Mashburn

Frontier Nursing University
Community-Based Nurse-Midwifery
Education Program
PO Box 528
Hyden, KY 41749-0528
(606) 672-2312
www.midwives.org
Director: Tonya Nicholson
Fully Distance

Georgetown University
School of Nursing and Health Studies
Graduate Program in Nurse-Midwifery
3700 Reservoir Road NW, Box 571107
Washington, DC 20057-0001
(202) 687-1563
http://nhs.georgetown.edu/nursing/masters/nm/
Director: Carolyn Gegor
Fully Distance

Marquette University
College of Nursing
Nurse-Midwifery Program
PO Box 1881
Milwaukee, WI 53201-1881
(414) 288-3810
www.marquette.edu/nursing/index.shtml
Director: Leona VandeVusse
BA/BS to RN/CNM/Graduate Option
Partially Distance

Midwifery Institute of Philadelphia University
222 Hayward Hall
4201 Henry Avenue
Philadelphia, PA 19144
(215) 951-2525
www.philau.edu/midwifery/
Director: Katherine L. Dawley
CM Option
Fully Distance
Foreign-Educated Midwife Transfer Credits

New York University
College of Nursing at the College of Dentistry
Midwifery Program
246 Greene Street
New York, NY 10003-6677
(212) 998-5895
www.nyu.edu/nursing
Program directed by: Julia Lange Kessler

Ohio State University
College of Nursing
Nurse-Midwifery Graduate Program
1585 Neil Avenue
Columbus, OH 43210-1216
(614) 292-4041
www.con.ohio-state.edu
Director: Jeremy Neal
BA/BS to RN/CNM/Graduate Option
Partially Distance

Oregon Health Sciences University
School of Nursing
Nurse-Midwifery Program
3181 SW Sam Jackson Park Road
Portland, OR 97239-3011
(503) 494-3114
www.ohsu.edu/xd/education/schools/school-of-nursing/
programs/graduate/specialities/nurse-midwifery/
index.cfm
Director: Carol L. Howe
BA/BS to RN/CNM/Graduate Option

San Diego State University
School of Nursing
Nurse-Midwifery Graduate Education Program
5500 Campanile Drive
San Diego, CA 92182-0001
(619) 543-2540
www.nursing.sdsu.edu
Director: Lauren P. Hunter

Seattle University
College of Nursing
Nurse Midwifery Program
901 12th Avenue
Seattle, WA 98122-4411
(206) 296-5666
www.seattleu.edu/nursing
Director: Katherine Camacho Carr
BA/BS to RN/CNM/Graduate Option

Shenandoah University
Division of Nursing
Nurse-Midwifery Education Program
1775 N. Sector Court
Winchester, VA 22601-2859
(540) 678-4382
www.su.edu
Director: Juliana Fehr
Partially Distance

State University of New York
Downstate Medical Center
College of Health Related Professions
Midwifery Education Program
450 Clarkson Avenue, #1227
Brooklyn, NY 11203-2012
(718) 270-7740
www.downstate.edu/CHRP/midwifery/
Director: Ronnie Lichtman
CM Option
Partially Distance

Stony Brook University
School of Nursing
Pathways to Midwifery
Health Sciences Center
Stony Brook, NY 11794-0001
(631) 444-2867
www.nursing.stonybrookmedicine.edu
Director: Nicole Rouhana
BA/BS to RN/CNM/Graduate Option
Fully Distance

Texas Tech University Health Sciences Center
School of Nursing
Nurse-Midwifery Program
4800 Alberta Avenue
El Paso, TX 79905-2709
(915) 545-6710
www.ttuhsc.edu/son/nmw
Director: Elizabeth Portugal
Partially Distance

University of California, San Francisco at SFGH
Interdepartmental Nurse-Midwifery Ed Program
1001 Potrero Avenue, Room 6D-29
San Francisco, CA 94110
(415) 206-5106
www.nurseweb.ucsf.edu/www/spec-mwf.htm
Director: Amy Levi
BA/BS to RN/CNM/Graduate Option
Partially Distance

University of Cincinnati
College of Nursing
Nurse-Midwifery Education Program
PO Box 210038
Cincinnati, OH 45221-0001
(513) 558-5282
http://nursing.uc.edu
Director: Melissa Willmarth
BA/BS to RN/CNM/Graduate Option
Fully Distance

University of Colorado Denver
College of Nursing
Nurse-Midwifery Option
13120 E. 19th Avenue, #6511
Aurora, CO 80045-2567
(720) 971-1526
www.ucdenver.edu/academics/colleges/nursing
Director: Jennifer G. Hensley
Partially Distance

University of Florida
College of Nursing Jacksonville
653-1 W. 8th Street, LRC-3rd Floor, Box L-4
Jacksonville, FL 32209-6511
(904) 244-5171
www.nursing.ufl.edu
Director: Susan Salazar
Partially Distance

University of Illinois at Chicago
College of Nursing
Nurse-Midwifery Program
845 S. Damen Avenue, #MC802
Chicago, IL 60612-3727
(312) 355-3038
www.uic.edu/nursing
Director: Barbara Camune
BA/BS to RN/CNM/Graduate Option
Partially Distance

University of Indianapolis
School of Nursing
Nurse-Midwifery Program
1400 E. Hanna Avenue
Indianapolis, IN 46227-3630
(317) 788-3327
www.nursing.uindy.edu
Director: Barbara Winningham
Partially Distance

University of Kansas
School of Nursing
Nurse-Midwifery Education Program
3901 Rainbow Boulevard
Kansas City, KS 66160-0001
(913) 588-1683
www2.kumc.edu/midwife
Director: Cara Busenhart
Partially Distance

University of Medicine and Dentistry of New Jersey
School of Nursing
Women's Health and Nurse-Midwifery
65 Bergen Street
Newark, NJ 07107-3001
(973) 972-4298
http://sn.umdnj.edu/academics/masters/nursemidwifery
Director: Elaine Diegmann
BA/BS to RN/CNM/Graduate Option

University of Miami
School of Nursing and Health Studies
Nurse-Midwifery Program
PO Box 248153
Coral Gables, FL 33124-8153
(305) 284-3666
www.miami.edu/sonhs/index.php/sonhs/academics/
master_programs/nurse_midwifery
Director: Jeanne Gottlieb
BA/BS to RN/CNM/Graduate Option

University of Michigan
School of Nursing
400 N. Ingalls Street, Room 3320
Ann Arbor, MI 48109-2003
(734) 763-0016
www.nursing.umich.edu/academic-programs/
masters-programs/certified-nurse-midwife
Director: Lisa Kane Low
BA/BS to RN/CNM/Graduate Option
Partially Distance

University of Minnesota
School of Nursing
Nurse-Midwifery Program
308 Harvard Street SE, #6-101
Minneapolis, MN 55455-0353
(612) 624-5933
www.nursing.umn.edu/DNP/Specialties/
NurseMidwifery
Director: Melissa Hanner Frisvold
BA/BS to RN/CNM/Graduate Option
Partially Distance

University of New Mexico
College of Nursing
Nurse-Midwifery Program
MS C09 5350
Albuquerque, NM 87131-0001
(505) 272-6789
http://nursing.unm.edu/prospective-students/masters-
in-nursing/nurse-midwifery.html
Director: Julie Gorwoda

University of Pennsylvania
School of Nursing
Midwifery Program
Room 417 Fagin Hall
418 Curie Boulevard
Philadelphia, PA 19104-4217
(215) 573-7679
www.nursing.upenn.edu/whcs/pages/
MidwiferyProgram.aspx
Director: William McCool
BA/BS to RN/CNM/Graduate Option

University of Puerto Rico
Graduate School of Public Health
Nurse-Midwifery Education Program
Med Sci Camp
PO Box 5067
San Juan, PR 00936
(787) 281-7355
www.rcm.upr.edu/publichealth
Director: Irene de la Torre

University of Utah
College of Nursing
Nurse-Midwifery Program
10 South 2000 East
Salt Lake City, UT 84112-5880
(801) 585-7183
http://nursing.utah.edu
Director: Susanna Cohen

University of Washington
School of Nursing
Nurse-Midwifery Education Program
University of Washington
Seattle, WA 98195-0001
(206) 543-8736
http://nursing.uw.edu/node/371
Director: Ira Kantrowitz-Gordon
Partially Distance

Vanderbilt University
School of Nursing
Nurse-Midwifery Program
402 Godchaux Hall
461 21st Avenue South
Nashville, TN 37240
(615) 343-5876
www.nursing.vanderbilt.edu/msn/nmw.html
Director: Mavis Schorn
BA/BS to RN/CNM/Graduate Option

Wayne State University
College of Nursing
Nurse-Midwifery Option
5557 Cass Avenue, Room 248
Detroit, MI 48202-3615
(313) 577-5926
http://nursing.wayne.edu
Director: Deborah S. Walker
BA/BS to RN/CNM/Graduate Option
Partially Distance

Yale University
School of Nursing
Nurse-Midwifery Specialty
100 Church Street South
New Haven, CT 06519-1703
(203) 785-2389
http://nursing.yale.edu/nurse-midwifery-specialty
Director: Marianne T. Stone-Godena
BA/BS to RN/CNM/Graduate Option

NARM-Approved Clinical Sites outside the United States

Abundant Grace of God Maternity Center, Tabuk, Philippines
http://gthemidwife.com

Active Birth Unit, Mowbray Maternity Hospital, Cape Town, South Africa
http://activebirth.za.org

African Birth Collective, Kafoutine, Mboro, Darou Khoudous, Diamanguene-Senegal
www.africanbirthcollective.org

Al-Nisa Maternity Home, Capetown, South Africa
www.alnisamaternityhome.co.za

Bumi Sehat, Bali
www.bumisehatbali.org

Bus Fare Babies Birth Centre, South Africa
http://busfarebabies.blogspot.com

Luna Maya, San Cristobal, Mexico
http://lunamayamexico.blogspot.com

MamaBaby Haiti
www.mamababyhaiti.org

Mamatoto Resource and Birth Centre, Trinidad
www.mamatoto.net

Mercy in Action, Philippines
www.mercyinaction.com

Mercy Maternity Center, Davao, Philippines
www.midwifeschool.org/mercy.htm

Midwives on the Move, Abura Dunkwa District Hospital, Central Region, Ghana, West Africa
http://midwivesofcolor.wordpress.com/2011/07/23/midwives-on-the-move

Mother Health International, Haiti
http://motherhealthinternational.org

Shiprah Birthing Home, Philippines
www.helpintl.org/shiprah.html

Appendix O

HIPAA GUIDELINES

This is a summary of the Health Insurance Portability and Accountability Act (HIPAA) guidelines as applied to midwifery practice, which can be used to develop a Notice of Privacy Practices statement for clients to read and sign. (Personalize this document by changing the word *midwife* to *my* or *I* and the word *client* to *you* or *your*.)

Midwife's Legal Duty

1. To maintain privacy of client's health information
2. To provide clients written notice about midwife's privacy practices and their rights concerning their health information
3. To change privacy practices according to applicable law and make new written notice available to clients

Uses and Disclosures of Health Information

1. **Treatment.** The midwife may disclose health information to other health care providers providing client treatment.
2. **Payment.** The midwife may use or disclose information to obtain payment for services.
3. **Health care operations.** The midwife may use and disclose health information in connection with quality assessment and improvement activities; reviewing the competence or qualifications of the midwife and her associates; or conducting training, accreditation, certification, or licensing activities.
4. **Client authorization.** The client may give the midwife written authorization to use or disclose her health information to anyone for any purpose. Authorization may also be revoked, in writing, at any time.
5. **To family and friends.** The midwife will disclose information to family and friends only with the client's written consent.
6. **Persons involved in care.** In the event of an emergency or client incapacity, the midwife may use or disclose health information to notify, or assist in notifying, a family member, personal representative, or other person responsible for client's care, of client's location and general condition, disclosing only the health information directly relevant to that person's involvement in client's care.
7. **Marketing services.** The midwife will not use client information for marketing operations without the client's written authorization.
8. **Required by law.** The midwife may disclose the client's health information when required to do so by law.
9. **Abuse or neglect.** The midwife may disclose the client's health information to appropriate authorities if it reasonably appears the client is a possible victim of abuse or domestic violence, to the extent necessary to avert a threat to the client's health or safety.

Client Rights

1. **Access.** The client has the right to look at or get copies of her health information.
2. **Disclosure accounting.** The client has a right to receive a list of occasions in which the midwife has disclosed her information for purposes other than treatment, payment, or health care operations for the past six years, but not before April 14, 2003 (the date HIPAA guidelines became effective).
3. **Restriction.** The client has the right to request that additional restrictions be placed on the use and disclosure of her health care information. The midwife is not required to abide by these but may agree to do so (except in emergency).
4. **Alternative communication.** The client has a right to request that the midwife communicate with her by alternative means or at alternative locations, as necessary, to maintain confidentiality (request must be in writing).
5. **Amendment.** The client has the right to request that the midwife amend her health information (request must be in writing, and must explain why the information should be amended). Under certain circumstances, the midwife may deny this request.
6. **Questions.** The client may contact the midwife for information about privacy practices at any time.
7. **Complaints.** If the client has complaints about the midwife's use or disclosure of her health information, or the midwife's response to her request to amend health information or communicate with her by alternative means or at alternative locations, she may complain to the midwife and to the U.S. Department of Health and Human Services.

About the Author

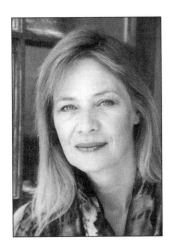

A renowned expert on women's issues, Elizabeth Davis, BA, CPM, has been a midwife, women's health practitioner, educator, and consultant for thirty-five years. She is cofounder and codirector of the National Midwifery Institute, Inc., a three-year, accredited midwifery program that qualifies graduates for national certification and licensure in California. A popular international lecturer and activist, she serves as academic advisor to many midwifery programs throughout Europe.

She was on the founding board of Midwives Alliance of North America (MANA) and served as Pacific regional representative for five years. As cofounder of the Certification Task Force (CTF), she was instrumental in developing national midwifery certification in the United States. In 1991, she was appointed president of the Midwifery Education Accreditation Council (MEAC). She also helped design and implement the *State of California Alternative Birthing Methods Study* and later spearheaded the California legalization effort. Since then, she has provided expert testimony to many states and countries on educational and legislative midwifery issues. She holds a degree in holistic maternity care from Antioch University and is certified by the North American Registry of Midwives.

Her books have been translated into nine languages and include *Women's Sexual Passages: Finding Pleasure and Intimacy at Every Stage of Life*, *The Women's Wheel of Life*, and *Orgasmic Birth: Your Guide to a Safe, Satisfying, and Pleasurable Birth Experience*. She is a popular television and radio guest, and her mission is to help women embrace an integrated view of birth, sexuality, family, and ecology.

She lives in Sebastopol, California, and is the mother of three children. Contact her at www.elizabethdavis.com.

INDEX

Cyanosis
circumoral, 137
prematurity and, 85
Cystic fibrosis, 42
Cystocele, 197
Cytomegalovirus, 15, 17, 21
Cytotec, 15, 164, 167

D

Dairy products, 34
D & C, 15, 168, 172
Dandelion
for anemia, 52
as liver tonic, 46
for pregnancy support, 52
Davis-Floyd, Robbie, 6, 222
Davis maneuver, 162
Death
of baby, 72, 183–84
certificate, 183
of mother, 1, 16
Debriefing, after birth, 61–62, 193, 199
Deflexion, 32, 145, 147
Dehydration
avoiding, 35
in baby, 197, 200
headache and, 47
hyperemesis and, 46
ketones and, 46
prematurity and, 85
DeLee mucus trap, 126, 127
Delivery, 125–29
assisting, 125–29
catching baby, 128–29
in the caul, 159
estimated date of, 20, 22, 25, 31
positions for, 125, 152, 161–62
precipitous, 124, 167, 171
See also Labor
Delivery Self-Attachment (video), 129
Demmin, Tish, 122, 243
Denominator, 31
Depo-Provera, 219
Depression, postpartum, 213–17
after cesarean birth, 210
disposing factors for, 215–16
emotional factors in, 193
frequency of, 214
onset of, 214
postpartum blues vs., 202, 213–14
treating, 216–17
Descent
cause of, 119
definition of, 58
promoting, 112

Desquamation, 137
Dexotrostix, 88, 204
Diabetes
as contraindication to homebirth, 15, 77
dangers of, 20, 76
gestational, 75–77
tests for, 39–40, 76
treatment for, 77
Diagonal conjugate, measuring, 25, 28
Diaper rash, 209
Diarrhea, 53
Diastolic reading, 23
DIC (disseminated intravascular coagulation), 72
Diet. *See* Food; Nutrition
Dieting, 71
Dilation of cervix
in active labor, 120
average rate of, 142
in early labor, 111–12
estimating, 118
in final six weeks, 58
visual indication of, 117, 118
Disseminated intravascular coagulation (DIC), 72
Dissociative disorder, 102
Distance learning programs, 229–30
Dizygotic twins, 82
Dizziness, 71
Domestic violence, 103
DONA International, 265
Donnely, Joan, 248
Double hip squeeze, 152
Douching, 40, 49
Doula work, 223–27
Doula World, 265
Down syndrome, 42–43
Dropping, 109
Drugs
addiction to, 15, 21
antipsychotic, 19
birth defects and, 18–19
for depression, 216
for herpes, 50
over-the-counter (OTCs), 18–19
oxytocic, 169, 235
purchasing, 235
for stopping labor, 86
See also individual drugs
Duck walking, 148
Due date. *See* Estimated date of delivery
Duncan mechanism, 134
Dycloxicillin, 213
Dystocia. *See* Shoulder dystocia

E

Early labor, 107–12
contractions of, 107, 108–9
homeopathy during, 130
infection prevention during, 108
intense, 130
length of, 142, 143–44
lightening or dropping, 108–9
midwife's involvement in, 109–11
physical assessments and duties in, 111–12
prolonged, 112
rest and, 107–8, 109
signs of, 107
vaginal exams in, 111
waters releasing, 107, 108, 157–58
Ears, checking baby's, 137–38
Eating disorders, 70–71, 102
Echinacea
in early labor, 108
for mastitis, 195
for vaginal health, 44
Eclampsia, 81
Ectopic pregnancy, 17, 73
Eczema, 204
EDD (estimated date of delivery), 20, 22, 25, 31
Edema
of ankles, 47
cervical, 145
of face, 105
generalized, 17, 80
pitting, 80
Effacement, 58, 111
Elderly primigravida, 96
Electrolyte imbalance, 116
Elephant walking, 84
Elevator exercise, 60, 197
El Halta, Valerie, 124
ELISA test, 42
Embolism
amniotic fluid, 164–65
definition of, 164
pulmonary, 211
Embryonic period, 45
EMDR (eye movement desensitization and reprocessing), 16
Emotional Intelligence (Goleman), 246
Emotional upsets, 91–92, 141
Endometritis, 210
Endorphins
in baby, 123
in mother, 109, 113
Engagement
checking for, 58, 59, 88
definition of, 119

Hemorrhage, prenatal
    from cervical polyps, 74
    discussion of, with client, 14
    placental abruption, 74–75
    placenta previa, 74–75
Hemorrhoids, 53, 209
Hemostats, 175
Hepatitis B (HBV), 21, 41, 42
Hepatitis C (HCV), 21, 41–42
Herbs
    buying, 51
    contraindicated during pregnancy, 51
    infusions of, 51–52
    during labor, 130–31
    for postpartum care, 194–96
    for pregnancy support, 51–52
    tinctures of, 51
    for vaginal douche, 50
    See also individual herbs and conditions
Hernia, umbilical, 138
Herpes
    as contraindication to homebirth,
        15, 18, 49
    dangers of, 21
    symptoms of, 49, 105
    treatment for, 50
HGB (hemoglobin), 38–39, 44, 69, 203
Hibiclens, 43–44
High blood pressure. *See* Hypertension
Hind leak, 108
HIPAA guidelines, 243, 299–300
Hips
    checking baby's, 139–40
    size of, as predictor of pelvic
        capacity, 26
HIV
    screening for, 42
    sperm donors and, 98
    universal precautions for, 114–15
HMOs (health maintenance
    organizations), effect of, on
    midwifery, 220
Holistic Midwifery (Frye), 19, 20, 27, 77,
    119, 222
Holistic model of health care, 6–7, 34
Homan's sign, 211
Homebirths
    breech births as, 83
    contraindications to, 15, 20–21, 38
    mother's commitment to, 20
    reasons for choosing, 12–13
    research on, 8, 10
    for twins, 83
Homeopathic Medicine for Women
    (Smith), 52

*Homeopathic Medicines for Pregnancy and
    Childbirth* (Moskowitz), 51, 52
Homeopathy
    during labor, 130–31
    for postpartum care, 194–96
    potencies of, 51
    during pregnancy, 51–53
    using, 51
Home visits
    advantages of, 235
    final, 60–61
    importance of, 60
    making notes during, 242–43
    minimum number of, 60
    scheduling time for, 236
Homophobia, 99
Honey, infant botulism from, 88
Hops
    for headaches, 47
    for hypertension, 78, 157
    for milk production, 195
Horowitz, Rob, 222
Hospitals
    backup at, 239
    birth assisting in, 224–27
    environment of, 225
    infant resuscitation at, 180
    labor and delivery personnel at, 239
    See also Transport
HPA (hypothalamic-pituitary-adrenal
    axis), 213
HPV (human papilloma virus), 41
Humanistic model of health care, 6, 7, 34
Human Labor & Birth (Oxorn and
    Foote), 90, 222
Human papilloma virus (HPV), 41
Hutchon, David, 127
Hydatidiform mole, 73–74
Hydramnios. *See* Polyhydramnios
Hydration
    constipation and, 209
    diarrhea and, 53
    oligohydramnios and, 82
    prematurity and, 85
    water requirements for, 35
Hydrocephaly, 42, 81, 182
Hydroxocobalamin, 36, 70
Hygiene, personal, 237
Hymenal ring, 176
Hyperactivity, 71
Hyperemesis
    description of, 18
    eating disorders and, 70
    molar pregnancy and, 70
    sexual abuse and, 102
    thyroid dysfunction and, 46

Hyperreflexia, 80, 157
Hypertension, 77–79
    borderline, 62, 110
    as contraindication to homebirth, 15
    dangers of, 77–78
    essential, 77
    gestational, 77–79, 156–57
    labor and, 156–57
    preeclampsia and, 80
    transport for, 157
    treating, 78–79
    undiagnosed, 23
Hyperthyroidism, 15, 20
Hyperventilation, 225
HypnoBirthing Institute, 265
Hypnotherapy, 16
Hypocalcemia, 34, 76, 204
Hypo-fibrinogenemia, 21
Hypoglycemia, 76, 87, 198, 204
Hypothalamic-pituitary-adrenal axis
    (HPA), 213
Hypothermia, 87
Hypothyroidism, 20, 214–15
Hypoxia
    apnea and, 178
    breech birth and, 83
    large for gestational age and, 89
    meconium staining and, 108, 121
Hysterotomy, 172

I

IAIM (International Association of Infant
    Massage), 266
ICAN (International Cesarean Awareness
    Network, Inc.), 266
ICEA (International Childbirth
    Educators Association), 266
ICM (International Confederation of
    Midwives), 246, 266
ICP (intrahepatic cholestasis of
    pregnancy), 47
ICTC (International Center for
    Traditional Childbearing), 266
Identical twins, 82
Ikenze, Ifeoma, 131
IMBCO (International MotherBaby
    Childbirth Organization), 266
Ina May's Guide to Childbirth
    (Gaskin), 222
Incoordinate labor, 58
Indigestion, 46, 69, 213
Induction of labor
    cervix condition and, 89
    natural methods of, 89
    postdatism and, 91
    PROM and, 157

310   *Heart & Hands*

Inevitable abortion, 72
Infant. *See* Baby
Infanticidal behaviors, 217
Infection
    bladder, 18, 40
    after circumcision, 207
    eye, 41
    neonatal, 205
    pelvic, 211
    preventing, in labor, 108, 157–58
    puerperal, 210–11
    thrush, 209
    trichomonias, 49
    urinary tract, 18
    uterine, 210–11
    vaginal, 47, 49, 102
    viral, 15, 17–18, 21
Influenza, 21
Informed choice, 7, 242
Infusions, herbal, 51–52
In His Hands Birth Supplies, 265
Injections
    of lidocaine, before suturing, 174,
        175–76
    technique for, 172
Inlet disproportion, 147, 148, 150
Insemination, artificial, 98
Instincts, social vs. biological, 12–13
Instruments
    care and preparation of, 291
    quality of, 235
Insulin therapy, 77
Insurance
    health, 237
    malpractice, 14
International Association of Infant
        Massage (IAIM), 266
International Birth and Wellness
        Project, 266
International Center for Traditional
        Childbearing (ICTC), 266
International Cesarean Awareness
        Network, Inc. (ICAN), 266
International Childbirth Educators
        Association (ICEA), 266
International Confederation of Midwives
        (ICM), 246, 266
International Definition of a Midwife, 4–5
International Federation of Gynecology
        and Obstetrics (FIGO), 4
International MotherBaby Childbirth
        Organization (IMBCO), 266
Intrahepatic cholestasis of pregnancy
        (ICP), 47
Intrauterine growth restriction (IUGR),
        87–88, 110

Intuition, development of, 251
Iron
    deficiency of, 68
    sources of, 36, 52, 69
    supplements, 34, 35, 69
Irritability, nervous, 207–9
Ischial spines
    assessing, 25–26
    finding, 29
Ischial tuberosities, 30, 60
Isoimmunization, 39
IUDs, 17, 219
IUGR (intrauterine growth restriction),
        87–88, 110

J

Jacquemier's maneuver, 162
Jaundice
    from ABO incompatibility, 206
    breast milk, 206
    checking for, 137, 197, 200
    pathological, 206
    physiologic, 205–6
    polycythemia and, 88
    treating, 196, 206–7
Jones, Ricardo Herbert, 110, 171
The Journal of Nurse-Midwifery, 223
Journals, 223
Judging vs. assessing, 249

K

Kalman, Janice, 93, 194, 199
Kamoroff, Bernard, 237
Kangaroo care, 86
Kegel exercise, 60
Kelp, for anemia, 52
Kernicterus, 206
Ketoacidosis, 144
Ketonuria, 76, 112, 144
Kick-counts, 77, 90
Kidney disease, 15, 21, 47
Kitzinger, Sheila, 62, 122, 222
Klaus, Phyllis, 103

L

Labial tears, 173
Labor
    active, 113, 115–20, 130, 142
    baby's movements during, 119
    back, 112, 152
    blood pressure during, 79
    brainwave frequencies in, 116, 120, 226
    breathing during, 113, 123, 225

    early, 107–12, 130, 142, 143–44
    environment for, 113, 115
    false, 58, 108
    fear in, 225
    herbs during, 130–31
    homeopathy during, 130–31
    incoordinate, 58
    induction of, 89, 91, 157
    length of, 142
    mother's position during, 115, 125,
        152, 161–62
    note-taking during, 243
    oxytocin and, 89, 109–10, 113, 116,
        120, 150
    partner helping during, 112
    plateau phenomenon, 118, 144
    premature, 53, 85–86, 105
    privacy and, 112, 113, 115, 146
    progress notes for, 111, 122, 281
    prolonged, 112, 116, 124, 142–47
    record of, 111, 280
    rest-and-be-thankful phase, 122
    second stage, 122–29, 130, 142,
        145–46
    surrender and, 113, 120
    third stage, 129, 132, 134–35
    transition, 120–22
    true, 109
    vaginal exams in, 111, 118
    walking during, 115, 116
    warm-up, 108–9
    See also Active labor; Birth;
        Contractions; Delivery; Early
        labor; Labor complications;
        Prolonged labor
Labor-aide, 116
Labor complications
    amniotic fluid embolism, 164–65
    art of handling, 141
    breech presentation, 163–64
    cephalopelvic disproportion, 147–51
    clinical exhaustion, 116, 142–47
    cord problems, 156
    fetal anomalies, 181–83
    fetal distress, 154–56
    hemorrhage, 165–71
    hypertension, 156–57
    maternal emotions and, 141
    neonatal death, 183–84
    nuchal arm, 159, 160
    posterior arrest, 152–54
    prolonged rupture of the membranes,
        157–58
    resuscitation, 173, 178, 180–82
    retained placenta, 171–73

certification process for, 3–4
challenges faced by, 249–52
clothing for, 237
enthusiasm of, 249
floundering by, 251
individual biases of, 19, 232
international definition of, 4–5
parents choosing, 9
personal development and, 252
personal hygiene and, 237
personal life of, 249–50
professional identity of, 252
as rebel, 7
relationship between mother and,
    5, 13, 54, 256
self-care for, 251–52
See also Midwifery; Midwifery
    practice; Midwifery training;
    Nurse-midwifery
Midwifery
advantages of, 5–8, 10
art of, 255
attacks against, 1–3
autonomy of, 4
as calling, 220
cultural/evolutionary aspect of, 7
in Europe, 1
feminism and, 7
history of, 1–2
legal status of, 2–5, 232, 237
maternal satisfaction with, 8
newsletters and journals, 223
parents supporting, 253
as personalized care, 5
professionalization of, 3–5
resources for, 264–67
values and ethics of, 254–57
as way of life, 249
See also Midwife; Midwifery practice;
    Midwifery training; Nurse-
    midwifery
*Midwifery Certification in the United
    States,* 3
Midwifery Education Accreditation
    Council (MEAC)
contact information for, 266
founding of, 5
programs accredited by, 228, 229,
    292–93
Midwifery Institute at Philadelphia
    University, 230
Midwifery practice
advertising of, 238
annual review of, 236
apprentices and, 227–29, 244–47
burnout and, 251

business meetings for, 236
challenges of, 231, 232
client confidentiality and, 14, 243,
    299–300
collectives, 233, 243
competition and, 233, 237
core competencies for, 258–61
equipment for, 234–35
fees for, 237, 253
filing system for, 236
group practice, 244
location of, 235
medical backup and consultation for,
    234, 239–41
medical records for, 241–43
partnerships, 243–44
peer review of, 248
philosophy of care for, 231–32
physical setup for, 235–36
principles of, 258
public relations and, 238
rural, 234
standards and qualifications for,
    262–63
supplies for, 236
taxes and, 237
urban, 232–33
vacations and, 251
Midwifery Today
contact information for, 266
magazine, 221, 223
role of, 5
Midwifery training
apprenticeships, 221, 227–29, 244–47
birth assisting, 223–27
core areas of study, 228
doula work, 223–27
formal schooling, 229–30, 292–98
instructor qualifications, 246
newsletters and journals, 223
nurse-midwifery programs, 220–21,
    230
study groups, 227
textbooks, 221–23
A Midwife's Handbook (Sinclair), 222
Midwives Alliance of North America
    (MANA)
contact information for, 266
Core Competencies for Midwifery
    Practice, 258–61
history of, 3
newsletter, 223
Standard and Qualifications for the
    Art and Practice of Midwifery,
    262–63

Statement of Values and Ethics,
    254–57
Student Section, 221
Midwives Information and Resource
    Service (MIDIRS), 266
Midwives Model of Care, 266
Military presentation, 159
Milk. *See* Breast milk
Miscarriage, 72–73
blood loss and, 72
emotional support for, 73
habitual, 73
history of, 15
preventing, 72
symptoms of, 72
technical terms for, 72
Misoprostrol, 15
Missed abortion, 72, 74
Molar pregnancy, 73–74
Moles, hairy, 137
Mongolian spots, 137, 138
Monilia, 47
Monitoring
external vs. internal, 154–55
intermittent, 154–55
Monozygotic twins, 82
MoonDragon Birthing, 266
Morning sickness, 46, 52
Moro reflex, 138, 139
Mortality rates
for infants, 1, 8, 10
maternal, 1, 16
Morula, 45
Moskowitz, Richard, 51, 52
Mosquito hemostats, 175
Mothering (magazine), 267
Mother(s)
adoptive, 95–96
birth as pivotal event for, 7
blood type of, 39
confidential worksheet for, 275–77
death of, 1, 16
debriefing with, after birth, 61–62,
    193, 199
with estranged partners, 97–98
first contact with, 12
first-time, 99
grand multipara, 97
initial interview with, 12–20
lesbian, 98–99
mirroring feelings of, 50
with new love relationship, 98
older, 96–97
personality of, 92
receiving baby, after birth, 129

U.S. Department of Agriculture, 34
U.S. Department of Education, 5
Uterine atony, 169
Uterine infection, 210–11
Uterine involution, 193, 196
Uterine rupture, 159
Uterine tone, promoting, 210
Uterus
  assessing size of, 25
  guarding, 132
  inverted, 172
  involution of, 193, 196
  ligaments supporting, 48
  after placental delivery, 134
  postpartum examination of, 196,
    200, 203
  prolapsed, 194
Uva ursi, for postpartum bath, 194

V

Vacations, 251
Vagina
  bacteria in, 43–44
  discharge from, 18, 47, 49
  douching, 40, 49
  gush of fluid from, 105
  toning, 60, 203
Vaginal awareness
  practices for, 60
  single mothers and, 94
Vaginal birth after cesarean (VBAC),
    15–16, 62
Vaginal exams
  bleeding and, 75
  in final six weeks, 58, 60
  in labor, 111, 118, 157–58
  permission for, 24
Vaginal infection, 47, 49, 102
Vaginal lacerations, 167, 169
Vaginal mucosa, 176
Vaginal muscles
  involuntary contraction of, 102
  massaging, 60, 147
  toning, 60
Vaginal ruggae, 176
Vaginal sores, painful, 18, 49
Vaginismus, 102
Valaclovir, 50
Valerian, for sleep difficulties, 52
Values, statement of, 254–56
Varicella. *See* Chicken pox
Varicose veins, 47
Varney, Helen, 20, 222
Varney's Midwifery (Varney), 20, 222
Vasa previa, 158–59

VBAC (vaginal birth after cesarean),
    15–16, 62
VDRL/RPR, 39
Vegan mothers, 36, 70
Velamentous cord insertion, 135
Vernix, 45, 137
Version, external, 84
Vertical transmission, 49
Vicodin, 19
Village pregnancy, 236
Viral infections, 15, 17–18, 21
Vitamin A, 34
Vitamin B-2, 216
Vitamin B-3, 216
Vitamin B-6, 216
Vitamin B-12
  deficiency of, 68, 69
  sources of, 70
  supplements of, 36, 70
  vegans and, 36
Vitamin C
  daily supplement of, 35
  in early labor, 108
  importance of, 68
  iron supplements and, 69
  large quantities of, 34
Vitamin D, 34
Vitamin E
  daily supplement of, 35
  for sore nipples, 200
  for varicose veins, 47
Vitamin K, 137, 139, 159, 163, 165, 207
Vomiting
  chronic, 18
  ginger tea for, 18, 46
  See also Nausea
Vulva, varicose veins of, 47

W

WABA (World Alliance for Breastfeeding
    Action), 267
Wagner, Marsden, 223
Waiting area, 236
Walking
  during active labor, 115, 116
  duck, 148
  elephant, 84
  groin pain during, 46
  hypertension and, 78
  postpartum, 151
  as prenatal exercise, 71
Walsh, John, 173, 174
Warm-up labor, 108–9
Water
  chlorine in, 35
  drinking, 35

Water birth
  for breech presentation, 62, 164
  catching baby, 128
  preparation for, 62–63
Waterbirth International, 267
Watermelon, for hypertension, 78
Weaning, 213
Weaver, Pam, 228
Weed, Susun, 51, 223
Weight (baby's)
  estimating fetal, 32
  fetal growth spurt, 70
Weight gain (mother's), 70–71
  average, 22, 70
  causes of, 70
  excessive, 70
  inadequate, 70–71
Western blot test, for HIV, 42
Wharton's jelly, 135
*What Every Pregnant Woman Should
    Know* (Brewer and Brewer), 78
Whiff test, 49
Whitson, June, 236
WHO (World Health Organization),
    4, 42, 267
Wickham, Sara, 39
Williams Obstetrics (Cunningham et al.),
    75, 172, 222
*The Wise Woman Herbal for the
    Childbearing Year* (Weed), 51, 223
Witch hazel
  for hemorrhoids, 53, 209
  for postpartum bath, 194
Working mothers, 94–95
World Alliance for Breastfeeding Action
    (WABA), 267
World Health Organization (WHO),
    4, 42, 267

Y

Yarrow, for postpartum bath, 194
Yeast infection, 47, 49
Yellow dock
  for anemia, 52, 69
  as liver tonic, 46
Yoga, 38, 101, 203, 227
YourWaterBirth.com, 267

Z

Zinc, 35
Zoloft, 216
Zovirax, 50
Zygote, 45
Zyprexa, 19